Low-Carb Diet

2nd Edition

by Katherine B. Chauncey, PhD, RDN

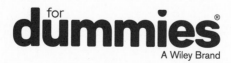

for dummies®

A Wiley Brand

Low-Carb Diet For Dummies®, 2nd Edition

Published by: **John Wiley & Sons, Inc.,** 111 River Street, Hoboken, NJ 07030-5774, www.wiley.com

Copyright © 2022 by John Wiley & Sons, Inc., Hoboken, New Jersey

Published simultaneously in Canada

For general information on our other products and services, please contact our Customer Care Department within the U.S. at 877-762-2974, outside the U.S. at 317-572-3993, or fax 317-572-4002. For technical support, please visit https://hub.wiley.com/community/support/dummies.

Wiley publishes in a variety of print and electronic formats and by print-on-demand. Some material included with standard print versions of this book may not be included in e-books or in print-on-demand. If this book refers to media such as a CD or DVD that is not included in the version you purchased, you may download this material at http://booksupport.wiley.com. For more information about Wiley products, visit www.wiley.com.

Library of Congress Control Number: 2021950165

ISBN: 978-1-119-83902-6

ISBN 978-1-119-83904-0 (ebk); ISBN 978-1-119-83906-4 (ebk)

SKY10031539_112221

Contents at a Glance

Recipes at a Glance

Main Dishes

Side Dishes

Desserts and Beverages

Table of Contents

Introduction

Welcome to the 2nd edition of *Low-Carb Diet For Dummies.* Nutrition and medical professionals have learned a lot about low-carbohydrate eating plans since the publication of the first book. When the first edition was published, two sides — the low-fat way of eating and the low-carb way of eating — were at odds with each other. Food was looked at as grams of fat or grams of carb. No one really looked at the quality of the food source. So, any food labeled "fat free" was considered healthy on one plan and anything labeled "carb free" was considered healthy on the other plan.

In this controversy the low-fat side had the favor of the scientific community and low-carb side had their ridicule. A lot has changed since then. Today nutritionists know more about the health benefits of a low-carb diet and the importance of the quality of the carbohydrates people include in their diet. Also, nutritionists know more about the health benefits of certain fats in a person's diet and the importance of including them in a person's eating.

Read on for a fully integrated diet plan that you can follow healthfully and deliciously for the rest of your life. Not only does it contribute to a healthy lifestyle, it will help you lose those extra pounds you may be carrying around.

About This Book

In this second edition of *Low-Carb Diet For Dummies,* I continue to address the differences in carbohydrate foods: the good, the bad, and the ugly. I delve a tad deeper into the nutrition aspects of eating a low-carb diet, discussing the differences between low-carb and very low-carbohydrate diets (VLCD) and which fats are healthy and need to be included in your diet and which ones aren't healthy and need to be excluded. Unlike many other popular low-carb eating plans available today, this plan helps you control, *but doesn't entirely eliminate,* the intake of refined sugars and flour, and it encourages you to eat whole, unprocessed food. You may be surprised to see that the plan contains moderate amounts of starch, protein, and fat. The plan allows your nutrition needs to be supplied *naturally.*

I help you focus your eating on natural, unprocessed foods whenever possible, particularly fresh fruits and vegetables, lean meat and protein, and low-fat dairy. I give you guidelines for appropriate serving sizes of carbohydrates. This is not the eat-all-the-fat-and-protein-you-can-stuff-in-your-face plan. You'll definitely feel full and energetic on this plan.

Carbohydrates are counted differently in the Whole Food Weight Loss Eating Plan than in other low-carb diets. Other low-carb diets count all the carbohydrate in a meal regardless of the food source. A new feature in this plan is you're given a range of one to five carbohydrate choices per day. You choose how many you want. For example, if you want to lose weight faster, you can choose one to three carb choices per day, although five carb choices per day will also yield a weight loss. Eliminating carbs completely is dangerous, so eat at least one carb choice a day.

A carbohydrate choice is approximately 15 grams of total carbohydrate and can be a bread, cereal, starchy vegetable, pasta, chips, sugar, or sweet. In recipes, you only count the carbohydrate that comes from starch or sugar, not the carbohydrate from fruit, vegetables, or low-fat dairy foods. Because of this difference, the recipes in this book have the number of carbohydrate choices calculated for you. That information will be stated in the recipe's Yield. The nutrition analysis of the recipes calculate the total carbohydrate, but if that carbohydrate is supplied by fruit or vegetables and not starch or sugar, the recipe is considered "free" and will be marked with a Green Light icon.

Here are a few other specs to keep in mind about the recipes in this book:

>> All butter is unsalted unless otherwise stated. Margarine isn't a suitable substitute for butter; instead you'll find plant butters or plant oils mixed with yogurt.

>> All eggs are large.

>> All onions are yellow unless otherwise specified.

>> All pepper is freshly ground black pepper unless otherwise specified.

>> All salt is kosher.

>> All dry ingredient measurements are level.

>> All temperatures are Fahrenheit (see Appendix D to convert Fahrenheit temperatures to Celsius).

>> All lemon and lime juice is freshly squeezed.

>> All sugar is white granulated sugar unless otherwise noted.

>> All flour is all-purpose white flour unless otherwise noted.

>> All Greek yogurt is full-fat yogurt unless otherwise noted.

>> When a recipe says to steam a vegetable, the amount of water you need to use in your pot or steamer depends on your steaming method, so I don't include the water in the ingredients list. As a general rule, if you're using a basket in a pot, the water level should be just below the basket.

>> When a recipe says sugar-substitute equivalent, the amount of sugar-substitute you use should be equal to the amount of sugar indicated in the recipe. In some recipes, a specific low-calorie sweetener and the amount is stated. Many good natural sweeteners weren't available when I wrote the first edition of this book.

Foolish Assumptions

When writing this book, I make a few assumptions about you:

>> You're overwhelmed by the number of dieting plans and books and just can't make a decision about which is best for you.

>> You're busy and want a simpler and healthier way to eat that you can apply to any situation such as home, office, restaurant, or fast food.

>> You want to model healthy eating for your family and serve easy and delicious meals.

>> You're tired of the stress that happens at mealtime in deciding what and/or where to eat.

>> You fear having to eat differently from your family while you prepare a "regular" meal for them.

>> You're tired of being overweight and unable to join in fun activities.

>> You're fearful of never being able to eat your favorite foods again.

Icons Used in This Book

Icons are those little pictures in the margins. Here's a key to what they mean:

TIP

The Tip icon is handy, and I use it extensively. It marks things that I've identified as being helpful in your journey to lifelong good health.

REMEMBER

This icon marks important points that are reinforced throughout a section of the book. You'll do well to remember what I point out here.

WARNING

Pay particular attention to the Warning icon to steer clear of situations that can be seriously dangerous or hazardous. Exercise some extra caution.

TECHNICAL STUFF

This icon marks interesting information that isn't essential to understand. You can even skip over the text if it doesn't appeal to you and still enjoy the book.

GREEN LIGHT

This icon points out recipes that use only Green Light foods, which are free foods you can eat anytime anywhere. They're primarily vegetables, fruits, lean meats, and low-fat cheeses. Any other recipe not marked with a Green Light icon is counted as one of your carb choices. Check the yield part of the recipe to see how much carb to count.

Beyond This Book

This book is chock-full of tips and other pieces of helpful advice you can use as you eat a low-carb diet. If you want some additional tidbits of wisdom, check out the book's Cheat Sheet at www.dummies.com. Just search for "Low-Carb Diet For Dummies Cheat Sheet."

Where to Go from Here

One of the best things about this book, or any *For Dummies* book for that matter, is the fact that you can start just about anywhere and find something that's interesting and relevant. Feel free to start wherever you want. If you want a little more guidance, try this handy list on for size:

>> If you want to get shopping right away and need a grocery list to get you started, go right to Appendix B.

>> If you're not sure if the plan is right for you, take a look at Chapter 4. It's full of information on discovering your own personal health history, assessing your current health situation, and helping you see why this plan can work for you.

>> To go straight to the recipes, focus on Part 3. For a quick list of which recipes I include in the book, take a look at the Recipes at a Glance at the front of the book.

>> If you want a quick overview of the plan, and why it's better than any other low-carb plan out there, take a look at Chapter 2.

1

Understanding the Carbohydrate Controversy

Chapter **1**

Mapping Out a Low-Carb Diet

Although eating in the United States has been changing since the beginning of the 20th century, it has dramatically changed in the last 50 years. Americans eat out more frequently, eat larger portions of food, and eat more foods with little resemblance to their form in nature. Everywhere Americans turn, they're inundated with refined and processed foods such as snack foods, chips, candies, cereals, cookies, and all other sorts of junk food. In addition, Americans are bombarded with best-selling diet books that just repackage fad diets to make them seem new and exciting. So, the old adage, "Eat less and exercise more" just seems dull and boring. As a result, more Americans than ever are overweight or obese and struggling to find a plan that helps them lose the extra pounds.

Americans unfortunately are exporting this dilemma around the world. Kuwait has more fast-food restaurants per capita than any other country in the world. And, yes, the incidence of diabetes, heart disease, and obesity are on the rise in Kuwait. So, does this mean fast foods are the culprit? Not exactly. Most people are overwhelmed with the availability of cheap, tasty foods and junk foods whose advertising barrages them in every media at every twist and turn.

My goal is to help you discover a better way of eating that is easy, healthy, and reasonable. In this chapter, I map out a low-carb eating plan that is healthy *and* satisfying. I show you how to remove *refined carbohydrates* (carbohydrates with lots of sugar and very little fiber) from your diet, to make your diet healthier. By improving the quality of the carbohydrates you eat, and by controlling your daily intake of starchy carbs (like breads, pasta, and starchy vegetables), you'll lose weight and experience many other healthy benefits including increased energy, improved mood, and better sleeping.

How Low Is Low Carb? That's the Question

If you've looked into low-carb diets, you've probably found more than a few that require you to banish carbs from your diet entirely. And if you like carbs the way most people do, you've probably thrown down those books with a mixture of fear and frustration. Low-carb diets include a variety of carbohydrate levels, and not one specific level is accepted by all. The end result is confusion and a barrier in communicating the real risks and benefits of low-carb eating.

Americans are eating more food than ever, and carbs have replaced much of the fat. That increased food intake means an increased carbohydrate intake, which is largely sugars, sweeteners, and processed flour. That increase has had a direct impact on the health (and waistlines) of Americans. In working with patients at Texas Tech Medical Center, I found the low-carb eating plan approach referred to as the Whole Foods Weight Loss Eating Plan as more effective than a low-fat diet approach. Patients watching their fat intake were eating a lot of fat-free food products that weren't any healthier than the fat they had been eating.

This Whole Foods Weight Loss Eating Plan doesn't reduce carbohydrate so much that it induces *ketosis* (a process that happens when you don't have enough carbs to burn for energy so you burn fat, which makes ketones to use for fuel). The Whole Foods Weight Loss Eating Plan not only reduces your intake of processed carbs, but it also shows you how to control your intake of those foods for a more permanent weight loss. The following sections delve deeper into the world of low-carb diets and explain what a low-carb diet is and isn't.

Defining a low-carb diet: Not as easy as you'd think

Although the term "low carb" is bandied around freely in general conversation and most everyone using the term assumes that they're using the term in the same way, unfortunately no clear definition of the term exists.

REMEMBER

In an attempt to overcome this barrier to communication, researchers have suggested four definitions:

>> **Very-low carbohydrate ketogenic diet (VLCKD):** Carbohydrates are limited to 20 to 50 grams per day or less than 10 percent of a 2,000 kcal/day diet, whether or not ketosis occurs. It's derived from levels of carbohydrate required to induce ketosis in most people. VLCKD is the recommended early phase (induction) of popular diets such as Atkins Diet or Protein Power and is the basis for the Keto Diet.

>> **Low-carbohydrate diet:** This diet limits carbohydrates to less than 130 grams per day or less than 26 percent of total energy. The Dietary Reference Intake (DRI) defines 130 grams per day as its recommended minimum. The Whole Foods Weight Loss Eating Plan promoted in this book adheres to this carbohydrate level. See Appendix C for more on the DRIs.

>> **Moderate-carbohydrate diet:** This diet sets carbohydrate limits at 130 to 225 grams per day or 26 to 45 percent of your total calorie intake. This was the prevailing upper limit of carbohydrate intake in the western diet before the obesity epidemic (43 percent) began.

>> **High-carbohydrate diet:** Carbohydrate intake is more than 225 grams per day or greater than 45 percent of total calorie intake on this diet. More recent surveys estimate that the current American diet is 53 percent refined and processed carbohydrate.

The Whole Foods Weight Loss Eating Plan that I describe in this book provides 130 grams of carbohydrate and fits the definition of a low-carbohydrate diet. But don't worry — the guidelines I give don't ask you to remove carbs from your diet completely. Instead, I want to get you thinking about the *quality* of the foods you consume, rather than the number of carb grams those foods contain. For more details about this, turn to Chapter 2.

Clarifying what this low-carb diet is about

The Whole Foods Weight Loss Eating Plan isn't an eat-all-the-fat-and-protein-you-can-possibly-consume diet. It's really focused on enjoying *whole* or *unprocessed foods* and enjoying the healthy side effects, including having more energy, stabilizing your blood-sugar levels, losing weight, and improving your self-confidence. *Whole foods* are fruits, vegetables, grains, beans, nuts, and seeds that haven't been processed to remove vitamins, minerals, fiber, and so on. They're foods that are sold to consumers as close to the same state that nature provided them.

Most foods contain some carbohydrates. Even an 8-ounce glass of skim milk contains 12 grams of carbs. A cup of broccoli contains 8 carb grams. And yet, both milk and broccoli are packed full of other nutritional benefits, including vitamins, nutrients, fiber, and phytochemicals. If you strictly limit the number of carb grams in your diet without considering the quality of the carbs you eat, you'll be missing out on some key foods that will enhance your overall good health.

These sections clarify which carbs you can eat as much as you want on the Whole Foods Weight Loss Eating Plan and with which carbs you need to be more selective.

Identifying free foods — eat all you want

Even though you're limited to five carbohydrate servings a day on the Whole Foods Weight Loss Eating Plan, many foods that contain carbohydrates are absolutely *free* (which means you can have as many of them as you want, without counting them toward your daily carb allowance).

Here are some quick tips on which foods to focus your attention on and which to pass by (Chapter 5 has more details about free foods):

>> **Don't be afraid of fruit.** Fruit does contain carbohydrates, but the carbs in fruit give it a delicious *natural* sweetness, which is partnered with a ton of vitamins, fiber, and relatively few calories. Increasing your fruit intake is a great way to help you wean yourself off refined sugars. (*Refined sugars* are sugars like table sugar and high-fructose corn syrup that are added to processed foods.) Fruits make a great dessert option and, because they come pre-portioned in their own natural package, they're a great choice for grab-and-go snacks. On this diet plan, almost all fruits are free The recipes in Chapter 16 offer a wide array of healthy, fruit-filled desserts.

>> **Look at leafy green and non-starchy vegetables.** Leafy greens, like spinach, watercress, cabbage, and romaine lettuce, and non-starchy vegetables, like green beans, broccoli, carrots, and tomatoes, come in an almost limitless variety. You can further vary your diet by trying new preparations of old favorites and partnering them with new choices. Check out some great recipes for salads and other greens in Chapter 12.

>> **Remove refined sugars from your life.** Refined sugars provide calories, but lack vitamins, minerals, and fiber. They're also high on the glycemic index table. See Chapter 3 and Appendix A for more on the glycemic index. The amount of refined sugar in the American diet is a disastrous, but fairly recent, development. Watch out for hidden sugars in breads, lunch meat, and salad dressings. Pay attention to the not-hidden sugars in non-diet sodas, cookies, and candy. For more on reducing the amount of sugar in your diet, see Chapter 6.

Eyeing what five carb servings you can eat

A carbohydrate serving is a portion of a carbohydrate food that provides 15 grams of carb per serving. On the Whole Foods Weight Loss Eating Plan you're allowed up to five servings a day, although you do have some flexibility. You can eat as few as one to three servings per day or three to five servings per day based on your weight loss goals. After all, *you* are in control. *You* decide. That's why the quality of the carbohydrate food you eat is so important.

REMEMBER

For those five carbohydrate servings you're allowed to eat each day on the Whole Foods Weight Loss Eating Plan, choose wisely and consider the following:

>> **Check out legumes.** *Legumes* (leh-*gooms*) are foods like peas, beans, and peanuts. They're nutritional powerhouses that add fiber to your diet, are naturally low in fat, are a great source of protein, and are very inexpensive. Look for several varieties at your market including canned, dried, and fresh. Legumes make great additions to salads, serve as excellent side dishes, and make healthy delicious entrees in their own right. Look for great recipes for legumes throughout the recipes in Part 3.

>> **Choose whole grains whenever possible.** Look for *whole grains* (grains that still have their bran and nutrients intact) as the first ingredient on a food nutrition label's ingredients list. Items made from whole grains tend to be higher in fiber and lower in sugar, and have a stabilizing affect on blood sugar levels compared to their refined-grain counterparts. For more on the benefits of fiber and whole grains, look at Chapter 6.

>> **Introduce more soy products into your diet.** Soy foods contain both carbs and protein, making them off-limits on many low-carb eating plans. Not so with my plan. In fact, if you're a vegetarian, you can substitute soy products for lean proteins and still get many of the nutritional benefits this plan has to offer. Regardless of whether you're a vegetarian, adding more soy to your diet can offer tremendous health benefits, including a reduced risk of several types of cancer and heart disease, as well as more-balanced hormone levels.

CONSIDERING HOW A LOW-CARB DIET DIFFERS FROM OTHER POPULAR DIETS

This sidebar describes several popular diet plans that are currently promoted. This information can help you appreciate the benefits of the Whole Foods Weight Loss Eating Plan:

- **Very-low-carb diet:** This eating plan significantly restricts carbs and is intended to induce ketosis in most people. The Whole Foods Weight Loss Eating Plan doesn't induce ketosis.

- **Atkins Diet:** This diet, which resurfaces about every 25 years, starts with an induction phase designed to induce ketosis and then gradually moves the person to higher carbs.

- **Keto Diet:** The Ketogenic Diet or Keto Diet as it's commonly known is a low-carbohydrate, high-fat dieting plan that has been used for centuries to treat hard-to-control epilepsy in children. The diet forces the body to burn fats (*ketones*) rather than carbs, which forces the body into ketosis.

- **Paleo Diet:** The Paleolithic Diet or Paleo Diet as it's commonly known states that because humanity's genetics and anatomy have changed very little since the Stone Age, people should eat foods available during that time to promote good health. Your diet should be based on whole, unprocessed foods. Meats, nuts, seeds, fruits and vegetables are all acceptable in the Paleo Diet. Grains aren't.

- **Intermittent fasting:** This eating pattern cycles between brief periods of fasting and eating. The fasting period consists of no food or significant calorie reduction alternating with periods of unrestricted eating. The most common regimens are fasting on alternate days, for whole days with a specific frequency per week, or during a set time frame such as eating only within an eight-hour window each day.

These weight-loss plans have a common feature. Even though their starting points tend to vary, *they all restrict refined and processed carbs.* So, your weight loss is not only from your carb intake, but it's also from the absence of refined and processed carbs. Even though these plans can yield a significant weight loss in the beginning, they all eventually fail. Why? Because refined and processed carbs are so pervasive in the western diet and so persuasively advertised, they'll eventually creep back into your daily eating. Before you know it, you've lost control and your hunger has become ravenous. None of the given plans have taught you how to *control* those processed foods. That's where the Whole Foods Weight Loss Eating Plan differs. It not only shows you how to reduce your intake of those foods, but also how to keep them at bay.

Figuring out whether low-carb eating is right for you

The following are *all* good reasons to follow this low-carb plan:

>> If your personal health history includes the precursors to diabetes, high blood pressure, heart disease, or obesity

>> If you're concerned about stabilizing your blood sugar levels

>> If you're tired of the way convenience foods and prepackaged, sugar-laden foods make you feel

>> If your Body Mass Index (BMI) is 30 or above

REMEMBER

Check with your healthcare provider before beginning any exercise or diet regimen. Chapter 4 provides more details in determining whether this plan is right for you.

Discovering Whole Foods

The most important element of the Whole Foods Weight Loss Eating Plan is the introduction of whole foods into your diet. A *whole food* is any food that's not refined or processed. Fresh, frozen, or canned fruits and vegetables are whole foods; french fries aren't. A sirloin steak is a whole food; a breaded veal cutlet isn't. Whole-grain bread is a whole food; white bread isn't. Apple juice is a whole food; a fruit roll-up isn't. A baked potato is a whole food; potato chips aren't.

REMEMBER

The more refined a food is, the fewer vitamins and nutrients, the less fiber the food has, and the higher the glycemic index. If you see a food that's refined but has been fortified with vitamins and minerals, like sugary breakfast cereal, be wary. Those vitamins aren't as easily used by your body for all of its vital processes as their naturally occurring counterparts. And 99 times out of 100, the food contains more sugar than your body needs. Check out Part 2 for the skinny on using whole foods to their best dietary advantage.

Living the Low-Carb Way

Low-carb dieting quickly will become second nature. The key to your success is planning. Plan your meals and plan your shopping trips to fit with your low-carb lifestyle.

TIP

Be aware of the layout of your grocery store. Food manufacturers want to lure you toward the center aisles where the shelves are stocked with expensive prepared dinners and other refined foods. Stick to the perimeter for most whole-food choices (such as fresh produce, low-fat dairy products, and lean meats). When you do take the plunge into the center aisles for dried beans, canned vegetables, or whole oats, avoid the temptation to toss prepackaged dinner helpers, chips, cookies, or sugary cereals into your cart. For more shopping tips, take a look at Chapter 9.

With a little effort, you'll be able to navigate your way around a low-carb kitchen. Find your own shortcuts to make your life easier *and* low-carb friendly.

TIP

When dining out, don't be afraid to ask for substitutions. If your steak comes with french fries, ask for an extra side of veggies instead. If the pasta special sounds very tempting, the chef can likely make it for you without the pasta. Just think of that chunky seafood in a hearty marinara sauce — it's fantastic without the white pasta. Most restaurants, even fast-food restaurants, have a house or green salad that's a great addition to any meal and totally free on this eating plan. Just get your dressing on the side, so you don't eat unwanted fat and calories. For more tips on dining out, read Chapter 17.

Beyond the Scale: Identifying Other Factors for Overall Health

For most people, weight loss and dieting go hand in hand. In fact, when you hear someone say, "I'm on a diet," it usually means, "I'm trying to lose weight." But the word *diet* (coming from the Latin *dieta,* or "daily regimen") can also refer simply to the food you eat day in and day out. I want to change your daily food plan for the rest of your life, not just help you lose weight now. So, considering factors other than a number on the scale is important when you're charting your progress.

REMEMBER

Lowering your BMI by as few as two points can have a profoundly positive effect on your overall health. Check out Chapter 3 for details.

TIP

Your body shape, genetics, and age have as much to do with your physical appearance as your weight. So, set realistic expectations for what you expect your body to look like. An unrealistic self-image can be devastating to your health and self-esteem. For more details, take a look at Chapter 22.

Exercise and low-carb dieting:
Your partners in fitness

Exercise isn't just a necessary part of life, it's fun! With so many different forms of exercise available, you're sure to find one that matches your interests and lifestyle. You don't have to run out and buy workout clothes, join a gym, and attend a Pilates class this week. Just pulling weeds in the garden or mowing the lawn can get your heart pumping. Walk around the block with your dog. Find a friend to walk with you during your lunch break. Volunteer to coach a Little League team in the sport of your choice. Anything that gets you moving is a great addition to your lifestyle.

REMEMBER

The effects of exercise are cumulative, which means that you don't have to get your 30 minutes a day in one shot. You can take a 15-minute walk around the block in the morning and another 15-minute walk after dinner.

Daily exercise stabilizes your blood sugar levels, improves your cardiovascular health, increases your strength and stamina, and helps you get a better night of sleep. You may feel more tired immediately after beginning a new exercise program, but you should quickly enjoy increased energy levels, as well as an improved mood because of the *endorphins* (chemical signals in your blood that act like your body's own version of morphine or painkillers) running rampant in your bloodstream.

The more you exercise, the more lean muscle you develop. And the more lean muscle you develop, the higher your resting metabolism. (Your *metabolism* is sort of your internal rhythm, or the rate at which you burn calories when completely at rest.) With a higher resting metabolism, you burn more calories while you're sleeping, working at your desk, or even just breathing. How's that for efficiency?

Exploring vitamins and supplements

On the Whole Foods Weight Loss Eating Plan, you're encouraged to take in most of your vitamins and minerals through the whole foods that you consume. However, a few important exceptions may exist. If you're at risk for osteoporosis, you'll want to calculate your calcium intake, and if it doesn't meet your daily need, add a calcium supplement to your daily regimen. Certain health conditions and certain stages in life may make considering a vitamin or mineral supplement appropriate as well. Antioxidant nutrients like vitamins C, E, and beta-carotene and the minerals zinc, copper, selenium, and manganese may help lower your risk of disease and the ravages of aging. New guidelines for supplements and information on upper limits can help you to know the amounts to take and still stay within safe levels. For more on incorporating vitamins and supplements into your low-carb lifestyle, take a look at Chapter 21 and Appendix C.

Maintaining Your Low-Carb Lifestyle

As with making any long-term change to your diet, the key to enjoying the ultimate benefits of your low-carb lifestyle is sticking with the plan. Part 5 is loaded with tips and tricks to help you set yourself up to succeed.

Making the commitment

The first step in making the low-carb commitment is mental or psychological. Customize your food habits to meet the demands of your lifestyle and your low-carb diet. If you can get your family, roommates, or other housemates to follow the diet with you, you'll definitely have a better shot at success, because you can completely remove tempting foods and sweets from your cabinets and fridge. But don't stress if others aren't interested in the plan. You can still cook for the whole family with the plan and adjust your own portion sizes to coincide with it. You'll just need to be careful not to indulge in cookies or snacks. For more on getting (and staying) committed to the plan, check out Chapters 18 and 19.

Planning ahead

Let your lifestyle help determine your food-plan strategy. If you know that you have no time in the mornings, prepare your healthy breakfast and lunch the night before. Plan your meals before you're hungry. Making healthy choices is much more difficult when you're hungry and refined foods are handy.

REMEMBER

The rise of prepackaged, convenience foods has increased the amount of refined sugar in the American diet, but your busy schedule doesn't have to be a barrier to healthy eating. Keep healthy snacks on hand in snack-size resealable plastic bags for easy treats. You'll eliminate the urge to grab cookies, chips, and crackers.

Picking yourself up when you fall

I wish I could say that no one ever slips up on this plan, that no one ever gives in to temptation and succumbs to that extra baked potato or slice of cake. But the fact is giving in to temptation is part of life. You're human and, therefore, you aren't perfect. However, don't beat up on yourself when you slip up, and more importantly, don't use it as an excuse to throw all your progress out the window. So, you had a piece of cake and didn't save any carb choices for it? Analyze what went wrong in your plan and resolve to have a better day tomorrow. These small setbacks can be the gateway to long-term success. If you can learn from them and make better choices next time, you can have better overall health and weight control. Refer to Chapter 20 for more details.

Chapter **2**

Delving Deeper into Carbohydrates

Nothing has polarized the nutrition world as much as the low-carbohydrate diet, but this diet isn't new. It's been around for more than 100 years — and for most of that time, it has been controversial. The quick-weight-loss effect of the low-carb diet, its permission to eat as much meat and fat as you want, and the lack of hunger in those who follow it has always attracted many fans. However, very-low-carb diets were hard to maintain.

In this chapter, I show you why the low-carb diet is controversial. I discuss the migration of the American diet toward more calories from increased snacks, sugars, soft drinks, and bigger portions of all foods. I give you ways to evaluate low-carb diet plans to help you make the best choice for you. And most importantly, I give you an overview of the Whole Foods Weight Loss Eating Plan — my version of the low-carb diet — which is healthy for a lifetime and will also help you lose excess pounds.

Evaluating the Controversy

The low-carb diet gained modern-day popularity about 50 years ago only to later be squelched by the fully accepted and heavily promoted low-fat diet. Cholesterol was implicated as a major determinant of heart disease, and diets high in saturated fat were found to raise blood cholesterol levels. Lowering fat intake in the diet enjoyed approval by the scientific community and was embraced by national health organizations and public policy. There was a halo-effect over the low-fat diet and horns and a devil's fork over fat. Fat was branded as the ultimate dietary villain, for several reasons:

>> Heart disease was increasing and was correlated with high cholesterol. Scientists discovered that saturated fat increased cholesterol levels in the blood. Scientists also sensed that people were slowly becoming a little fatter. A fat gram contained twice the number of calories of protein or carbohydrate grams, so a good way to reduce the number of calories people ate was to reduce the number of fat grams consumed.

>> Fat was also blamed for cancer and a host of other diseases.

The low-fat diet approach enjoyed almost universal acceptance and respect from the scientific community and the public. Fat in any form was demonized. And, the concept of low fat being healthy became deeply ingrained in society. Along with the lowering of fat in the diet was the recommendation to replace the fat with carbohydrate foods that were virtually devoid of fat.

Then the low-carbohydrate diet started making another comeback with not only its good results in blood glucose and weight loss, but also good results in blood cholesterol parameters. Media headlines questioned the honesty of the low-fat diet, and nutrition scientists were accused of waffling on their nutrition advice. Obesity was worse than ever, now at epidemic proportions; cancer was also just as bad as ever, accompanied by increases in diabetes, high blood pressure, joint pain, and heartburn. Heartburn became more sophisticated and was renamed gastro-esophageal reflux disease (GERD). And a "new" disease phenomena appeared on the scene dastardly labeled at first as *Syndrome X* and later as *metabolic syndrome.* Metabolic syndrome is actually the manifestation of *insulin resistance* and is considered a strong risk factor for heart disease. (Check out Chapter 4 for more information on metabolic syndrome.) Accusers pointed directly at carbohydrate as the villain. The low-fat diet, which recommended carbohydrate as a substitute for fat, was dealt a blow. Even the United States Department of Agriculture's Food Pyramid was included as an enabler and was eventually eliminated.

So, where is the truth? Is it the very-low-fat diet? No. Is it the very-low-carb diet? No. Do people need to eat less fat? Yes. Do people need to eat less carbohydrate? Yes. In fact, people need to eat less of just about everything. In the era of the very-low-fat-diet or very-low-carb diet, eating was relegated to math. You were allowed 20 grams of fat or 30 grams of carbohydrate depending on which plan you followed. So, the only important thing was how many grams of fat or carbohydrate were in the food. The quality of the food didn't matter.

Two other factors played a role in this nutritional thinking:

» **Scientists discovered the glycemic index to evaluate carbohydrate quality.** The *glycemic index* measures equal quantities of carbohydrates on blood glucose levels. Refer to Chapter 3 and Appendix A for more information.

» **Healthcare providers now use not only total cholesterol value to assess heart disease risk, but also a lipid profile to evaluate other cholesterol factors in the blood.** A lipid profile includes the following:

- Total cholesterol

- Low density cholesterol (LDL)

- High density cholesterol (HDL)

- Triglycerides (TG)

Flip to Chapter 4 for more about cholesterol and triglycerides. The following sections discuss the fallacies in the low-fat and low-carb dietary approaches. They encourage you to start looking at the quality of the food you eat and not just how many grams of fat or carb the food contains.

The low-fat, high-carb diet

Americans are heavier than ever before, despite the fact that they're reducing the percentage of calories consumed from fat. Popular diet books and the media immediately targeted carbohydrates as the bad guys and labeled them fattening. What was ignored is the fact that the average American consumes 40,000 calories more (over the course of a year) than they did previously. The real message should be that excess calories from *any* source will result in increased body weight. High-carbohydrate diets recommend that the carbohydrate comes from fruits, vegetables, beans, whole grains, and dairy, but high-carb diets also impose a tight restriction on fat, which leads to a higher consumption of fat-free and reduced-fat snack foods.

One thing the advocates of the low-fat diet didn't plan on was the abundance of fat-free foods that would become available. The low-fat message became distorted into counting fat grams. Therefore, *fat-free* foods just became *free* foods in people's minds. The fat in sweet rolls, cookies, cake, and crackers was replaced with sugar or other refined sweeteners. Intake of fruits, vegetables, beans, and grains, the preferred replacement for fat, increased some, but it still fell short of the recommended goals.

THE HISTORY OF THE LOW-CARB DIET

The low-carb diet isn't new. In fact, a London coffin maker and undertaker named William Banting devised it to treat his own obesity. He had become so obese that he had to walk downstairs backwards to keep from falling. He lost 50 pounds on the diet and published a pamphlet, *Letter on Corpulence, Addressed to the Public,* in 1864. Banting declared the diet a "cure for extreme corpulence."

His cure became so popular that the word banting became a synonym for dieting in the English language. The diet also caught the interest of Americans in the late 1800s and became popular. However, in the next century, it was labeled the "Banting Scheme" because it was full of unproven medical lingo and followers of the plan often developed gout. Since those early days, the low-carb diet approach has resurfaced about every 25 years and is always controversial.

The low-carb, high-protein diet

With carbohydrate at an all-time high and the health of the country as bad as ever, the low-carb diet rose in favor. People following the low-carb diet attest to its effectiveness and proudly proclaim the number of pounds lost. So if it's effective in losing weight as so many contend, then what's the problem?

Most low-carb diets count grams of carbohydrate regardless of the food source. So "good" carbs, such as fruit, vegetables, whole grains, and dairy, are eliminated solely because they contain carbohydrate. If you follow these restrictions, you're eliminating vital nutrients, phytochemicals, and fiber (see Chapter 3). Certainly, everyone needs to eat less carbohydrate, but the decrease needs to come mainly from refined flour and sugar products. You must take into consideration the *quality* of the carbohydrate you eat.

Another problem is that low-carb diets tend to be high in fat and protein. Many interpret the low-carb diet as a license to load up on bun-less burgers, steaks, sausages, eggs, and bacon. Unfortunately, this approach can have potentially negative health effects.

Whether you count grams of fat or count grams of carbohydrate, you're still using a calculator to make your food choices. Give me a break! Who wants to eat a calculator? Counting all fats the same and counting all carbohydrates the same is misleading. You should definitely include some fats in your diet and you should definitely include some carbohydrates. For the full story on fats, take a peek at Chapter 8. For the lowdown on quality carbs, see Chapters 5 and 6.

Deconstructing the Typical (Bad) Diet

The modern western diet includes more calories, larger portion sizes, and increased frequency of eating. The modern western diet is characterized by all the following:

>> More soft drinks and sweeteners

>> More salty snacks

>> More cookies and snack foods

>> Eating out more often, especially in fast-food restaurants

>> Larger portion sizes, especially of soft drinks and french fries

>> Increased convenience, microwaveable, and processed foods

Instead of the USDA Food Guide Pyramid, which was in use at the time, the modern diet turned the Pyramid upside-down with refined grains, potatoes and sweets, and meats in greater quantity than fruits and vegetables. Today pyramid guides to depict healthy eating have been abandoned completely. Although some evidence suggests that the Food Guide Pyramid enhanced nutrition knowledge, it did nothing to change people's eating habits. The USDA replaced the pyramid with a plate diagram (MyPlate.gov) with a glass of milk set off to the side. Even though the USDA feels the plate diagram better reflects their recommendations for healthy diet, the current American diet still has lots of room for improvement.

Based on data from the USDA, the modern American diet is made up of the following:

>> 53 percent processed foods

>> 32 percent animal products

>> 11 percent veggies, fruits, beans, nuts

>> 4 percent whole grains

Of the measly 11 percent attributed to fruits and vegetables almost half of that consisted of french fries and ketchup. Combine that with the large intake of processed foods and animal products, and it's no wonder Americans are plagued with obesity, diabetes, and heart disease.

Eating more refined sugars

Most of the increase in sugar in the American diet has come from added sugars. *Added sugars* are sugars and syrups added to foods in processing or preparation, not the naturally occurring sugars in foods like fructose in fruit or lactose in milk. Sugar (including sucrose, corn sweeteners, honey, maple syrup, and molasses) is everywhere in the foods people eat — and it's often hidden. Sugar is the number-one food additive and turns up in some unlikely places like pizza, bread, hot dogs, boxed mixed rice, soup, crackers, spaghetti sauce, lunchmeat, canned vegetables, fruit drinks, flavored yogurt, ketchup, salad dressings, mayonnaise, and some peanut butter.

The number-one food source containing added sugar consumed in the United States is sugar-sweetened beverages and soft drinks. In fact, sweetened beverages provide 47 percent of the refined and added sugars in the American food supply. More than 50 percent of American adults, 65 percent of teenage girls, and 74 percent of teenage boys consume soft drinks daily, most of which are sugar-sweetened. Liquid calories are strictly additive to the diet and add nothing nutritionally. Consuming a lot of foods high in added sugars, especially soft drinks, is of concern especially in children, teenagers, and women because, when people are drinking soft drinks, they're not drinking as much water and other more nutritious foods like dairy and dairy alternatives. See Chapter 7 for more on dairy foods.

Eating more salty snacks

According to a recent report from Mintel, nearly all Americans (94 percent) snack at least once a day. And half (50 percent) of adults snack two to three times per day with 70 percent agreeing that anything can be considered a snack these days. That means everyone is eating the equivalent of a small bag of chips every day. If I don't eat any, that means someone else is eating two small bags of chips every day.

Today snack foods make up about 23 percent of the diet. That's more than double the amount eaten in the last century. In addition to extra salt, snack foods provide calories from refined grains and sugar. They contribute little nutritional value and displace more nutritious fruits and vegetables in the diet. In 2021, the Food and Drug Administration (FDA) issued new guidelines directed toward food companies to use less salt in their food products. A majority of the sodium in the U.S. diet comes from packaged or restaurant foods, not the salt added to meals at home. The FDA is allowing this change to happen gradually, but at least it's a step in the right direction.

Eating more fast foods

Eating in fast-food restaurants is so pervasive that, to increase profits, fast-food companies have to work to get customers away from other fast-food restaurants rather than bring in customers who are completely new to fast food. What does this mean? Virtually everyone eats at fast-food restaurants at least occasionally. The average American eats fast food at least three times per week according to the Centers for Disease Control and Prevention. Fast food is associated with poor diet and increased risk of obesity.

THE FRUCTOSE STORY

Americans and their children have become high consumers of sugar and sweet-tasting foods and beverages. Caloric sweeteners, most notably high-fructose corn syrup, have dramatically increased in the past 40 or so years. High fructose corn syrup is predominantly used in soft drinks (check the label the next time you drink one), but it's also found in frozen foods, bakery foods, and vending machine products.

Before 1970, high-fructose corn syrup was unknown in the food supply. However, in the 1970s scientists developed it as an economical way to produce a cheaper sweetener for commercial use. In fact, it's actually six times sweeter than cane sugar and is produced from corn, which gives food manufacturers a way to sweeten food products at a significant cost savings. By the end of the 1970s, mass-production techniques had been developed to make its use widespread.

Currently, high-fructose corn syrup makes up more than 40 percent of people's excessively high sugar intake. Fructose was once thought to be used by the body just like sucrose (table sugar). Scientists now know that the body metabolizes high concentrations of fructose differently. Due to this difference, ingesting high concentrations of fructose can increase the likelihood of weight gain and its associated insulin resistance. In addition to obesity, insulin resistance results in glucose intolerance, high triglyceride levels, high blood pressure, fatty liver, and increased risk of diabetes and heart disease.

The current levels of soft drink and sweetened food intake is an aspect of the modern lifestyle unknown in the past. The inclusion of high fructose corn syrup in the food supply parallels the dramatic increase in obesity, diabetes, and insulin resistance. Sweet-tasting foods in the diet stimulate a craving for more sweet foods, which can lead to overconsumption. Low-carbohydrate diets have the advantage of reducing the intake of soft drinks and foods with high-fructose corn sweeteners, but they don't deal with the desire many Americans have for sweet tastes.

The average American eats nearly 30 pounds of french fries (the size of a small child), almost 50 billion hamburgers, and 2.5 billion servings of chicken nuggets per year. A low-fat hamburger was dropped from a popular fast-food chain due to poor sales — so apparently Americans aren't buying the low-fat approach when they're eating fast food.

Eating larger portion sizes

A recent study compared the portions of popular foods to USDA and Food and Drug Administration (FDA) standards. The typical cookie is *700 percent larger* than the USDA suggested size. Most people eat a single serving of pasta that is 480 percent larger than recommended. And the average muffin exceeds the standard by 333 percent.

Portion sizes in restaurants started to increase in the 1970s, grew dramatically in the 1980s, and currently continue to rise in parallel to increases in average American body weight. Restaurants long ago switched to a 12-inch dinner plate from the standard 10-inch plate. Studies show that Americans ignore portion sizes even when attempting to follow a healthy diet and will eat as much food as they're given. As a rule, they won't leave food on their plates. Today Americans eat out in restaurants much more than they used to.

Portion sizes have grown dramatically over the last 50 years. When a popular fast-food chain opened in 1950, it sold only one size of regular fries, containing 200 calories. In 1970, the regular fries were then called "small" and a new "large" fries containing 320 calories appeared on the menu. In 1980, the 320-calorie french fries were called "regular" and a newer "large" fries containing 400 calories appeared on the menu. In 1990, the "large" fries had grown to 450 calories and a new "super-size" fries containing 540 calories appeared on the menu. And in 2000, the 540-calorie fry became "large" and a newer "super-size" French fries containing 610 calories appeared on the menu. Small and regular French fries are nowhere to be found on the menu. You can choose from medium, large, or super-sized. The kid meals come with the 320-calorie-sized fries.

Value meals and super-sized meals are a financial incentive for many eating establishments. They can add large-sized drinks and fries to a meal at minimal cost to them but increased cost to the consumer. So, in terms of nutritional quality, who gets the value from the "value" meal? Not you.

Eating more calories

Americans are consuming more food and several hundred more calories per person per day than did their counterparts in the late 1950s when calorie consumption was at the lowest level in the last century. A study from 2017 found that the average American eats 3,600 calories per day — almost 1,000 calories *more per day* than they did in 2000. About 54 percent of this increase comes from refined carbohydrates like processed grains and sugars, 32 percent from fats, and the remaining 1 percent from fruits, vegetables, meats, nuts, dairy products, and eggs.

Getting a lower percentage of calories from fat

The USDA food consumption survey revealed that the *percent of calories* from fat in the American diet has leveled off: 40 percent in the 1970s, 34 percent in 1990, 33 percent in 1994, and 34 percent today. That's in line with American Heart Association's recommendation to have no more than 25 to 35 percent of calories from fat. However, the total number of calories consumed, primarily from refined-carbohydrate foods, has increased. When the calories increase and the fat intake stays the same, the percent of calories from fat goes down. But the total amount in terms of actual grams of fat consumed per day has stayed about the same.

Even though the amount of fat consumed is about the same, more of the fat intake was represented by *trans fats.* Many processed carbohydrate foods contain trans fats from partially hydrogenated vegetable oils. Trans fats act like saturated fat by boosting levels of bad cholesterol and increasing the risk of heart disease. Trans fats are commonly found in carbohydrate foods such as cookies, crackers, chips, french fries, and fast foods. Since 2015 the FDA has taken steps to remove trans fats in processed foods entirely, and it's working. The FDA started regulating trans fats by identifying the adverse effects of trans fats. Soon after, labeling laws were enacted to identify trans fats on the nutrition facts food label. Trans fat intake in the American diet is decreasing.

Eating fewer fruits and vegetables

Fruit and vegetable consumption has increased but still falls below recommended levels. Less than 10 percent of the American population eat the recommended five fruits and vegetables each day. Interestingly, the popularity of pizza has boosted the average consumption of canned tomato products, but consumption of other canned vegetables declined. The popularity of french fries, eaten mainly in fast-food restaurants, caused a 63 percent increase in the average consumption of frozen potatoes. And the introduction of precut and prepackaged items has boosted the intake of fresh fruits and vegetables.

Highly publicized medical research linking compounds in fruits and vegetables to anticancer activity has provided a powerful incentive to consumption. However, in general, individual fast-food companies can spend multimillions of dollars to promote their products, whereas the national health organizations such as the National Cancer Institute is only able to spend a fraction of that amount to promote fruits and vegetables. And consider the fact that that applies to only *one* fast-food company! Go to Chapter 3 to find out more about the great diversity in carbohydrate foods.

Eating fewer whole grains

Individual use of flour and cereal products was 174 pounds per person in 2019 up from 138 pounds in 1970, but down from the 200 pounds per person in 2000. Some experts feel this may be the result of the avoidance of grains due to certain health conditions such as gluten sensitivity or the popularity of certain diets such as the Paleo Diet. The fact is that modern grains aren't the same as they used to be. Most of this change was in the form of refined flour food products.

Refined flour products can quickly spike your blood sugar and overstimulate your insulin production. Whole-grain food products raise blood-sugar levels gradually without overstimulating insulin. This effect is important in controlling obesity, diabetes, and heart disease. However, the USDA indicates consumption of whole grains is below guidelines. Evidence indicates that eating whole grains can reduce the risk of heart disease and some cancers. Current nutrition guidelines carry a strong recommendation to include at least three to five servings of whole-grain food products per day. However, that recommendation isn't being met in the United States.

Looking at the Nation's Health

With the changes that have occurred in the American food intake, the deterioration in the nation's health should come as no surprise. But food intake is not the only thing to blame; lack of exercise is a major contributor as well (see Chapter 22 for more on exercise). The American lifestyle is killing us — check out the following sections for information on how. Chapter 4 addresses many of these diseases in greater detail as you look at your own personal history and risk factors.

Obesity

Obesity has been growing rapidly, but health officials were shocked by a recent study that revealed that 71 percent of the population is either overweight or obese. Obesity is linked to diabetes, heart disease, hypertension, osteoarthritis, and cancer. The effects of obesity cost Americans billions of dollars per year.

Diabetes

Obesity is a worldwide epidemic and is being followed by a worldwide epidemic of diabetes. Thirty-four million Americans have diabetes and 88 million more have prediabetes and are at increased risk of developing the disease. Many of those with prediabetes are unaware that they have it. People who are obese have a five times greater risk of developing diabetes than people who are of a normal weight. Diabetes is a major health problem in the United States. It's characterized by an inability to keep blood-sugar levels consistent.

Metabolic syndrome

Metabolic syndrome is a name coined for a modern disease characterized by obesity, glucose intolerance, high triglycerides, and high blood pressure. It has also been called *Syndrome X, the Deadly Quartet, insulin resistance syndrome,* and *prediabetes. Insulin resistance* is the condition that causes this cluster of symptoms where the body doesn't respond very well to the insulin it produces. (*Insulin* is a hormone that moves glucose out of the blood and into the tissues where it can be used.)

If a person is insulin resistant, then they have to produce a greater amount of insulin in order to move the glucose into the tissue. High levels of insulin not only promote storage of fat but can cause serious harm to body organs. High levels of insulin cause high blood pressure, abnormal cholesterol levels, *atherosclerosis* (hardening of the arteries), and blood-clotting disorders. This can result in heart attacks and strokes. Eating high-carb foods — especially refined starchy and sugary foods — produces higher-than-normal amounts of insulin. The low-fat, high-carb diet universally recommended for high cholesterol is the worst diet for people who are insulin resistant.

Non-alcoholic fatty liver disease or non-alcoholic steatohepatitis

Cirrhosis of the liver is commonly associated with excess alcohol intake. However, many non-drinkers have been diagnosed with cirrhosis due to a fatty liver from excess calorie intake. This condition known as non-alcoholic fatty liver disease

(NAFLD) or as advanced disease of nonalcoholic steatohepatitis (NASH) is rising in prevalence due to the obesity epidemic. As the first step in treatment, health-care providers recommend lifestyle modification (diet and exercise).

Polycystic ovarian syndrome (PCOS)

Polycystic ovarian syndrome (PCOS) is an insulin-resistant disease in women that has become increasingly more prevalent. PCOS is characterized by elevated levels of male hormone, increased facial hair, irregular menstrual periods, and infertility. It's the most common cause of female hormone dysfunction and infertility. Women with PCOS may benefit from a low-carb diet.

Heart disease

The importance of insulin resistance as a heart disease risk factor has been recognized. New treatment guidelines for the prevention of heart disease identify the cluster of abnormalities associated with insulin resistance as risk factors. Specifically, levels of *triglycerides* (a fat in the blood) have been added to the list of risk factors. High levels of triglycerides in your blood are not only related to your fat intake, but also to your intake of excess calories and carbohydrate.

High blood pressure

High blood pressure (*hypertension*) is one of the nation's leading health problems. Forty-seven percent of adults are known to have high blood pressure and an estimated 100 million are at risk of developing it. High blood pressure greatly raises the risk of stroke, heart failure, and kidney disease. Current guidelines urge Americans to make diet and exercise changes designed to lower their blood pressure. Obesity is a major cause of hypertension. Approximately 78 percent of the high blood pressure cases in men and 65 percent in women can be directly attributed to obesity.

Compared with individuals with normal blood pressure, people with high blood pressure are relatively glucose intolerant. Insulin resistance is also a contributing factor to high blood pressure.

Inflammatory disease

Studies suggest that abdominal fat causes fat cells to release pro-inflammatory chemicals, which can make the body less sensitive to the insulin it produces by disrupting the function of insulin-responsive cells and their ability to respond to insulin. This is known as insulin resistance — the hallmark of type 2 diabetes.

Having excess abdominal fat (that is, a large waistline) is known as central or abdominal obesity, a particularly high-risk form of obesity. *Metaflammation* is the metabolic inflammatory state associated with obesity. The condition is defined by low-grade chronic inflammation in metabolic tissues, including adipose (fat) cells, liver, brain, and pancreas. Weight loss and calorie restriction have shown to decrease inflammation and increase insulin sensitivity in people who have been medically advised to lose excess weight.

Arthritis and related conditions

Arthritis is a very common degenerative joint disease. It commonly affects the weight-bearing joints in the knees, hips, and lower back. The most common risk factors are obesity and a family history of the condition. Being obese causes increase wear and tear on the joints, which decreases your ability to walk or get up and down out of a chair. There are different forms of arthritis and excess weight affects them all. Arthritis and joint conditions related to obesity are estimated to cost more than $128 billion a year in healthcare.

Cancer

Consumption of excess calories, regardless of the source, increases the risk of breast, prostate, and colon cancer. But just as important is what you *don't* eat. Diets full of whole foods such as fruits, vegetables, beans, whole grains, and low-fat dairy products are known to lower cancer risk. Dietary patterns that provide only the minimum servings of these foods increase cancer risk.

Gastroesophageal reflux disease (GERD)

Sometimes referred to as *heartburn*, gastroesophageal reflux disease (GERD) is much more extensive than heartburn. It has increased in incidence primarily due to obesity and the overconsumption of food. The intake of carbonated beverages and fatty and spicy foods aggravate the condition.

Determining Whether Low-Carb Dieting Is Dangerous

The question of safety has always arisen in regard to low-carb diets. That's because some low-carb diet plans restrict *all* carbohydrate foods from the diet. Eliminating carbohydrate from your diet is almost impossible, but some diets require you to get down to 10 or 20 grams of carbs per day. These kinds of severe carbohydrate diets not only restrict vital nutrients from the diet but the body also loses vital nutrients. And as you can guess, when you lose vital nutrients, you can end up in poor health. Modern-day proponents of very-low-carb diets recognize this problem and are adamant in recommending vitamin and mineral supplements to cover the losses. Now think about it: Can a diet plan that requires supplements to replace lost nutrients from food be good?

The Whole Foods Weight Loss Eating Plan doesn't completely eliminate carbs from your diet. In fact, you must eat some carbohydrates, like those found in fresh fruits and vegetables, to maintain good health. There's no way to get the necessary fiber, vitamins, and minerals, on a regular basis without some carbs. Here I show you how to pick the best and leave the rest.

Evaluating limits on carbs

Eating a healthy diet on a very-low-carb diet that restricts you to fewer than 50 grams of carbohydrate is impossible. If you tried, you'd be eliminating too many foods rich in vitamins, minerals, fiber, and cancer-fighters. Getting essential nutrients from foods is always better than getting it from supplements.

A moderately low-carbohydrate diet — such as the Whole Foods Weight Loss Eating Plan — includes 100 to 150 grams of carbohydrate per day. Recent nutrition guidelines say that 130 grams of carbohydrate per day is the minimum level needed for adequate brain function in children and adults. This level — also in-line with what the American Diabetes Association recommends — is the minimum to prevent loss of lean tissue from muscles and organs.

If you count the carbohydrate in milk, fruits, vegetables, legumes, breads, and cereals, you'd have 130 grams of carbohydrate from two servings of milk, two servings of fruit, three servings of vegetables, and four servings of legumes, breads, or cereals.

A high-carb diet, on the other hand, includes more than 250 grams of carbohydrate each day. That diet is appropriate for active people who are at a healthy weight (with a BMI between 20 and 25 — see Chapter 4 for more on BMI). No matter how many grams of carbs you eat every day, fruits, vegetables, whole grains, and legumes should be the main food sources of carbohydrates, with added sugar sources kept to a minimum.

The potential physical consequences of very-low-carbohydrate diets range from mild to serious to life-threatening. Because the Whole Foods Weight Loss Eating Plan I recommend is a modified low-carbohydrate diet, you shouldn't experience any of these problems. But, as with any diet plan, consult your healthcare provider for advice before beginning the plan. Check out Chapter 3 for the physical consequences of very-low-carbohydrate diets.

To evaluate your own lifestyle and health risks to determine if a lower-carbohydrate diet may be good for you, turn to Chapter 4.

Getting Back to Basics: The Whole Foods Weight Loss Eating Plan

Very-low-carb diets, allowing no more than 15 to 30 grams of total carbohydrate per day, restrict many healthy foods and do not represent balanced lifetime nutrition. However, *moderate* restriction of carbohydrates — below the 60 percent recommended by the USDA, but not to the extreme — can produce positive benefits in many individuals.

REMEMBER

Not all carbohydrates are created equally. Certain types of carbohydrates can keep you satisfied longer, and eating a variety of foods keeps you interested in the diet. So which carbs are good and which are bad, and how can you tell the difference? It all depends on the glycemic load of the food. Check out Chapter 3 and Appendix A for more information on glycemic load.

Looking at the changes in food intake and the increase in obesity in the past 20 to 30 years, it's pretty obvious that Americans have gotten away from eating basic whole foods. Much of what Americans eat is processed, refined, or somehow changed from its original form. The intake of fruits, vegetables, whole grains, lean protein sources, and good fats is severely lacking.

Unveiling the plan

The Whole Foods Weight Loss Eating Plan is designed to help you get back to eating basic healthy foods in a satisfying way. The plan shows you how to lower your total carbohydrate intake in a safe and satisfying way, and it explains how you can replace the refined sugars and flour products in your diet with whole, unprocessed fruits and vegetables. Not only do you discover how to eat quality lean proteins and protective fats, but your appetite needs will be met naturally, and you won't be hungry. Your body will thrive on the nutrients you're feeding it rather than wilting on empty calories. You'll naturally start to lose your surplus fat and your health and energy will soar.

The Whole Foods Weight Loss Eating Plan consists of the following:

>> Vegetables and whole fruits

>> Lean protein, fish, and poultry

>> Low-fat cheese, low-fat milk (or dairy alternatives), and yogurt

>> Moderate amounts of fat, especially monounsaturated and polyunsaturated fats such as avocados, olives, olive oil, peanut oil, canola oil, flaxseed oil, and sesame seeds; and nuts and seeds

>> Whole grains, and starchy vegetables such as legumes and corn

Sugar, white flour, and other refined grains are limited on the Whole Foods Weight Loss Eating Plan, as are fried foods, processed snack foods and processed meats. The following sections discuss the three categories on the plan.

Green Light foods

The green light means go. You can move around *freely* in this section and eat as much as you need to satisfy your hunger. Green Light foods include lean meat, fish, poultry, eggs, low-fat cheese, low-fat cottage cheese, salads, nonstarchy vegetables, and fresh whole fruits.

For a full list of Green Light foods, check out Chapter 5. You can also find a great shopping list in Appendix B — don't miss it!

Yellow Light foods

The yellow light is the control feature of the Whole Foods Weight Loss Eating Plan. It allows for your weight loss and lowers your triglycerides and blood sugar if they're elevated. You're allowed five carbohydrate choices per day from the Yellow Light group.

A carbohydrate choice is a food that supplies 15 grams of total carbohydrate per serving. (Green Light foods don't count toward this number.) Your five carb choices should ideally be whole grains, beans, or starchy vegetables, but they can be a piece of cake or candy, or a cookie. (Everyone needs a sweet now and then.)

REMEMBER

You're allowed to vary your Yellow Light foods to one to three carb choices or no carb choices if you want to speed up your weight loss. However, you'll find these levels hard to maintain long term, so you'll be glad to have that maximum of five carbs.

Examples of Yellow Light carb choices include the following:

>> One slice of regular bread

>> ½ cup pasta or cereal

>> ½ cup potatoes, beans, or corn

>> One serving (15 grams carbohydrate) chips, cookies, cake, or candy

Check out Chapter 6 for the real deal on using your carb choices each day.

In addition to the five carbohydrate choices, you're allowed the following every day:

>> Two to three servings from the dairy group, which includes skim or low-fat milk, and low-fat yogurt. The carbohydrate in these foods isn't counted.

>> Eight monounsaturated or polyunsaturated fat choices like avocados, almonds, cashews, peanuts, olives, canola oil, olive oil, or peanut oil; or polyunsaturated fats such as tub or squeeze margarine, reduced-fat mayonnaise, Miracle Whip, salad dressing, corn oil, safflower oil, soybean oil, or sunflower or pumpkin seeds.

For the full scoop on fats, take a look at Chapter 8. Track down the dairy story in Chapter 7.

Red Light foods

Although the Whole Foods Weight Loss Eating Plan doesn't have foods in the Red Light category, red is important because it simply means, "Stop and think! You're about to exceed the limit." No food is absolutely forbidden on the Whole Foods Weight Loss Eating Plan. You just want to make sure that most of the time your five carbohydrate choices per day come from legumes, whole grains, and starchy vegetables in the Yellow Light category. But, if you must have a treat, you can trade it for an equivalent amount of Yellow Light food.

Stopping is what you should do when you're faced with breads, cookies, cakes, pastries, cereals, gravies, thickened soups, sugar, syrup, chocolate, or soft drinks that can cause you to exceed your carbohydrate limit. These highly refined carbohydrate foods can spike your blood sugar and stimulate your insulin response. You'll find yourself with hard-to-control hunger the rest of the day. When you do occasionally indulge in these foods be sure to make them part of the five carb choices and you'll not experience erratic blood sugar and insulin levels.

Knowing who can benefit from the plan

If any of the following describes you, you can benefit from the Whole Foods Weight Loss Eating Plan

>> You've tried other weight-loss plans and have been unsuccessful.

>> You're overweight or obese (BMI 25 or over for overweight; BMI 30 or over for obesity).

>> You have or are at risk of developing type 2 diabetes or insulin resistance.

>> You have high triglyceride concentrations in your blood.

>> You have borderline or high blood pressure.

Check out Chapter 4 to determine if lower-carb eating is for you.

Chapter **3**

All Carbs Aren't Equal: Looking at the Differences

Where is carbohydrate? It's in sugar, bread, potatoes, cereal, pasta, beans, chips, cookies, cake, soft drinks, fruit, vegetables, and dairy. It's even a substance in your blood that your body depends on for fuel. Carbohydrate is everywhere except in meats and animal fats, and most of it is pretty tasty. Carbohydrate as a nutrient source is an important part of a healthy diet. To restrict all dietary intake of carbohydrate, the way some low-carb diets prescribe, regardless of its food source is short-sighted. Dismissing fruits, vegetables, whole grains, and beans simply because they contain carbohydrates can be disastrous to your health, in both the short run and the long run.

The intake of *refined* carbohydrate foods (foods that have been stripped of their nutritional value during processing), yielding little nutritive value except calories, has overwhelmed this sedentary nation. (For more on this situation, take a look at Chapter 2.) Children and athletes can consume larger amounts of starches and sugars with less harm than can relatively inactive people, but many people tend to eat a greater amount of these kinds of carbohydrates than they can handle. So, before you start to lower your carbohydrate intake, you need to get a sense of the various forms and functions of carbohydrates. This chapter can help you decide which ones to keep and which ones to control.

TECHNICAL STUFF

All dietary carbohydrates, from starch to table sugar, can be converted into glucose to be used as fuel for the body, especially the brain. How active you are governs your need for this fuel. So, if you're not very active and all your body's reserved carbohydrate fuel is full, you'll store the surplus as fat. Refer to Appendix A for more details.

Understanding Carbohydrates

The primary role of carbohydrates in human nutrition is to supply an indispensable commodity — energy. When carbohydrates yield energy at the rate of 4 calories per gram, they spare proteins from being used for energy so that proteins can do the building and repairing of body tissues that they are uniquely suited for.

Without sufficient carbohydrate, your body will burn its protein for fuel. Carbohydrates appear in virtually all plant foods and in only one food taken from animals — namely, milk. Choosing good sources of carbs can help you control your blood sugar and your weight.

To understand carbohydrates you need to appreciate the various roles they play in the body and the various ways they appear in food. The following sections describe the diverse names and functions of the foodstuffs called carbohydrate.

Identifying the sugar connection

Carbohydrates come in three main sizes:

>> **Monosaccharides:** Sugars whose atoms are arranged in a single ring

>> **Disaccharides:** Sugars made from pairs of rings

>> **Polysaccharides:** Long chains of single-ring carbohydrates

The monosaccharides and disaccharides are known as *simple carbohydrates*; the polysaccharides are known as *complex carbohydrates.* Your body almost invariably converts carbohydrates, whatever form they come in (except dietary fibers), to its own energy source, commonly referred to as *blood sugar.*

What carbs give you beyond nutrition

Six essential nutrients are necessary for good health and for life: protein, carbohydrate, fat, vitamins, minerals, and water. Only protein, carbohydrate, and fat provide energy in the form of calories. Your body needs all these nutrients in order to stay alive. Scientists are discovering, however, that other components are essential for *good health.* These components don't yield energy either (in other words, they don't have calories), but their role in disease prevention is vital. I cover these non-nutrient components in the following sections.

Fiber

Dietary *fiber* is found in plant foods and is mainly the fiber component of a plant's cell walls, which aren't digested by the enzymes in your intestinal tract and, therefore, don't provide you with any energy. There are two types of dietary fiber:

>> **Soluble:** *Soluble* fiber helps to lower your LDL ("bad") cholesterol and lowers your rate of glucose absorption.

>> **Insoluble:** *Insoluble* fiber helps to soften your stool and lowers your risk of some kinds of cancer.

As with anything in nutrition, you need a balance of both types of fiber. Each type of fiber performs a distinct function and is necessary for good health. (For specifics on working more fiber into your diet, sneak a peek at Chapter 6.)

EXPLAINING NET CARBS

The concept of *net carbs* is based on the fact that not all carbohydrates affect the body in the same manner. Fiber is important in calculating net carbs, but fiber doesn't carry any caloric value. The Nutrition Facts food label lists Total Carbohydrate followed by Dietary Fiber and Total Sugars. The sugars are the natural and added sugars in the food product and are included in the Total Carbohydrate.

For example, if a food has 15 grams of Total Carbohydrate and 6 grams of Dietary Fiber, then subtract the 6 from the 15 to equal 9, which is how much Net Carbohydrate the food has, making it half of a carbohydrate choice. Check out Chapter 6 for more on counting carbohydrate choices and Chapter 9 for more on the Nutrition Facts food label.

Traditionally, soluble fiber got the credit for lowering cholesterol, whereas improvement of bowel regularity was attributed to insoluble fiber. The truth is that both fiber sources improve regularity and lower blood cholesterol.

Phytochemicals

Phytochemicals are compounds that exist naturally in all plant foods (*phyto* comes from the Greek word for "plant"). Scientists have identified about 10,000 different phytochemicals (*or plant chemicals*) in the foods you eat, and many still remain unknown. An apple alone has hundreds of phytochemicals. Carbohydrate foods such as fruits, vegetables, grains, legumes, seeds, licorice root, soy, and green tea all contain these plant chemicals. Phytochemicals are best supplied from fruits and vegetables — not from supplements.

Phytochemicals contain protective, disease-preventing compounds. Thousands of different phytochemicals have been identified as components of food, and many more phytochemicals continue to be discovered every day. Just one serving of vegetables gives you more than 100 different phytochemicals. See Chapter 25 for more information on phytochemicals.

REMEMBER

Think of *phyto* as "fight-o." Every mouthful puts disease fighters in your body. Phytochemicals occur to protect the plant from disease and destruction and continue to protect the humans who eat the plants.

Phytochemicals are associated with the prevention and/or treatment of at least four of the leading causes of death in the United States — cancer, diabetes, cardiovascular disease, and hypertension. They're involved in many processes including those that help prevent cell damage, prevent cancer cell replication, and decrease cholesterol levels.

Table 3-1 lists a few phytochemicals and their sources in carbohydrate foods.

TABLE 3-1 ## Noteworthy Phytochemicals and Food Sources

Phytochemical	Sources
Allyl sulfides	Garlic, onions, leeks, and chives
Capsaicin	Hot peppers
Carotenoids	Dark green and yellow fruits and vegetables
Coumarins	Citrus fruit, tomatoes
Ellagic acid, phenols	Grapes, berries, cherries, apples, cantaloupe, watermelon
Flavonoids	Citrus fruit, tomatoes, berries, peppers, carrots
Genistein	Beans, peas, lentils
Indoles	Broccoli, cabbage
Isoflavones	Soybeans, dried beans
Lignans	Flaxseed, barley, wheat
Lutein, zeaxanthin	Spinach, kale, collard greens, romaine lettuce, leeks, peas
Lycopene	Tomatoes, red peppers, red grapefruit
Phytic acid	Whole grains (barley, corn, oats, rye, wheat)
Saponins	Soybeans, dried beans

GOT GAS? FODMAP CARBS

Fermentable, oligosaccharides, disaccharides and monosaccharides, and polyols (FODMAPs) are short-chain carbohydrates (sugars) that can induce abdominal symptoms that are similar to people with irritable bowel syndrome (IBS). Some people's small intestines poorly absorb this group of carbohydrates.

The FODMAP food list is extensive and includes milk, dairy products, legumes, cruciferous vegetables such as cabbage and cauliflower, some fruits, and grains, especially wheat and rye. Many of these foods are gas-producing foods. Other symptoms of carbohydrate malabsorption are diarrhea, pain, and bloating. In 2005, a low FODMAP diet was introduced as a therapy for IBS. Since then the mechanisms of action, food content of FODMAPs, and efficacy of the diet have been extensively studied. In many parts of the world, the low FODMAP diet is now considered a frontline therapy for IBS. Before you consider the FODMAP diet, consult with your healthcare provider and a registered dietitian nutritionist (RDN).

Discovering How Carbs Affect Your Blood Sugar Levels

The glycemic index measures the effects of equal quantities of different carbohydrates on blood glucose levels. Since introduced more than 40 years ago, the glycemic index challenged traditional thinking about carbohydrate effects on blood sugar; the scientific community was slow to embrace the index. Traditional theory stated that simple carbohydrates, such as orange juice, raised blood glucose levels quickly, whereas complex carbs, such as crackers, raised blood glucose levels more slowly. Researchers now realize the distinction between sugar and starch is largely useless from a biological viewpoint. Research on glycemic index values showed some simple carbohydrates raise blood glucose slowly and some complex carbohydrates raise blood glucose quickly.

REMEMBER

The *glycemic load* is a measurement that is calculated from the glycemic index and is used to evaluate the glucose response in a normal serving of a particular food. The formula is the glycemic index multiplied by the number of grams of carbohydrate in a serving, divided by 100.

Don't worry about the mathematical formulas though: Appendix A lists more information on the glycemic index and glycemic load of foods. You can use glycemic load to evaluate the kinds of foods in your diet. If most of your foods are on the high glycemic load level and those foods are low in nutritive factors, then I recommend exchanging some of those high glycemic choices for low glycemic choices. If most of your foods fall into the low glycemic category, then chances are you're eating a very healthy diet.

Carbohydrate foods that are low in glycemic load seem to increase *satiety* (feeling of fullness after eating) and maintain consistent blood glucose and insulin levels. Non-starchy vegetables, fruits, legumes, and high-fiber whole-grain products tend to have a low glycemic load. These foods have a proven record of health benefits such as lower risk of heart disease and cancer and less gastrointestinal diseases and are a component of any reasonable diet. Such slowly absorbed carbohydrates can contribute greatly to overall health, satiety, and weight loss.

Understanding Refined and Processed Carbs

A *refined* food is a food that doesn't contain all its original nutrients. For example, a grain of wheat to make white flour has 16 essential nutrients refined out of it. Five of those (iron, thiamin, niacin, riboflavin, and folic acid) are added back in by the government enrichment program to prevent nutritional deficiencies. All refined foods are processed foods; you can't pick a refined food out of your garden and eat it. On the other hand, a healthy whole food is considered processed if it has simply been sliced, chopped, rolled, or ground. That is, it has gone through a process, but its original nutrition content is intact.

Most refined and processed carbs are high in glycemic load and may result in hunger soon after their rapid digestion. Refined and processed carbs such as those found in cookies, crackers, rice cakes, bagels, cakes, doughnuts, croissants, chips, pastries, pretzels, most packaged breakfast cereals, white bread, and white rice have a high glycemic load; their easy digestion causes a rapid elevation in blood glucose and insulin levels. After a couple of hours, the blood glucose levels quickly decline, resulting in cravings for more food in some people. This phenomenon may have led to the coining of the phrase *carbohydrate addiction*.

You don't have to totally avoid high-glycemic-load foods. You can eat some high-glycemic foods in the presence of low-glycemic foods and the effect on your blood sugar wouldn't be as great as it would be with high-glycemic foods alone. What you need to be aware of is the percentage of high-glycemic load foods to low-glycemic-load foods. Try to include more low-glycemic-load foods in your diet than high. See Appendix A for more information on glycemic load and glycemic index.

Replacing the Food Pyramid with a Healthy Eating Plate

Even though the Food Guide Pyramid was around for many years and increased nutrition knowledge in the United States, it did little to change the eating habits of consumers. The Food Guide Pyramid emphasized lowering fat in the diet and replacing it with bread, cereals, grains, fruits, and vegetables. Fat is a calorie-dense fuel and provides 9 calories per gram, whereas carbohydrate and protein each supply 4 calories per gram.

Current wisdom would say if you cut out something that gives 9 calories and replace it with something that gives 4 calories, you'd reduce your total calorie intake. Sounds reasonable, right? Take away high-fat foods and replace them with fruits, vegetables, and whole grains, but that's not what happened.

Unfortunately, along with the reduced-fat message came fat-free cookies, cakes, chips, snacks, and desserts that displaced the intended healthier choices of fruits, veggies, and whole grains. After all, fat tastes good, so to trick consumers' taste buds into thinking that fat-free foods tasted good, manufacturers loaded the food with sugar. So, they didn't just replace a fat gram with a carbohydrate gram in an even swap; they replaced the fat with double, triple, and quadruple the carbohydrate! Many consumers saw a box of fat-free cookies as a free food and ate the whole box rather than just a serving.

Scientists realized a change needed to happen to provide guidance to consumers to help them eat healthier. That's how the Healthy Eating Plate came about. Designed by experts at Harvard School of Public Health and Harvard Medical School, the Healthy Eating Plate (see Figure 3-1) directs consumers to the healthiest choices in major food groups.

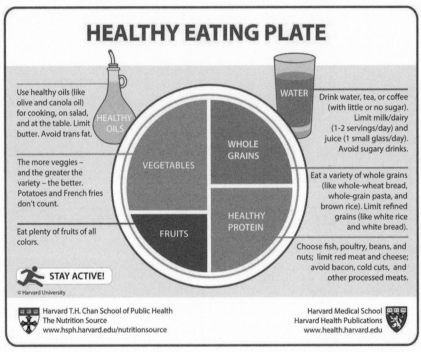

HEALTHY EATING PLATE

Use healthy oils (like olive and canola oil) for cooking, on salad, and at the table. Limit butter. Avoid trans fat.

HEALTHY OILS

WATER Drink water, tea, or coffee (with little or no sugar). Limit milk/dairy (1-2 servings/day) and juice (1 small glass/day). Avoid sugary drinks.

The more veggies – and the greater the variety – the better. Potatoes and French fries don't count.

VEGETABLES

WHOLE GRAINS

Eat a variety of whole grains (like whole-wheat bread, whole-grain pasta, and brown rice). Limit refined grains (like white rice and white bread).

Eat plenty of fruits of all colors.

FRUITS

HEALTHY PROTEIN

Choose fish, poultry, beans, and nuts; limit red meat and cheese; avoid bacon, cold cuts, and other processed meats.

STAY ACTIVE!

© Harvard University

Harvard T.H. Chan School of Public Health
The Nutrition Source
www.hsph.harvard.edu/nutritionsource

Harvard Medical School
Harvard Health Publications
www.health.harvard.edu

FIGURE 3-1: The Healthy Eating Plate.

Copyright © 2011 Harvard University.

TIP

For more information about The Healthy Eating Plate, see The Nutrition Source, Department of Nutrition, Harvard T.H. Chan School of Public Health, www.thenutritionsource.org and health.harvard.edu.

A number of research studies suggest that diets designed to lower the insulin response to ingested carbohydrate (such as a low-glycemic-index diet) may improve utilization of stored energy (body fat), decrease hunger, and promote weight loss. The Healthy Eating Plate demonstrates that such a diet would have as its base abundant quantities of low- to moderate-glycemic vegetables and fruits, moderate amounts of protein, legumes, reduced-fat dairy, and healthy fats (like olive and canola oil), and an emphasis of whole grains over refined-grain products, potatoes, french fries, and concentrated sugars. The Whole Foods Weight Loss Eating Plan closely approximates the recommendations of Harvard's Healthy Eating Plate (refer to Chapter 2 for more about this plan).

Going Low-Carb without Going Extreme

Following any diet that doesn't allow you to get the minimum requirements of key nutritional benchmarks, including fiber, calcium, fat, protein, and carbohydrate can have disastrous long-term health complications. Always seek input from your healthcare provider before altering your diet or beginning an exercise program.

WARNING

If you go too low in restricting carbs — say 20 to 30 grams daily —you can encounter several immediate side effects (refer to Chapter 1 for more about Very Low Carbohydrate Ketogenic Diet (VLCKD). Here's a quick list of a few of the most common ones:

>> **Constipation:** Severe carbohydrate restriction eliminates fruit, vegetables, and grains. The resulting low fiber intake can lead to constipation and gastrointestinal problems.

>> **Dehydration and low blood pressure:** This results from the excessive water loss in the early stages of the diet.

>> **Dizziness and fainting:** This can result from low blood pressure due to the dehydration. It's often felt when standing up too quickly.

>> **Nausea and fatigue:** Both are often associated with *ketosis* (burning fat for fuel) and low blood-sugar levels.

>> **Halitosis:** *Halitosis* is bad breath. It's also associated with an excess amount of *ketones* (a byproduct of burning fat for fuel) in your body. This occurs when someone is in ketosis. It has been described as smelling like a cross between nail polish and overripe pineapple. (Just the kind of thing you're striving for, right?)

>> **Ketosis:** Ketosis is a condition resulting from switching from using carbs to fat as the primary energy source. As your body metabolizes fat, it gives off ketones; excess ketones show up in your urine. Although ketosis is your body's natural backup survival system, when it occurs over an extended period of time, it can cause light-headedness and fogginess. In some medical conditions, prolonged ketosis can cause coma and even death. Being in ketosis continually isn't normal or healthy, and the long-term safety of this condition is unknown. Ketosis definitely isn't good for children.

>> **Short-term weight loss:** Initial weight loss is due to water loss and levels off in about 7 to 14 weeks. Permanent weight loss occurs more slowly and only if you stay on the diet. When you stop following a low-carb diet and you return to normal eating, the weight usually returns.

WARNING

Possible *long-term effects* of a very low-carb diet include the following:

>> **Loss of muscle mass:** Your body needs a source of glucose. In diets with too low a restriction in carbohydrate (below 130 grams), your body starts to metabolize the protein in muscle tissue in order to get carbohydrate. This eventually weakens your body.

>> **Increased workload on your kidneys:** Very low-carbohydrate diets are associated with excess protein and fat intake. High protein intake puts an added burden on the kidneys and liver. If you have diabetes, you already have an increased risk of kidney disease, so be sure to check with your healthcare provider before following a high-protein diet. If you already have kidney disease, then a very low-carb diet definitely isn't for you.

>> **Kidney stones and gout:** A high protein, ketosis-inducing diet, can lead to high uric acid levels in the blood, increasing the risk of kidney stones and gout.

>> **Increased risk of heart disease:** Diets very low in carbohydrate are usually high in saturated fat and high in animal protein. High saturated fat increases the risk of heart disease and some forms of cancer.

>> **Increased risk of some cancers:** The risk of many cancers is likely to be increased when most fruits, vegetables, whole grains, and beans are eliminated from the diet.

>> **Osteoporosis:** High animal protein intake combined with the ketosis from a very low carbohydrate intake is thought to draw calcium from the bones, leading to calcium depletion and increasing the risk of osteoporosis and hip fractures. Also, rapid weight loss can accelerate bone deterioration and cause osteoporosis.

>> **Vitamin and mineral deficiencies:** When entire food groups are eliminated from a diet, such as fruits, vegetables, grains, and dairy, vitamin and mineral deficiencies can occur. High-protein, very low-carbohydrate diets usually lack several vitamins and minerals such as vitamins A, C, D, the B vitamins, antioxidants that can slow the effects of aging, and calcium.

REMEMBER

None of these complications should occur on the Whole Foods Weight Loss Eating Plan. On the Whole Foods Weight Loss Eating Plan, you're allowed five carbohydrate choices per day, because this amount allows for a healthy 1 to 2 pounds of weight loss per week. Carbohydrate from fruits and vegetables isn't restricted because fruits and vegetables are so essential to good health and disease prevention, and they have a low glycemic index/load.

Chapter **4**

Determining Whether Low-Carb Eating Is Right for You

Not every diet is beneficial to every person. Some people are in perfect health and likely also have nearly perfect diets. Others may need very strict limits or restrictions on foods due to allergies or other conditions. Still others with existing health conditions may need to cut out refined sugars but can enjoy artificially or naturally sweetened foods.

So how do you know if a low-carb diet can benefit you personally? One way is to talk with your healthcare provider about the plan I outline in this book. But before you do, consider reading this chapter to get your low-carb ducks in a row. You'll likely be a step ahead when you actually do talk to your provider, because they'll probably want you to complete some version of this assessment.

REMEMBER

This chapter isn't intended to diagnose your health problems. Its only intent is to make you aware of your risk factors. Healthy adults should have complete physical exams at least every five years beginning at age 20. Check with your healthcare provider to find out what's appropriate for you.

What's Your Story? Assessing Your Personal Health Risks

People metabolize carbohydrates in different ways. Some carbohydrates are beneficial to your health and others can actually be harmful to your health, depending on your own health history. Before you make a change in your diet, you need to take a look at yourself, your family, and your lifestyle.

Grab a pencil to record the information on your history or open your Notes app on your phone.

REMEMBER

Knowing your body mass index (BMI), blood glucose (sugar) level, total cholesterol level, HDL cholesterol, LDL cholesterol, triglycerides, and blood pressure is important. If you haven't seen your healthcare provider in a while, call and make an appointment to discuss the plan with them and get much of this information. (Refer to the section, "Looking at your body mass index," later in this chapter for more information. You may be able to get your blood pressure and cholesterol tested in your community. YMCAs and even some grocery stores often offer inexpensive blood pressure and cholesterol testing from time to time, so check around.)

Playing detective: Uncovering your family medical history

What kinds of diseases or health problems are in your family? Did Grandma have diabetes? Did Uncle Joe have a heart attack in his forties? Is Uncle Joe Grandma's brother? And, how about Mom and Dad? Are they in good health? If you're like most people, you probably go through life not really thinking about how your family members' health affects you — but I'm here to tell you it does.

Your family's health is part of your own personal health history. That's why your healthcare provider asks you to fill out pages and pages of questions about others in your family (and you thought it was just to keep you occupied while you were waiting to finally get in to see the doctor). Your own health destiny rests, at least in part, in your genes. The sooner you know what you face, the better.

REMEMBER

Just because you have a family member who had diabetes or died of a heart attack or cancer doesn't necessarily mean you're destined to have diabetes or heart disease or cancer. But knowing your family's health history does let you know if you're at risk for developing those diseases — and it empowers you to do whatever you can to prevent that from happening.

Start by collecting information from your first-degree relatives. A *first-degree relative* is your brother, your sister, your parents, or your children. Record each disease, illness, or surgery each person has had. Especially ask about chronic illness such as diabetes, heart disease, high blood pressure, cancer, and obesity. If one of your first-degree relatives has died, record the person's age at death and what they died of and as much information as you can about any diseases, illnesses, or surgeries they had. Especially make note of any disease such as heart disease, cancer, or diabetes that occurred at an unusually early age.

After you've collected all the information you can find on your first-degree relatives, move on to your *extended family*. Your extended family includes grandparents, aunts, uncles, and cousins. If possible, trace your family history back at least three or four generations.

The American Medical Association (AMA) can get you started with their online Adult Family History Form (`www.ama-assn.org`) and type "Family History Form" into the search. You can fill out the form online and then print it for your records. You can also email it to family members for their input.

However you gather the information, keep it up to date and share it with your healthcare provider and family. After gathering information on your family's health, share it with your provider. Especially tell them if you discover two first-degree relatives with the same cancer or one first-degree relative younger than the age of 50 with an illness usually associated with older people, such as cancer or heart disease.

If you're adopted or have no contact with a biological family, then start keeping a record of what you know about yourself for your current or future offspring.

Figuring out how your age is affecting your health

When it comes to your health, you have control over many, many factors. But one factor you can't control is your age. And as you age, you face increased risk of developing certain diseases. So read on to determine what role your age is playing in your health.

If you get a group of 25-year-olds together, chances are you'll have a very healthy group of people. If you get that same group together 35 years later when they're 60 years old, you'll have a very diverse group in terms of their health status. As people age, they reap the benefits or destruction of their lifestyle, genetics, and exposure. Everyone wants to live long, healthy lives. But that doesn't start at 60 — it starts when you're young. If you're older than 25, don't worry: A healthy lifestyle can start today.

SMOKING AND YOUR HEALTH

If you're a smoker, quitting smoking is the most important step you can take to improve your health. Smoking increases your risk of lung cancer, throat cancer, emphysema, heart disease, high blood pressure, ulcers, gum disease, and other conditions. Smoking can cause coughing, poor athletic ability, and sore throats. It can also cause face wrinkles, stained teeth, and dull skin.

Remember: It's never too late to quit smoking. Save your money, prolong your life, and quit today. Some people fear the weight gain that sometimes comes with quitting smoking, but it's usually no more than 5 pounds and is easily remedied. The smoking is far worse than the weight gain. Your healthcare provider can help you decide which smoking cessation method will work best for you.

Younger adults

You fall into this age bracket if you're a man between the ages of 20 and 35 or a woman between the ages of 20 and 45.

Heart disease is rare in this age bracket except in those individuals with severe risk factors, such as a genetic tendency for high cholesterol or high triglycerides, high blood pressure, or diabetes. Heavy smoking (more than a pack a day) can also be a significant risk factor (see the nearby sidebar for more on smoking's impact on your health). Even though heart disease is rare in young adults, *atherosclerosis* (hardening of the arteries) is in its early stages in this age bracket and may progress rapidly. Long-term studies show that high blood cholesterol in young adulthood predicts a higher rate of premature heart disease in middle age.

Middle-aged adults

You fall into this age bracket if you're a man between the ages of 35 and 65 or a woman between the ages of 45 and 75.

Men generally have a higher risk for heart disease than women. Middle-aged men especially have a tendency to gain weight around the waistline (referred to as *abdominal obesity*), which increases their tendency to become resistant to their own insulin (or suffer from a condition called *insulin resistance*). Insulin resistance can impair your ability to handle blood sugar properly, increase your triglycerides, and lower your HDL ("good") cholesterol. (Check out the section, "Recognizing the silent syndrome," later in this chapter for more details about insulin resistance.) These conditions lead to a dramatically increased risk of heart disease. A sizable portion of all heart disease in men occurs in middle age. Exercise and even a moderate weight loss can dramatically improve the condition.

Heart disease is generally delayed in women by 10 to 15 years compared with men. Therefore, most heart disease in women occurs after the age of 65. Yet, at this later age, heart disease accounts for a third of all deaths in women. Three million women die from stroke each year. These deaths are more than the deaths from all types of cancer. Heart disease can occur in women younger than 65 if they're heavy smokers, have high blood pressure, have insulin resistance, have diabetes, or if they have a family history of early heart disease. The good news is women can be proactive in their health education in preventive lifestyle choices such as diet and exercise.

Older adults

You fall into this age bracket if you're a man older than 65 or a woman older than 75.

Most new heart disease events and most heart attack deaths occur in older adults. High blood cholesterol — especially high LDL (or "bad") cholesterol — increases the risk for heart disease in older adults.

Your chances of developing high blood pressure increase with age. Information from the long-running Framingham Heart Study shows that a 55-year-old with normal blood pressure today has a 90 percent chance of developing high blood pressure in the next 25 years.

Looking at your body mass index

In the past, height and weight tables developed by insurance companies classified weights by frame size (small, medium, or large), with one table for men and one for women. BMI is now used as an assessment of body size. BMI looks at what people weigh and classifies their weight by degree of medical risk. The BMI is a close measurement of body fat in most people. The same table is used for men and women.

Figuring out your BMI

Go to www.nhibi.nih.gov/bmicalc.htm for an easy-to-use calculator to determine your BMI. Or, you can download one of the many BMI apps to your smartphone. *Note:* BMI is a screening tool and not necessarily a hard and fast rule. A person's body type, muscle mass, and health status should be factored into determining a healthy weight.

TIP

You use the same calculation to figure the BMI for a child older than 2 years of age, but the result isn't interpreted the same as in Table 4-1. Check with your pediatrician for the correct interpretation of a child's BMI.

GET MOVING: PHYSICAL ACTIVITY AND AGE

You never outgrow your need for physical activity. As you age, you need to be even more dedicated to being active. Normal aging results in a gradual decline in heart and lung function, nerve function, and muscle and bone strength. Being active improves your heart and lungs and allows you to do more work without feeling tired. Physically active older adults have faster reaction times, better balance, and better hand-eye coordination for performing manual tasks. Physical activity can reduce the number of fractures in older adults as well.

A BMI of 20 to 24.9 is considered a healthy weight. A BMI of 25 to 29.9 is considered overweight, but not obese. And a BMI of 30 or greater is obesity. Refer to Table 4-1 to determine your medical risk based on your BMI.

TABLE 4-1   **Your Medical Risk Based on Your BMI**

BMI	Degree of Obesity	Degree of Medical Risk
20 to 24.9	None	None
25 to 29.9	Mild	Low
30 to 34.9	Moderate	Moderate
35 to 40	High	High
Greater than 40	Severe	Severe

REMEMBER

In Table 4-1, medical risk is determined just by your weight. You may have an increased medical risk due to other conditions, such as high cholesterol, high blood pressure, diabetes, or some other condition.

Recognizing the limitations of the BMI

Because your BMI is based solely on weight and height, it may overestimate body fat in athletes and others who have a lot of muscle. If this applies to you, you'll need a measure of your body-fat percentage. (Most gyms and fitness centers have facilities and trained personnel to complete these tests.)

On the other hand, BMI may underestimate body fat in older people or others who have lost muscle. So just remember to use the BMI as a helpful tool and realize that its readings and scores aren't absolute.

Improving your BMI score

If your number is 30 or above, don't make the mistake of thinking you have to reach the 20 to 25 range before you'll see a benefit to your health. Research shows that if you reduce your weight by 10 percent or even lower your BMI number by 2 points, you'll significantly improve many health factors such as blood glucose, triglycerides, cholesterol, and blood pressure. Give yourself six months to lose 10 percent of your body weight.

If you aren't overweight or obese, but health problems run in your family, keeping your weight steady is important. If you have family members with weight-related health problems, you're more likely to develop them yourself. Talk to your health-care provider if you aren't sure of your risk. Developing a regular habit of physical exercise and eating a healthy diet is the best way to prevent weight gain.

Identifying your diabetes risk

People who have diabetes have a blood glucose level (often called *blood sugar level*) that is too high. Everyone's blood has some glucose in it because our bodies need it for energy. But too much glucose in the blood isn't good for your health.

These sections discuss the three main types of diabetes.

Type 1 diabetes

Formerly called *juvenile diabetes* or *insulin-dependent diabetes,* type 1 diabetes is usually diagnosed in children, teenagers, or young adults. In this form of diabetes, the body can no longer make insulin. Treatment for type 1 diabetes includes taking insulin shots or using an insulin pump, making wise food choices, exercising regularly, and controlling blood pressure and cholesterol.

Type 2 diabetes

Formerly called *adult-onset* or *non-insulin-dependent diabetes,* this is the most common form of diabetes. People can develop type 2 diabetes at any age — even during childhood. In type 2 diabetes, the body either doesn't make enough insulin or the body can't properly use the insulin it does make; this condition is called *insulin resistance.* Being overweight increases your chances of developing type 2 diabetes. Treatment includes using diabetes medications and sometimes insulin, making wise food choices, exercising regularly, and controlling blood pressure and cholesterol.

There is a genetic component to developing type 2 diabetes; however, environmental factors such as diet and exercise can influence whether genes express and diabetes develops. If you have several family members with the disease, you should be checked for the disease regularly by your healthcare provider. Age, inactivity, and having obesity are risk factors for type 2 diabetes.

Exercising, maintaining a healthy weight, and eating a healthy diet such as the Whole Foods Weight Loss Eating Plan can delay or prevent the onset of type 2 diabetes.

Watch out for these signs and symptoms:

>> Extreme thirst

>> Frequent urination

>> Extreme hunger or unusual tiredness

>> Unexplained weight loss

>> Frequent irritability

>> Blurry vision

>> Cuts or sores that heal slowly

>> Unexplained loss of feeling or tingling in your feet or hands

>> Frequent skin, gum, or bladder infections

>> Frequent yeast infections

According to the 2020 CDC report 34.2 million Americans of all ages have diabetes. That's just a little more than 1 in 10 people or 10.5 percent of the U.S. population. Most of them have type 2 diabetes, the most common form of the disease. It's estimated that nearly one third of these people aren't even aware they have the disease. One reason is that for a long time, you may not have any warning signs or symptoms. Sometimes the diagnosis may be made only after a serious complication occurs.

If you have one sign or symptom, that doesn't mean you have diabetes. But you should start to be concerned if you have several symptoms. A checkup with your healthcare provider now can start you on treatment to help prevent or reduce the heart, eye, kidney, nerve, and other serious complications diabetes can cause.

Gestational diabetes

Some women develop gestational diabetes in the late stages of pregnancy. This form of diabetes usually goes away after the baby is born. However, a woman who has had gestational diabetes has a greater chance of developing type 2 diabetes later in life.

Recognizing the silent syndrome

A key development in the treatment of diabetes has been an improved understanding by the medical community of one of its major underlying causes: insulin resistance, also called *metabolic syndrome.* This increased understanding of insulin resistance has resulted in more appropriate medical treatment options.

Insulin resistance occurs when the body fails to respond properly to the insulin it already produces. It is an underlying cluster of symptoms that often precedes the diagnosis of type 2 diabetes. Many people at risk for diabetes do not know what insulin resistance is or even realize that they have signs of diabetes development.

A family history of diabetes, being overweight or obese, and physical inactivity increase your chances of developing insulin resistance. Certain ethnic groups, such as Latinos, Blacks, and Native Americans, are twice as likely as Caucasians to develop insulin resistance and diabetes. Insulin resistance is associated with an increased risk of heart disease and stroke.

Unfortunately, there's no simple test for insulin resistance. It's usually marked by a cluster of characteristics. The presence of three or more characteristics can result in a diagnosis of insulin resistance or metabolic syndrome. The characteristics of insulin resistance syndrome are as follows:

>> Abdominal obesity (a waist measuring more than 35 inches in women or more than 40 inches in men)

>> Fasting glucose level of 110 mg/dl or greater

>> Triglycerides of 150 mg/dl or greater

>> HDL cholesterol less than 50 mg/dl in women or less than 40 mg/dl in men

>> Blood pressure of 130/85 or greater

Understanding lipids

Lipid is another name for fat, so blood lipids are fats in your blood. Your doctor can create a *profile* (a breakdown of the different types of fat in your blood) of your lipids to help determine the type of heart disease you're at risk for (if any) and also to help determine the dietary approach to best lower your lipids.

When your healthcare provider checks your lipids, you're likely to get a list of numbers in each of the following categories:

>> **Total cholesterol:** This is a measurement of your total blood fats. This includes the sum of the HDL, LDL, and VLDL cholesterol components.

>> **High-density lipoprotein (HDL) cholesterol:** This is commonly called "good" cholesterol because it carries excess cholesterol back to the liver, which processes and excretes the cholesterol. You want this number to be greater than 40 mg/dl.

>> **Low-density lipoprotein (LDL) cholesterol:** This is commonly called "bad" cholesterol because high levels are linked to increased risk for heart disease. Ideally, you want this number to be below 100 mg/dl.

>> **Very-low-density lipoprotein (VLDL) cholesterol:** This number is determined by dividing the triglyceride number by 5. VLDL cholesterol can be converted to LDL or "bad" cholesterol.

>> **Triglycerides:** Triglycerides are a blood fat that is not only affected by the fat in your diet but is also increased by excess calories in the diet and by excess carbohydrate in the diet. Triglycerides normally increase after eating a meal, and they usually fall back to normal in two to three hours. Chronically high triglycerides have recently been linked to heart disease. You want this number to be below 150 mg/dl.

Check out Table 4-2 for guidance on what blood lipid levels you should be shooting for.

TABLE 4-2

Blood Lipid Levels

Type of Cholesterol	Desirable	Borderline	Unacceptable
Total cholesterol	Less than 200	200 to 239	240 or above
HDL cholesterol	60 or above	40 to 59	Less than 40
LDL cholesterol	Less than 100	100 to 159	160 or above
Triglycerides	Less than 150	150 to 199	200 or above

Spotting early problems with blood pressure

Blood-pressure readings are expressed in two numbers that reflect the pressure on artery walls when the heart contracts. Turn to Table 4-3 for information on what your blood pressure reading means.

TABLE 4-3 ## Blood Pressure Reading

Blood Pressure Classification	Systolic (Top Number)		Diastolic (Bottom Number)
Normal	Less than 120	and	Less than 80
Elevated	120 to 129	and	Less than 80
High Blood Pressure (Hypertension) Stage 1	130 to 139	or	80 to 89
High Blood Pressure (Hypertension) Stage 2	140 or higher	or	90 or higher
Hypertensive Crisis (consult your doctor immediately)	Higher Than 180	and/or	Higher than 120

New guidelines for blood pressure readings were issued by the American Heart Association, the American College of Cardiology, and nine other health organizations in 2017. These new guidelines lowered the thresholds for blood pressure readings. Health officials recognize a category for blood pressure called *elevated*. If the top (or *systolic*) number in your blood pressure reading is between 120 and 129 and if the bottom (or *diastolic*) number is less than 80, you have elevated blood pressure. *Elevated* is a blood pressure that doesn't require treatment with medication but still can increase your risk of heart disease and stroke. These guidelines along with medication when indicated encourage you to make lifestyle changes such as losing weight, exercising, quitting smoking, or reducing alcohol intake. A dietary approach known as Dietary Approaches to Stop Hypertension (DASH) and the Mediterranean Diet have been shown to reduce blood pressure. The low-carb Whole Foods Weight Loss Eating Plan described in this book incorporates the principles of the DASH Diet and the Mediterranean Diet.

Understanding the relationships between ethnicity and health risks

Certain diseases seem to be more prevalent in some races than others. So, with no other issues in your family health history, you still may have risk factors for several diseases just by belonging to a particular ethnic group.

Here's a quick list of some ethnicity-related health concerns. If you belong to any of these groups, pay special attention to the health risks associated with them.

» Blacks:
  - Have an increased risk for diabetes and insulin resistance
  - Are five times more likely than Caucasians to develop kidney disease if diabetic
  - Have the highest heart-disease risk and an increased risk for high blood pressure

» Asians:
  - Have an increased risk for osteoporosis (especially women)

» Caucasians:
  - Have an increased risk for osteoporosis (especially women)

» Latinos:
  - Have an increased risk for diabetes and insulin resistance
  - Are over six times more likely to develop kidney disease if diabetic

» Native Americans:
  - Have an increased risk for diabetes and insulin resistance
  - Are six times more likely to develop kidney disease if diabetic

Be Honest! Examining Your Current Diet and Lifestyle

After you have an idea of your health status and history, look at your lifestyle. The good news here is that, unlike your age or your family history, you can make changes to your lifestyle. Some of the risk factors you can change include the foods you eat, how much physical activity you get, whether you smoke, and how much alcohol you drink. If you have family tendencies for diabetes, heart disease, cancer, high blood pressure, and obesity, or if you're starting to show early signs of the conditions yourself, your diet and lifestyle can make those conditions worse or better.

These sections help you evaluate what you eat, how much exercise you get, and what your stress levels are so you can begin to make positive changes.

Paying attention to what you eat

An important factor in determining whether a low-carb eating plan is right for you is your willingness to look at your current eating habits. But you can't figure out where you want to go if you don't know where you are. What you need to do is keep track of what you eat so you can then determine how healthy it is.

Recording it

How frequently do chips, crackers, cookies, fast foods, soft drinks, snack foods, cakes, or desserts appear in your food intake? You may not even know the answer to that question. Eating is such a normal daily activity that you may be unaware of what you put in your mouth on a regular basis.

TIP

To keep track, record everything you eat. Buy a little notebook and write down what you eat, open a new file on your laptop, or download an app that helps you keep an accurate record. Do it as soon as you eat and keep track for a week; make sure you're honest (you're only cheating yourself if you aren't). Eat as you normally would. Don't make any changes while keeping the record. If you aren't up to keeping a one-week record, then keep it for a day or two. Record the type of food eaten, the amount, where you were, and your current mood.

Another option is to sit down and recall what you've eaten in the last 24 hours. Start with your most recent meal and track back for 24 hours. (The only problem with this approach is that you can easily forget about small snack items you ate, like bread or crackers, as well as beverages, all of which should be counted.)

No matter how you do it, develop a picture of your eating pattern. Interestingly, even with all the variety in the food supply, most people eat the same seven to ten meals on a regular basis. So, what does your dietary pattern look like?

Evaluating it

After you have a record of what you've eaten, you need to evaluate how healthy it is. To determine the number of servings you consumed, you'll need to estimate portion sizes. You'll be surprised to see that normal portion sizes are a lot smaller than you think. Here are some examples:

Portion	Approximate Size
½ cup	About the size of a woman's tight fist, or a tennis or billiard ball
1 medium fruit	About the size of a man's tight fist
1 medium potato	About the size of a computer mouse
1 ounce cheese	About the size of your thumb
3 ounces meat	About the size of the palm of a woman's hand or a deck of cards
1 cup	A standard 8-ounce measuring cup

TIP

To assess your diet, follow these steps:

1. **Look for the basic foods known to be essential in a healthy diet.**

   Calculate your average daily intake by taking your totals and dividing them by the number of days you kept your food record. For example, if you've tallied seven fruits over a four-day period, you've consumed an average of 1.75 pieces of fruit each day (7 ÷ 4 = 1.75).

   Use a chart like Table 4-4 to track what you eat.

TABLE 4-4

Recording What You Eat

Foods	Recommended Daily Servings	Number of Servings You Consumed
Fruit	Medium piece or ½ cup	2
Vegetables, non-starchy	½ cup	3
Starchy vegetables	½ cup	3
Breads or cereals	1 slice or ½ cup	2
Whole-grain breads or cereals	1 slice or ½ cup	3
Lean meats, poultry, or fish	3 ounces	2
Egg or cheese, low-fat*	1 ounce*	1
Milk (skim, ½%, 1%) or yogurt	1 cup	2
Water or other Nonsweetened beverage	1 cup	8

You don't need foods from this category every day.

2. **Look for extra foods that contribute calories but don't contribute significant nutrients.**

   There are no recommended servings in this category so you just need to record your daily intake. Be honest in this assessment. Research indicates that the Western diet can contain more than 50 percent of refined and processed foods. These foods count as carbs and provide calories, sugar, and fat, but no significant nutrients.

   Use Table 4-5 to record your intake.

TABLE 4-5

Recording Your Refined and Processed Foods

Serving Sizes	Number You Consumed
Chips, 1-ounce snack size	
Cookies	
Dessert, cake, pie, pudding, ½ cup or 1 piece	
Ice cream or other frozen desserts, ½ cup	
Soft drink, regular, 8 ounces	
Meals away from home	
Fast-food meals	
Hamburger	
Cheeseburger	
Fried fish or fried chicken	
Burritos or tacos	
French fries, regular size	
Pizza, 1 medium slice	
Biscuits, 1 medium	
Rolls, 1 medium	
Gravy, ¼ cup	

3. **Answer the following questions about your food intake:**

- Did you meet the minimum servings for the basic foods in Step 1?

- Did your intake of the foods in Step 2 equal or exceed your intake of the foods in Step 1?

- Can you replace some of your Step 2 choices with Step 1 choices?

- Are you starting to get the picture of your food habits?

Step 2 food choices are okay if you're meeting your intake of the basic food groups and if your weight is in the normal range. If you're physically active, you can handle more Step 2 foods than people who aren't very active.

Determining your level of activity

Being active in today's environment doesn't come easy. Advances in the modern age have decreased the opportunities for exercise. Streaming services, video games, the Internet, smartphones, televisions, and so on have all pulled people indoors and gotten them sitting down. But your body is designed for physical output. You have large muscle groups in your legs, arms, back, chest, and abdomen, and smaller but very important muscles in your organ systems like your heart and lungs. If your muscles don't get the workout they're designed for, your whole body suffers.

The U.S. Department of Health and Human Services (DHHS) published its 2nd edition of *Physical Activity for Guidelines for Americans* in 2018. These recommendations for exercise are a mix of moderate-intensity aerobic activity at least 150 minutes up to 300 minutes per week *and* muscle-strengthening activity at least two days per week:

>> Moderate-intensity aerobic activity is any activity that gets your heart beating faster counts, such as, biking, swimming, gardening, or even walking the dog.

>> Muscle-strengthening activity is activity that makes your muscles work harder than usual such as lifting weight, wearing ankle weights, or working with resistance bands.

If those activities are more than you can do right now, then do what you can. Even 5 minutes of physical activity has real health benefits.

This recommendation stems from studies that indicate that physical activity is linked with even more positive health outcomes than researchers previously thought. The good news is that the exercise can be cumulative — you don't have to get in 30 minutes or one hour all at once. The recommendation means you have to look for opportunities throughout the day to be more active. Taking the stairs, parking farther away, walking to a coworker's desk rather than sending an e-mail, and walking short distances rather than driving a car are just some of the ways to build more exercise into your day. (You can find more on this in Chapter 22.)

Less than 30 percent of American adults are sufficiently active in their leisure time to achieve health benefits. Thirty-one million Americans aged 50 or older aren't physically active at all. Even light activities such as standing or walking around the house are better than no activity at all. If you aren't very active, start gradually and build up.

Look at the following categories of activity and mark the one that comes closest to describing how you spend your week. Unless you're in the active or very active category, plan to up your exercise by one level:

>> **Sedentary:** Watching television, driving a car, sitting at work, playing video games, sewing, reading, writing, texting, or talking on the phone. No program of regular exercise.

>> **Light exercise:** Ironing, dusting, doing laundry, loading/unloading the dishwasher, preparing and cooking food, walking 2 miles per hour for 10 to 20 minutes three to five times per week.

>> **Moderate exercise:** Dancing, gardening, doing carpentry work, mopping/scrubbing, bicycling, jogging or walking at 3 miles per hour for 20 to 40 minutes three to five times per week.

>> **Active:** Heavy work, aerobics, tennis, skating, skiing, racquetball, brisk walking at 4 miles per hour for 30 to 60 minutes three to five times per week.

>> **Very active:** Bicycling 15 miles per hour, running 6 miles per hour, swimming, or participating in martial arts, for 45 to 60 minutes three to five times per week.

Discovering the effects of stress

Stress is unavoidable, but it can be good or bad. Normal transitions in life like getting married or having a baby bring about stress. A job promotion that calls for a move to a new city brings about stress. Other kinds of stress can bring prolonged responses. An unpleasant coworker or difficult job situation is there every day. You have to manage a decrease in your finances every day. Significant stress events like the death of a spouse or child never fully go away. Stress is part of living.

ALCOHOL: MODERATION IS THE KEY

Many people drink alcohol at some point in their lives. Some only drink during social occasions and others may have an evening glass of wine. Moderate alcohol consumption of no more than one drink per day can offer some heart benefits. The following figure shows what qualifies as a drink. However, the benefit is not so great that a nondrinker should consider drinking alcohol. About one-third of individuals who drink alcohol will develop problems with alcohol. Drinking problems can increase your risk of serious health problems (both physical and behavioral) and accidents or injuries.

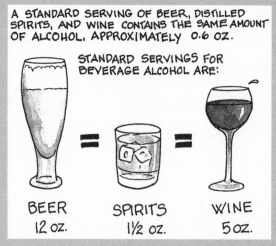

Illustration by Liz Kurtzman

If you want to drink alcohol, moderate consumption is considered safe. Moderate drinking is considered two drinks a day for men, and one drink a day for women or lighter-weight men. A drink is 12 ounces of beer, 5 ounces of wine, or 1½ ounces of hard liquor. Be sure to count these beverages in your daily five carbohydrate choices. Each one counts as one carbohydrate choice.

How you deal with the stress is what's important. Some people respond to stress by eating poorly, being physically inactive, smoking, or drinking alcohol. Others criticize their spouses, yell at their kids, and kick their dogs. And some employ the silent treatment — keeping everything bottled up inside when they're about to explode. All these reactions take their toll on your body.

Short-term responses to stress can be a headache, stomachache, diarrhea, constipation, or vomiting. Longer-term responses affect blood pressure and sleeping and increase your risk for depression, heart disease, and susceptibility to colds and infections.

Eating and bingeing just compound the stress. The temporary comfort provided by the food is followed by guilt for overeating. Stress is pent-up energy that needs to be released. When stress comes, step back, take a deep breath, and go for a walk. Buy yourself some time to relax and decompress.

If your problems with stress are far more serious, talk to a trusted friend, your religious leader, your healthcare provider, or a professional therapist.

Deciding Whether a Low-Carb Diet Can Help

A low-carb diet, especially one like the Whole Foods Weight Loss Eating Plan, can help the following conditions:

>> Overweight (BMI of 25 to 29.9)

>> Obesity (BMI of 30 or greater)

>> Type 2 diabetes

>> Insulin resistance

>> Heart disease

>> High triglycerides

>> Low HDL cholesterol

>> High blood pressure (but only if the low-carb plan allows fruits, vegetables, low-fat dairy, whole grains, nuts, and seeds)

>> Polycystic ovarian syndrome (PCOS), a disease in women associated with insulin resistance

If you suffer from any of the preceding conditions, going the healthy low-carb route may be exactly what your body needs. However, if you have kidney problems, you may want to find another eating plan.

REMEMBER

As with any diet plan, be sure to consult your healthcare provider or registered dietitian nutritionist (RDN) to determine if this plan is safe for you to follow given your specific health situation. (For the full story on the Whole Foods Weight Loss Eating Plan, check out Part 2.)

2

Steering Yourself Back to Whole Foods

Chapter **5**

Falling in Love with Whole Foods

About 25 years ago, I began to take a look at the fad diets that people found so appealing. Simplicity and the quick weight-loss results they promised were very attractive. But restrictive food choices and the inability to sustain the weight loss round out the fad-diet story. I saw people who were overwhelmed by the modern diet of super-sized fast foods, soft drinks, and salty and fat-free snacks — and their health was suffering. I also saw them struggling to lose weight by following a fad diet.

Since then the struggle hasn't changed. In fact, eating meals outside the home has increased — not always in a fast food restaurant, but in restaurants in general. In fact, the proliferation of fast food restaurants has grown exponentially internationally, and the United States has been and continues to export its "tasty" fast foods around the world. The associated health problems have also gone with them.

However, some evidence shows that Americans are becoming more health conscious in their eating. A Pew research survey indicated that 54 percent of Americans are paying more attention to eating healthy foods today compared with 20 years ago. On the other hand, the same survey said the same percentage (54 percent) of Americans' actual eating habits are less healthy today than they were 20 years ago. Even though Americans are more aware of what is healthy food and what isn't, this awareness hasn't resulted in better eating habits for everyone.

Little by little some Americans are starting to eat healthier, although it takes time to change eating patterns. The allure of fad diets is still evident: Individuals are aware they aren't eating well so they're tempted by simple weight-loss methods that promise quick weight loss results to achieve their weight "magic number" and then they can return to "normal." That mind-set over time sadly results in regaining the lost weight and frustration for the individual.

This brings me to the Whole Foods Weight Loss Eating Plan. In my review of fad diets, a friend gave me a fad diet for my collection that had one particularly appealing feature: It allowed you to eat as much as you wanted of certain fruits and vegetables. Other aspects of the diet weren't healthy — like allowing free intake of high-fat meats and dairy items, including bacon, sausage, butter, and whole milk — but I was intrigued by the idea of "free" foods. People don't like to be restricted in their eating, but maybe they can be redirected?

If you hate counting calories and grams, this chapter is definitely for you. Here, I show you the fruits, vegetables, and lean protein that are yours for the taking as free foods. (You can eat free foods in unlimited quantities — they're free because you don't pay for them by counting calories or using food-group choices like you may on another diet plan.) This "food freeway" is the first leg of your journey to your destination of the Whole Foods Weight Loss Eating Plan. The plan isn't a quick fix for getting rid of some extra pounds; it's a journey that can steer you back to healthy eating without forcing you to think much about quantities. But don't worry — on this trip, you'll also drop some excess baggage (in the form of unwanted pounds) along the way.

Even if you decide that the Whole Foods Weight Loss Eating Plan isn't for you, you can likely benefit from the information in the chapter and create your own low-carb plan. Removing processed foods, or at least reducing the amount of processed foods, from your diet is a fantastic change to just about anyone's diet. Just knowing which foods are the healthiest for you can help shape your eating in a healthier direction for the rest of your life.

Green-Light Foods: Identifying Foods You Can Eat without Thinking Twice

Knowing how far the American diet had drifted from the basics of good health, allowing convenient refined and processed foods to replace simple, nutritional food, I used the free-food idea to develop a plan that would turn people back to basic *whole foods* (foods with little processing). Essentially, I let the foods I wanted people to eat become *free foods.* The participants could eat as many of the free foods as they wanted, whenever they wanted, without restrictions. The results of the experiment were encouraging. People not only lost weight but told me how easy following the plan was. They were eating a lot healthier, and they didn't feel deprived!

REMEMBER

The Whole Foods Weight Loss Eating Plan is paved with fruits, vegetables, and protein foods, such as lean meat, fish, poultry, and low-fat cheeses — I refer to these foods as *Green Light foods.* I don't want you to be hungry on this eating plan. Instead, I want you to satisfy your hunger with fruits, vegetables, and lean protein foods. I mark each list of free foods in this chapter and in the recipes in Part 3 with a Green Light icon, which means "Go ahead and make your choice."

Green Light foods are the heart and soul of this low-carb diet. You don't have to weigh or measure Green Light foods — you can eat as much as you want whenever you want. Understanding portion sizes is important, of course, and I discuss portions in Chapters 6, 7, and 8. But in this chapter, I help you replace the highly refined carbohydrates in your diet with Green Light foods.

TIP

A winning strategy is to swap low-quality carbs for higher-quality carbs, replace saturated fat like in fatty meats with unsaturated fats in nuts and fish, and reduce calories from carbs overall by eating fewer snacks and drinks with added sugars and refined grains (refer to Chapter 3 for information about the Healthy Eating Plate, a good tool to use).

Exploring the Free Carbs: Fruits and Vegetables

Fruits and vegetables are as good as it gets, so don't hold back! You can eat and drink as much of the carbohydrates listed in this section as you need to satisfy your hunger. The fruits and vegetables in this group do contain carbohydrates, but they're low on glycemic load, which ranks foods according to how they affect your blood-sugar level. The fruits and vegetables on this list are whole foods, packed with nutrients!

TECHNICAL STUFF

The *glycemic load* of foods shows how rapidly a food is digested, thus driving up the blood sugar. Insulin, which lowers your blood sugar, is also stimulated. Foods with a high glycemic load cause a spike in your blood-sugar level, and then insulin quickly lowers it. This sudden change in your blood-sugar level can actually *cause* hunger. (Imagine, you can be even hungrier after you eat these foods than you were before!) Foods with a low glycemic load cause a gradual, moderate increase in blood sugar without overstimulating insulin and are more satisfying to your appetite. See Chapter 3 and Appendix A for more details on the glycemic load.

Eat and be merry with as many of the carbohydrates listed in the following sections as you need to satisfy your hunger. And remember, *free* really does mean free. You don't have to weigh or measure these foods.

TIP

To make eating fruits and vegetables more convenient, I suggest these strategies:

>> **Select fruits and vegetables that require little peeling and chopping.** Good options include baby carrots, cherry tomatoes, asparagus, grapes, apples, and broccoli spears.

>> **Shop the supermarket salad bars.** They offer many favorite raw vegetables and fresh fruits already cleaned and sliced.

>> **Put fruits that don't need refrigeration where you can see them.** Make a habit of grabbing a few pieces on your way out the door.

>> **Shop seasonal specials for better prices.** Check out nearby farmers' markets for the freshest fruits and veggies and best prices. Support your local farmers!

Making fruit choices — fresh is best

Fruit is the original fast food. Nature has nicely packaged it for easy take-out. When possible, choose fresh, whole, naturally ripe fruit. But if fresh isn't available, you can buy frozen fruit year-round. If you use canned, choose fruit in 100-percent fruit juice instead of sugary syrup. If you have to buy canned fruit in a light syrup, drain it before eating. In most cases, frozen and canned fruits are just as nutritious as fresh. Besides, eating canned and frozen fruits is better than eating no fruit at all!

WARNING

Bananas aren't on the Green Light food list. It's not that I don't want you to eat bananas — you can find them in Chapter 6 on a Yellow Light list signaling caution. Bananas are a very good food and the number-one fruit sold in the United States. However, they're starchier than other fruits, so I count them like bread. People who eat bananas tend to eat a lot of them. So, if I gave bananas a Green Light, some people would only eat bananas and no other fruit! *Remember:* Always eat a variety of fruits.

Wash fruit as soon as you get home from the store (even those with heavy peels like oranges). Then you can grab some directly from the fruit bowl or crisper on your way out. Berries and grapes are the only exceptions; wash them the day you eat them and not before.

Here's a list of the Green Light, or free, fruits, so, go, go, go, and eat them up:

>> **Apples, dried:** Dried apples make a great snack food and are easy to transport.

>> **Apples, fresh:** The variety of apple you choose makes no difference. My favorite is Golden Delicious. Availability changes with the seasons, though.

>> **Applesauce, unsweetened:** Applesauce isn't just for kids! Grownups love this tart sauce, too.

>> **Apricots, dried:** Dried apricots make a nice snack — the dense, sweet-tart apricot taste can be quite addictive.

>> **Apricots, fresh:** Apricots are a smooth, sweet summer fruit chock-full of nutritional goodness.

>> **Blackberries:** Blackberries are as big as your thumb, purple and black and thick with juice. I remember picking these as a kid while catching June bugs and watching for snakes.

>> **Blueberries:** Blueberries are late-summer berries with a very rich taste. They're great sprinkled in a salad!

>> **Cantaloupe:** Cantaloupe comes with its own bowl — just cut it in half and scoop out each half with a spoon.

>> **Cherries, sweet, canned:** When you buy canned cherries, you're getting two for the price of one — the fruit and the canned juice.

>> **Cherries, sweet, fresh:** Go for fresh cherries when possible, and use frozen ones in a pinch. Canned syrupy pie filling is overloaded with sugar and corn starch, so avoid it.

>> **Dates:** A few dates are all you need to fill up.

>> **Figs, dried:** Dried figs are readily available year-round. The easiest way to chop them is to snip them with scissors.

>> **Figs, fresh:** Fresh figs are a healthy fruit that can satisfy a craving for sweetness.

>> **Fruit cocktail:** When was the last time you had a serving of this pitch-in dinner specialty? Be sure to drain it.

>> **Grapefruit:** America's wake-up fruit, this eye-opener may be rosy-fleshed or white.

>> **Grapefruit sections, canned:** Keep canned grapefruit in the pantry, always ready to go.

>> **Grapes:** Good nutrition comes in small packages.

>> **Honeydew melons:** "Honey, dew try this!" (I couldn't resist.)

>> **Kiwis:** Don't let the hairy green skin turn you off this exotic little gem — just don't forget to peel it! One kiwi has more vitamin C than ½ cup of orange juice.

>> **Lemons:** You can use lemon to add flavor to any beverage. They're great to keep in the fridge for salad dressings, as a quick flavor for fish, or to give the flavors of your other fruits a twist.

>> **Limes:** Limes are highly underrated in the United States. I use lime to flavor everything from water and diet sodas to anything with cilantro, including salsa. Its crisp, fresh flavor makes just about everything taste better.

>> **Mandarin oranges, canned:** Mandarin oranges are Chinese oranges that are very sweet! Drain them well and add to any dish.

>> **Mangos:** Mango is delicious by itself or paired with other tropical fruits, like papaya. Their flavor is something like a tangy peach.

>> **Nectarines:** Nectarines are a smooth-skinned variety of peach. They taste best at the height of the season (in late June and July).

>> **Oranges:** Oranges are a fall and winter fruit. When eaten raw, none of its precious vitamin C is lost.

>> **Papaya:** You can bake unripe papayas like squash. They contain *papain,* the predominant ingredient in meat tenderizer.

>> **Peaches, canned:** Canned peaches make a quick dessert for any meal.

>> **Peaches, fresh:** Don't let a little peach fuzz keep you away. Peaches are delicious and loaded with nutrients.

>> **Pears, canned:** Cut up canned pears and add them to a salad.

>> **Pears, fresh:** You can purchase pears green and they'll continue to ripen. They get sweeter as they ripen!

>> **Pineapple, canned:** Always buy canned pineapple in its own juice instead of syrup.

>> **Pineapple, fresh:** Known as a symbol of hospitality in the South, fresh pineapple makes a sweet dessert.

>> **Plums, canned:** Canned plums are a readily available treat.

>> **Plums, fresh:** Plums come from trees found in every continent in the world except Antarctica.

- **Prunes, dried:** Prunes are dried, small, purplish-black, freestone plums. They're very rich in flavor. You can also find them infused with essence of orange and lemon.

- **Raisins:** Raisins are just dried grapes. They make a handy snack.

- **Raspberries:** When they are fully ripe, raspberries' caps detach. Midsummer is their prime season.

- **Strawberries:** Strawberries are a super food chock-full of health-giving nutrients.

- **Tangerines:** Tangerines are small, sweet, Chinese oranges. They peel so easily it's as if they have a zipper.

- **Watermelon:** Watermelon is a summertime treat that can't be beat! Try freezing watermelon juice in ice-cube trays and adding the cubes to drinks.

WARNING

Go easy on fruit juices! Don't let all your fruit servings come from juice. Try to eat at least one piece of whole fruit every day. But when you do reach for a glass of juice, make it ½ cup to 1 cup of 100–percent fruit juice with no sugar added.

To increase your fruit intake, try these suggestions:

- Nibble on grapes or raisins.

- Blend fresh fruit with your morning yogurt. Add a splash of orange juice and crushed ice for a homemade smoothie.

- Add strawberries or blueberries to your green salad.

- Try frozen Bing cherries for an instant treat.

- Make your own sorbet or granita with sweet, fresh berries.

Eating your veggies, the superstars

Vegetables are nutrition superstars! They're low in calories and fat, cholesterol free, and high in vitamins, minerals, cancer fighters, and heart protection. Veggies are nature's defense mechanism, protecting you against disease — and in the American diet, they're neglected.

Be adventurous and get acquainted with a new vegetable each week. You're in for a pleasant surprise.

TIP

JUICES, JUICES EVERYWHERE, BUT HOW MANY DROPS (OR OUNCES) TO DRINK?

Choose real fruit juice, not fruit drink. Fruit drink is only 10 percent real fruit juice or less — the rest is sugar water! Drink fruit juice instead of sodas or coffee in the car. You can keep 8- to 12-ounce bottles in your refrigerator chilled and ready to go. Or you can buy them at gas stations and fast-food chains. If you need a big gulp, combine a 6-ounce juice with a 12-ounce can of diet lemon-lime or ginger ale soda.

Give these healthy juices a try:

- **Apple juice/cider:** Apple juice beats a can of soda any time and doesn't take as much to satisfy your hunger.

- **Cranberry juice cocktail, reduced-calorie, light:** Cranberries lessen bladder infections by preventing bacteria from clinging to the inside of the bladder and urinary tract. To avoid too much sugar, always buy the light version of cranberry juice.

- **Fruit juice blends, 100-percent juice:** Fruit-juice blends are a delicious drink of pure juice.

- **Grape juice:** Grape juice is healthy for the heart.

- **Grapefruit juice:** Grapefruit juice makes a great snack between meals.

- **Orange juice:** Make it fresh whenever possible. It's worth the extra effort.

- **Pineapple juice:** You can use pineapple juice to sweeten less-sweet fruits.

- **Prune juice:** Prune juice improves your bowel regularity. Don't be afraid to try it.

Don't let your juice intake interfere with your intake of whole fresh fruit.

GREEN LIGHT

You may have these vegetables cooked, raw, canned, frozen, microwaved, steamed, or stir-fried (but not deep-fried, breaded, or creamed), with no limits on amounts:

» **Artichokes:** I don't recommend eating artichokes raw — not even in Texas. Take a look at Figure 5-1 for instructions on cleaning and trimming an artichoke.

» **Artichoke hearts:** Artichoke hearts make delicious salad material.

» **Asparagus:** Asparagus is a special, delicious vegetable, once only available to kings.

» **Bean sprouts:** Bean sprouts are the basis of a good stir-fry.

Cleaning an Artichoke

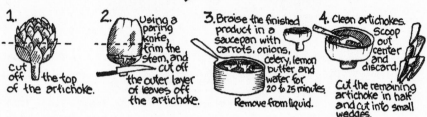

FIGURE 5-1:
Cleaning and trimming an artichoke.

1. Cut off the top of the artichoke.

2. Using a paring knife, trim the stem, and cut off the outer layer of leaves off the artichoke.

3. Braise the finished product in a saucepan with carrots, onions, celery, lemon butter and water for 20 to 25 minutes. Remove from liquid.

4. Clean artichokes. Scoop out center and discard. Cut the remaining artichoke in half and cut into small wedges.

Illustration by Liz Kurtzman

>> **Beans (green, wax, Italian):** Beans are a go-with-anything vegetable.

>> **Beets:** Plain or pickled, you can use the tops of beets as greens.

>> **Bok choy:** This delicious Chinese cabbage (see Figure 5-2) comes in several varieties but is most commonly found in the United States in regular and baby varieties. Baby bok choy, prized for its tender delicate texture, can be cooked whole. The larger variety needs to be cut before cooking.

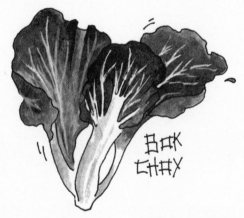

FIGURE 5-2:
Add bok choy to your stir-frys and soups.

Illustration by Liz Kurtzman

>> **Broccoli:** Broccoli is America's favorite vegetable — despite what the first President Bush thinks. Try broccoli sprouts, too, for a punch of nutrition in salads and on sandwiches.

>> **Brussels sprouts:** This tiny, green, cabbage-like vegetable is a big defender of good health.

>> **Cabbage:** Cabbage is a big cousin to the Brussels sprout. It packs a wallop against cancer and is a nutrition powerhouse. Choose red cabbage for its abundance of vitamin C. Savoy cabbage has extra beta carotene. And even the common green cabbage can't be beat for its wealth of nutrients.

TIP

You can make sauerkraut from cabbage. To retain its full flavor, sauerkraut should be served raw or barely heated through. Cooking makes kraut milder.

>> **Carrots:** It's true — carrots are good for your eyes.

>> **Cauliflower:** The "flower of the cabbage" is a nutritious bouquet.

>> **Celery:** Often seen on the relish tray, you can combine celery with anything.

>> **Cucumbers:** The cucumbers you find in the supermarket are often waxed, which means you have to peel them before eating. If the skin isn't waxed, however, it's edible.

>> **Daikon:** A daikon (refer to Figure 5-3) is a jumbo-sized Japanese radish sometimes exceeding 3 feet in length! The size typically used in the kitchen is about the size of a carrot.

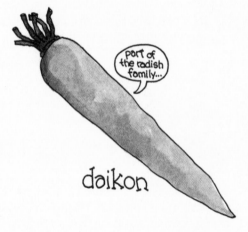

FIGURE 5-3:
A daikon tastes kind of like a radish, but hotter.

Illustration by Liz Kurtzman

>> **Eggplant:** A purple powerhouse of prevention, eggplant should always be eaten cooked.

>> **Green onions or scallions:** Green onions are sweetest when the bulbs are thinnest.

>> **Greens (collard, kale, mustard, turnip):** Greens are versatile vegetables of many virtues. Vary the way you serve greens, just to shake things up.

>> **Jicama:** Many people describe it as being a cross between an apple and a turnip, and it's also referred to as a Mexican yam bean or Mexican turnip. It adds a nice crunch and a lightly sweet and nutty flavor to your salad. Check out Chapter 13 for the simple Jicama Chips recipe.

>> **Kohlrabi:** Sometimes called the cabbage turnip, this cabbage has a swollen stem, resembling a root. It is crisp and juicy, with a surprising mixture of sweetness, much like an apple, with a slight peppery bite like a radish. Both the leaves and stems can be eaten fresh, steamed, braised, sautéed . . . you name it.

>> **Leeks:** A cousin to the onion, leeks are good heart medicine and may help prevent cancer. Be sure to soak and wash leeks thoroughly in order to remove dirt and sand deep down in the bulb. Figure 5-4 shows you how to clean and trim leeks.

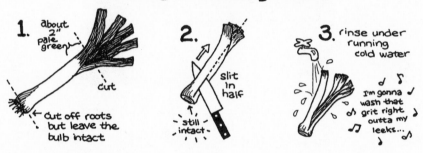

FIGURE 5-4:
Cleaning and trimming leeks.

Illustration by Liz Kurtzman

>> **Mushrooms:** Unless you're a mushroom expert, buy your mushrooms in a market. Those nice-looking mushrooms that pop up in your yard after a rain can be deadly. Cremini or cremini mushrooms are a slightly more mature version of the white button mushroom and are often referred to as a baby bella (baby portobella).

>> **Napa cabbage:** Napa cabbage (see Figure 5-5) is a Chinese cabbage that is normally formed with an oblong, rather than round head. It's a crisp, but delicate cabbage that will keep about four days in the refrigerator. Don't cut or wash it until you're ready to use it, or you'll diminish the nutritive value.

>> **Okra:** When included in stews, okra's gluey sap helps thicken the sauce.

>> **Onions:** The old-time cough medicine of onion juice and honey was nothing to sneeze at. The substance in onions that makes you cry also breaks up mucous congestion.

>> **Pepper (all varieties):** Sweet or hot, peppers are full of zesty nutrition. Figure 5-6 shows you how to core and seed a bell pepper.

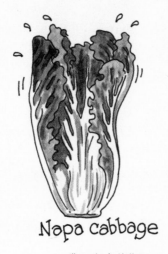

Napa cabbage

Illustration by Liz Kurtzman

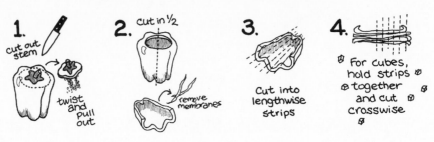

How to Core and Seed a Pepper

1. cut out stem

twist and pull out

2. cut in ½

remove membranes

3. Cut into lengthwise strips

4. For cubes, hold strips together and cut crosswise

Illustration by Liz Kurtzman

>> **Radishes:** Often transformed into a clever garnish, radishes are good to eat.

>> **Salad greens (arugula, endive, escarole, lettuce, romaine, rutabaga):** I'm not talking anemic iceberg lettuce here, but dark, leafy greens that are full of compounds to help you resist disease. Use several varieties together in your salad.

>> **Salsa and picante sauce:** Okay, not exactly a true veggie, but salsa adds pizzazz to anything!

>> **Snow peas:** Snow peas are excellent in salads, stir-fry, or featured on a veggie platter.

>> **Spinach:** Tender young spinach works best in salads, either alone or mixed with other greens. Even a greens-hating child may enjoy spinach in salads.

- **Squash, summer:** Summer squash is delicious raw or cooked.

- **Tomatoes, fresh:** The red color of tomatoes signals the presence of *lycopene*, a phytochemical that protects against cancer. Look for other tomato varieties in your market as well, including green zebra, yellow teardrop, pear, grape, and cherry. So many choices, so little time!

- **Tomato sauce:** Cooking doesn't destroy lycopene. It actually makes it better. So tomato sauce is a good source of the cancer fighter.

- **Tomato/vegetable juice:** Tomato juice, whether alone or combined with other vegetables juices, makes a great healthy drink — any time, any place.

- **Tomatoes, canned:** Canned tomatoes fill in nicely when fresh tomatoes are out of season.

Strictly speaking, a tomato is a fruit, not a vegetable (some nonsense about it having internal seeds that can later germinate into fruit berry plants, yada yada yada). But for the purposes of this book, I'm just going to keep it in the vegetable category, where everyone expects it.

- **Turnips:** Peel turnips before cooking; the peel gives a bitter flavor to the vegetable.

CRUCIFEROUS CABBAGE TO THE RESCUE!

The term *cruciferous* simply means vegetables in the cabbage family whose leaves form a crucifix or cross. This includes bok choy, broccoli, Brussels sprouts, cabbage, cauliflower, kale, mustard, and turnip greens, among others. Cabbage-family vegetables contain compounds that stop processes in the body that can develop into cancer. Check out Chapter 25 for more information.

The cabbage-family vegetables include the following:

- Bok choy
- Broccoli
- Brussels sprouts
- Cabbage
- Cauliflower
- Daikon
- Kale
- Kohlrabi
- Mustard greens
- Napa cabbage
- Radish
- Rutabaga
- Turnip
- Watercress

>> **Water chestnuts:** Combine the crunchy, crisp vegetable with other veggies.

>> **Watercress:** Watercress adds a distinctive flavor to salads, sandwiches, soups, and vegetables. Never overcook it — it becomes stringy when overcooked.

>> **Zucchini:** Zucchini is a versatile green squash — cooked or raw.

TIP

To increase your vegetable intake, try these suggestions:

>> Pile lettuce, sprouts, and tomatoes on your sandwich.

>> Enjoy soup or salad with a variety of vegetables.

>> Pack zucchini slices, baby carrots, or celery sticks in your lunch.

>> Chop raw veggies and add them to your green salad.

>> Steam your own mixed veggie combinations with a variety of seasonings. Vary the combinations by the day (carrots, cauliflower, and snow peas on Monday; zucchini, yellow squash, and red onions on Tuesday; and so on).

>> Sautee spinach in a tiny bit of olive oil with garlic for a super quick, warm salad.

Indulging in Free Proteins

Protein is an important part of a healthy diet. Its function is to build and repair body tissues. Proteins from animal sources like meat, fish, dairy, and egg products are valued because their total protein content is high. They're referred to as *complete proteins* because they contain all the essential *amino acids* (the building blocks for constructing and repairing body tissues) required from your diet. However, many animal protein sources are also associated with saturated fat. Saturated fat contributes to heart disease by raising your cholesterol level. Choose animal proteins that are low in saturated fat.

TECHNICAL
STUFF

Scientific studies show that in some people replacing some of the carbohydrate in a diet with lean protein lowers triglyceride levels and raises HDL cholesterol levels. That's good, because high triglycerides and low HDL cholesterol have been identified as risk factors for heart disease. Plus, if you eat some protein instead of carbs, you feel satisfied sooner!

The following sections identify some of the best options for getting protein in a low-carb diet.

Meat and cheese choices

Meat and cheese contain many good nutrients, but the fat in these foods is mostly saturated fat, and you need to limit your intake of saturated fat. Meat and cheese choices should have no more than 5 grams of fat per ounce. In the following sections, the number listed in brackets after each food is the number of grams of fat per ounce. To reduce saturated fat even further, choose the foods with 3 grams of fat per ounce, such as beef sirloin, or 0 to 1 gram of fat per ounce, such as chicken.

Beef

Lean beef is an excellent protein choice. You can eat it several times per week. Choose USDA Choice or Select grades of lean meat. Avoid heavily marbled (high-fat) meats because they're high in saturated fat. These beef options are great low-carb options:

- Corned beef [5 grams of fat per ounce]
- Flank steak [3]
- Ground beef, lean [3]
- Ground beef, regular [5]
- Prime rib [5]
- Roast (rib, chuck, rump) [3]
- Round [3]
- Short ribs [5]
- Sirloin [3]
- Steak (T-bone, porterhouse) [3]
- Tenderloin [3]

Pork

Pork is a lot leaner these days, and you can include it in a healthy diet. Prepackaged hams usually have only a fraction of the fat of a whole ham. Here are some great low-carb pork options:

- Boston butt [5 grams of fat per ounce]
- Canadian bacon [3]
- Center loin chop [3]
- Cutlet, unbreaded [3]
- Ham (fresh, canned, cured) [3]
- Tenderloin [3]

MAKING THE GRADE

Beef grading is conducted by the U.S. Department of Agriculture (USDA). Inspectors grade, or rate, meat based on the amount of *marbling* (flecks of fat within the lean portion of the meat) and the age of the animal. These quality grades are an indication of tenderness, juiciness, and flavor.

The most readily available grades are as follows:

- **Prime** has the most marbling (and the most fat and flavor). It's produced in limited quantities and usually sold to fine restaurants and specialty meat markets.

- **Choice** falls between Prime and Select.

- **Select** has the least amount of marbling, making it leaner than, but often not as tender, juicy, and flavorful as, the other two top grades.

Most markets today offer a selection of Choice and Select cuts.

Lamb

A favorite meat around the world, the leanest cuts of lamb are leg, arm, shank, and loin. The following are your best choices:

>> Chop [3 grams of fat per ounce]

>> Leg [3]

>> Roast [5]

Veal

Veal is a favorite meat in Italy. All cuts of veal are lean; it's what people tend to do to them — breading, like Veal Parmigiana, thick butter sauces, like Veal Picatta, and so on — that make veal not so healthy. Here are the healthy cuts:

>> Chop, trimmed of visible fat [3 grams of fat per ounce]

>> Cutlet (unbreaded) [3]

>> Roast [3]

Game

Game meats are leaner than domestic meats. Some wild game, such as venison and rabbit, are very lean. Some exotic "new" meats also low in fat are ostrich, emu, and buffalo. Check out the following:

- » Alligator [0–1 gram of fat per ounce]
- » Buffalo [0–1]
- » Emu [0–1]

- » Ostrich [0–1]
- » Rabbit [0–1]
- » Venison [0–1]

Poultry

Lower in saturated fat than many cuts of red meat, poultry is popular and easy to prepare. Much of the fat in poultry is in the skin, so you need to remove it or buy skinless, boneless chicken or turkey. You can cook poultry with skin on and remove it before eating. Consider these options:

- » Chicken, dark meat [3 grams of fat per ounce]
- » Chicken, white meat [0–1]
- » Cornish hen [0–1]
- » Duck, domestic [3]

- » Goose, domestic [3]
- » Pheasant (no skin) [0–1]
- » Turkey, dark meat [3]
- » Turkey, white meat [0–1]

TIP

Cholesterol in foods isn't the same as cholesterol in your blood. High levels of blood cholesterol can lead to heart disease. The saturated fat in your diet leads to high blood cholesterol more than the cholesterol in foods does.

Eggs

In the past, three eggs a week was the maximum allotted amount because egg yolks were believed to contain as much as 274 mg of cholesterol, practically filling up the daily allotment of 300 mg in one gulp. Today, an egg is known to have around 214 to 220 mg of cholesterol, allowing room in the diet for one egg a day — provided egg-lovers can keep their remaining cholesterol intake below the 300-mg-per-day benchmark.

REMEMBER

When eating eggs, keep the rest of your diet low in saturated fat. Eggs have 5 grams of fat per ounce.

If this still seems like too much cholesterol for your diet, you may want to check out some new cholesterol-friendly egg-based products like Eggland's Best and Egg Beaters. Eggland's Best are eggs from hens that are deliberately fed a diet that lowers the eggs' cholesterol significantly, to around 180 mg per egg. Egg Beaters are made primarily from seasoned egg whites (no yolks), making them a handy choice.

TIP

The cholesterol is all in the yolk; there is none in the white. If you have the time (and don't want to spend the extra cash for the premade products), you can make your own cholesterol-free egg products. Use two egg whites and 1 teaspoon of oil in place of a whole egg in a recipe. If you're making an omelet or frittata, you can probably get away without using the extra oil.

Cheese

Cheese is a nutritious food, but not a low-fat one. Most supermarkets carry reduced-fat cheeses. Try combining cheese with fresh fruit for a healthy snack or dessert. Consider these options:

>> Cheddar, reduced-fat [5 grams of fat per ounce]

>> Colby, reduced-fat [5]

>> Cottage cheese, low-fat [0-1]

>> Cottage cheese, regular [3]

>> Feta [5]

>> Mozzarella [5]

>> Parmesan [3]

>> Ricotta [5]

Note: Regular cheddar and Colby cheese have 10 grams of fat per ounce! Make sure to choose the reduced-fat variety.

Seafood

Seafood is a terrific source of protein, low in calories and low in fat. Whether you choose fish or shellfish, you're bound to get a dose of concentrated protein, all wrapped up in a light and delicate package.

TIP

If you're not familiar with including fish in your diet, start with canned tuna and salmon. Then try broiled orange roughy, flounder, tilapia, or grilled salmon. Start ordering grilled, broiled, or baked fish and seafood in restaurants to become familiar with nonfried choices.

REMEMBER

Current guidelines from the American Heart Association recommend two seafood-based meals a week for all Americans. Fish is a heart-healthy food because it's high in omega-3 fatty acids.

Omega-3 fatty acids are good fats that make your blood less likely to form clots that can cause a heart attack. Experts recommend that healthy people eat omega-3 fatty acids from fish and plant sources to protect their hearts. The fatty acids also protect against irregular heartbeat that causes sudden cardiac death. Check out Chapter 8 for more about omega-3s and other fatty acids.

Fish

Fresh fish contains less saturated fat than red meat. Try to eat fish two to three times a week. Most markets have significantly expanded their seafood offerings. Check with your local fishmonger for their recommendations about the following:

- Catfish [3 grams of fat per ounce]
- Cod, fresh or frozen [0-1]
- Flounder [0-1]
- Grouper [0-1]
- Haddock [0-1]
- Halibut [0-1]
- Herring, uncreamed or smoked [3]
- Mahimahi [0-1]
- Mackerel [3]
- Pompano [3]
- Orange roughy [0-1]
- Salmon, fresh or canned [3]
- Sardines, canned [3]
- Scrod [0-1]
- Snapper [0-1]
- Sole [0-1]
- Swordfish [3]
- Trout [0-1]
- Tuna, ahi [0-1]
- Tuna, albacore [0-1]
- Tuna, canned in oil [3]
- Tuna, canned in water [0-1]
- Tuna, yellowfin [0-1]

Healthy adults should eat two servings a week of fish such as mackerel, lake trout, herring, sardines, albacore tuna, and salmon.

Shellfish and mollusks

Most shellfish, if not fried, is very low in fat. Shrimp is higher in cholesterol than most other seafood but low in fat. Include the following in your diet:

- Clams [0-1 grams of fat per ounce]
- Crab [0-1]
- Crawfish [0-1]
- Lobster [0-1]
- Mussels [0-1]
- Oysters, raw [0-1]
- Scallops [0-1]
- Shrimp [0-1]

Making Meals from Whole-Food Choices

Let Green Light foods be the focus of your meals. Each meal should have a lean meat, fish, or poultry, at least one serving of the free veggies, and at least one serving of the free fruits. *Remember:* You aren't held to a specific amount. You can eat grilled chicken, a large leafy green salad, green beans, and a bowl of cantaloupe, and you're still in the Green Light section! Another meal selection can be baked cod, a mixed fresh fruit cup, steamed broccoli and carrots, and fresh spinach and orange salad.

To get you started, use the easy recipes of Marilyn's Orange Pineapple Delight in Chapter 13, and Vegetable Salad and Hearty Vegetable Soup in Chapters 12 as examples of ways to incorporate the Green Light foods listed in this chapter into a varied, delicious diet. Did I mention these are free foods? That means you can eat them any time you feel like it!

TIP

If you like a savory cottage cheese treat, try the Sharon's Zesty Cottage Cheese recipe in Chapter 13.

Soup tends to taste much better the second or third day, giving flavors time to fully develop. Most soups can be frozen in airtight containers for up to three months. For quick serving, freeze soup in serving-size portions.

Letting Green Light Foods Satisfy Your Appetite

The trick to eating well is knowing when you've had enough but not too much. You probably recognize that stuffed feeling, and you certainly know when you're still hungry. You also know that both of these states are uncomfortable. The trick is recognizing that just-right state and the feeling of satisfaction that goes with it.

TIP

To get a better sense of when you've had enough to eat, but not too much, follow these suggestions:

>> **Slow it down.** Your stomach needs 15 minutes to tell your brain that you're full. Eat slowly and let your brain catch up!

>> **Forget counting calories.** Focus on feeling satisfied with proper foods instead of targeting a specific calorie value. If you don't feel full, eat more fruits, non-starchy vegetables, or lean protein foods rather than sweets and junk foods.

>> **Prepare yourself mentally for making changes in your diet, then set a start date.** Be sure to have the right foods together for a good start.

>> **Eat regular meals — three meals, three to four hours apart, with three food groups at each meal.** Don't skip meals! Regular meals keep your blood sugar stable without peaks and valleys.

>> **Plan snacks of Green Light foods.** Have those grab-and-go fruits and veggies readily available.

>> **Divide your plate into quarters and fill three quarters with Green Light foods.** Leave that fourth quarter for starches and sweets.

>> **Drink six to eight 8-ounce glasses of water per day.** Staying hydrated helps to keep you feeling full.

>> **Follow this plan 90 percent of the time, and treat yourself to a favorite food 10 percent of the time.** That 10 percent keeps you from feeling deprived.

THE HEALTH BENEFITS OF EATING MORE FRUITS AND VEGETABLES

You can reduce your risk of coronary heart disease, stroke, and obesity by increasing your consumption of vegetables and fruit. In addition, some scientific studies have demonstrated that greater fruit and vegetable consumption is consistent with a reduced risk of some types of cancers, including cancer of the stomach, esophagus, and lungs. The types of vegetables that most often appear to be protective against cancer are raw vegetables, followed by *allium* vegetables (onions, garlic, scallions, leeks, chives), carrots, green vegetables, *cruciferous* vegetables (broccoli, cauliflower, Brussels sprouts, cabbage), and tomatoes.

This protective power of fruits and vegetables is due to the phytochemicals they contain. *Phyto* means plant; therefore, phytochemicals refer to any of various biologically active compounds found in all plant foods such as fruits, veggies, and cereal grains. Many of these phytochemicals are responsible for the plant's ability to resist disease and destruction, and these mechanisms of protection are passed on to the humans who eat them.

(continued)

(continued)

Although scientists have identified about 10,000 different phytochemicals, many still remain unknown. They tend to fall into four main categories:

- Carotenoids

- Flavonoids

- Ellagic acid

- Allium compounds

New knowledge of phytochemical benefits emerges every day. Just know that plant foods are very beneficial to your diet and overall health. You don't have to go full-throttle vegetarian (unless you want to), but incorporating more plant foods in your diet is a good thing to do.

Dietary antioxidants are phytochemicals that have an antioxidant function in the body. According to Rachel Link, MS, RDN, the term "antioxidant" doesn't actually refer to one specific compound but rather the activity of specific compounds in the body.

The organization Health Research Funding describes some interesting tidbits about antioxidants:

- Antioxidants prevent cell destruction caused by the action of free radicals. *Free radicals* are unstable molecules that take away electrons from other molecules and damage them. They're the result of the breakdown of food or environmental exposure to tobacco smoke, pollution, and UV radiation. If left unchecked, free radicals trigger a chain reaction that can damage your healthy cells causing heart disease, cancer, and many other diseases.

- Antioxidants donate electrons to free radicals to stabilize them, which prevents free radicals from invading other cells and causing diseases.

- Your body can produce antioxidant enzymes on its own, which work along with the antioxidants that come from the food you eat.

- Antioxidants play a vital role in anti-aging.

- Spices are highly rich in antioxidant content among all the food groups.

Chapter **6**

Navigating Your Way through Starchy Carbs

P oor misunderstood carbohydrate. First it was good, and then it was bad. Will these nutrition people make up their minds? I don't blame you if you're frustrated and confused when it comes to carbs. Nutrition science can actually be pretty complex. And to add insult to injury, when nutrition messages are simplified, very important facts often get left out. So, in this chapter I skip the nutrition talk and fast-forward to food. (If you want more details about the science of carbohydrates, check out Chapter 3.)

Of all the many functions of carbohydrate foods, in this chapter I want you to keep one main function in mind: Carbohydrate is fuel. You've probably heard carbs described as a quick-energy food. A lot of people think what that means is, "If I eat carbs, I'll feel more energetic." For most people, that's not exactly true. Marathon runners often eat a lot of pasta before a big race. Why? Because they need a quick energy source to fuel their muscles for their long run ahead. If you're going to sit or stand on the sidelines to cheer them on, do you need a lot of pasta? No. And if you aren't going to burn the fuel, then you'll store the fuel. And guess how that fuel is stored? You got it — as the dreaded body fat.

Any person who is overweight or obese needs to eat less refined carbohydrate. *Refined* carbohydrates are carbs that have been processed to the point of oblivion — well, at least to the point where their nutritive value is diminished and their glycemic index is usually high. Only lean and active people can tolerate a lot of carbohydrate. After you lose weight, if you want to eat more carbs, then you must become more active.

REMEMBER

If you sit around all day, you don't need many carbs. If you run around all day, then you can eat more of them.

In this chapter, I show you how to lower the carbohydrate in your diet from refined and starchy food sources to allow for weight loss without sacrificing good nutrition.

Yellow Light: Putting Starchy Carbs on Cruise Control

In the Whole Foods Weight Loss Eating Plan, certain fruits and vegetables are classified as Green Light, meaning "Go, go, go, and eat all you want." Chapter 5 lists these foods in detail. Those foods do have carbohydrate in them, but the carbohydrate isn't counted in the Whole Foods Weight Loss Eating Plan, because it's usually low on the glycemic load index and is very healthy for you. Carbohydrate that comes from starchy food sources is called Yellow Light, meaning "Exercise caution." Be careful not to eat too much of these foods, because you can only have five choices a day. Occasionally, you can substitute a refined or sweet carb for one or two of your starchy carbs.

Controlling your intake of the starchy carbs outlined in this section is a key component of the Whole Foods Weight Loss Eating Plan. This feature of the diet will allow for weight loss and will lower your triglycerides, blood sugar, and blood pressure if they're elevated. You may have five carbohydrate choices per day. If you want to speed up your weight loss, you can restrict your carb choices to one to three per day, but don't eliminate them entirely. A carbohydrate choice is a serving that supplies 15 grams of total carbohydrate — for example, 3 cups of low-fat microwave popcorn or ½ cup of beans. Try to choose the healthiest foods in this category (for example, whole-grain breads and cereals or dried beans and peas).

Because you live in the real world and not just in the pages of this book, the plan is designed to also let you have an occasional sweet treat or snack food. Don't fall into the trap of saying, "I won't eat any of the Yellow Light foods. I can just eat the Green Light foods and lose weight faster." Doing so will put you at risk of insufficient carbohydrate for your needs. Plus, you'll be eliminating some very important healthy foods from your diet.

In the recipes in Part 3, I use the Green Light icon to indicate these recipes. If I don't use the Green Light icon on the recipe, then by default the recipe falls into Yellow Light category.

The goal is to eat well *and* lose weight. Always eat at least one to three servings of carbs, but no more than five servings from this group per day. Check out the next section for information on how much constitutes a serving.

Controlling Portion Sizes

The key to enjoying carbohydrates while maintaining a low-carb lifestyle is portion control. The Yellow Light foods aren't free foods like the delicious cornucopia detailed in Chapter 5. They're categorized as Yellow Light because you need to exercise caution and keep them under control. Exceeding the serving size of a lot of the foods in this category is easy to do. The following sections detail the portion sizes of common starchy carbs and emphasizes the healthiest choices such as whole grains and starchy veggies.

Breads

Bread is an important part of any healthy diet, even a low-carb one. Over the years, many people have increased their intake of bread because it's low in fat, despite being fairly high in carbs. But the important thing to consider when choosing bread is the type of grain used to make it. Refined-grain breads, like every day white bread, are soft, smooth-textured, and very tasty. However, refining the grain eliminates a lot of nutrients and increases the glycemic load of the bread, meaning your body converts these carbs to glucose very quickly; thus, you aren't satisfied for long and get hungrier quicker. Whole-grain breads are more nutritious and lower on the glycemic index chart; they affect your blood sugar more slowly and leave you feeling full longer.

Choose whole-grain rolls, muffins, and bread products to stay fuller longer. For more on glycemic index and glycemic load, see Chapter 3 and Appendix A. For more information on the benefits of whole grains and fiber in your diet, take a look at "Choosing the Best, Leaving the Rest," later in this chapter.

Each serving of the following bread items in Table 6-1 equals approximately 15 grams of total carbohydrate (or one serving).

TABLE 6-1

Portion Size of Breads to Equal One Carb Choice

Food	Amount to Equal One Serving
Bagel, small	1
Bread, reduced-calorie (40 calories/slice)	2 slices
Bread, white, whole-wheat, pumpernickel, rye	1 slice
Breadsticks, crisp, 4 inches long by ½ inch thick	2
English muffin	½
Hot dog or hamburger bun	½
Pita, 6 inches across	½
Raisin bread, unfrosted	1 slice
Roll, plain, small	1
Tortilla, corn, 6 inches across	1
Tortilla, flour, 7 to 8 inches across	1
Waffle, 4½ inch square, reduced-fat	1

Note: One carbohydrate choice equals 15g carbohydrates.

REMEMBER

The more refined a grain is, the fewer the vitamins and minerals and the higher the glycemic load. When you eat these refined foods, they quickly turn to blood sugar. Choose whole, intact grain foods, such as wheat, rye, and barley. They're a major source of cereal fiber and contain numerous phytochemicals that can lower your risk of heart disease, diabetes, and cancer.

Cereals, grains, and pasta

The principle of whole grains applies here. Choose whole-grain cereals with no added sugar and whole-wheat pasta. Each serving of the foods in Table 6-2 equals approximately 15 grams of total carbohydrate (or one serving).

TABLE 6-2 **Portion Size of Cereals, Grains, and Pastas Equal to One Carb Choice**

Food	Amount to Equal One Serving
Bran cereals, ready-to-eat	½ cup
Bulgur, cooked	½ cup
Cereals, cooked	½ cup
Cereals, unsweetened, ready-to-eat	¾ cup
Cornmeal, dry	3 tablespoons
Couscous, cooked	⅓ cup
Flour, dry	3 tablespoons
Granola, low-fat, ready-to-eat	¼ cup
Grape-Nuts, ready-to-eat	¼ cup
Grits, cooked	½ cup
Kasha, ready-to-eat	½ cup
Millet, dry	¼ cup
Muesli, ready-to-eat	¼ cup
Oats, dry	½ cup
Pasta, macaroni, spaghetti, cooked	½ cup
Puffed cereal, ready-to-eat	½ cups
Quinoa, cooked	½ cup
Rice, white or brown cooked	⅓ cup
Shredded Wheat, ready-to-eat	½ cup
Sugar-frosted cereal, ready-to-eat	½ cup
Wheat germ, dry	3 tablespoons

Note: One carbohydrate choice equals 15g carbohydrates.

TIP

To bump up your intake of whole-grain foods, look for one of the following ingredients *first* on the food label's ingredient list:

>> Brown rice
>> Bulgur
>> Cracked wheat

>> Graham flour
>> Oatmeal
>> Popcorn

- » Whole barley
- » Whole cornmeal
- » Whole oats

- » Whole rye
- » Whole wheat

Try some of these whole-grain foods:

- » Corn tortillas
- » Low-fat whole-wheat crackers
- » Oatmeal
- » Tabouli salad

- » Whole barley in soup
- » Whole-grain ready-to-eat cereal
- » Whole-wheat bread
- » Whole-wheat pasta

But remember to count each serving of 15 grams of total carbohydrate as one of your five carbohydrate choices.

WARNING

Wheat flour, enriched flour, and degerminated corn meal aren't whole grains. Most basic all-purpose or white flour comes from wheat; it's just refined and less healthy. And just because the bread is brown doesn't mean it's whole-grain. Some food manufacturers just add color to white bread to make it look like whole wheat.

Vegetables and fruit

Starchy vegetables are delicious and you're not alone if you love them. The white Russet potato, a big crowd-pleaser, is particularly high in glycemic load. Enjoy the vegetables in Table 6-3, but watch the portion size and count them appropriately as part of your five carbohydrate choices.

The banana is one fruit I put on the starch list, because it has a higher starch content than other fruits. The more ripe the banana, the higher the glycemic index. Bananas are the number-one fruit sold in the United States, and many people who eat bananas tend to eat a lot of them. If that's you, enjoy them occasionally, but be sure to count them as a carbohydrate choice. If you have been told by your healthcare provider to eat bananas for potassium, be aware that you can get just as much potassium from your Green Light fruits and vegetables, such as cantaloupe, orange or grapefruit juice, honeydew, watermelon, raisins, broccoli, spinach, summer squash, and tomatoes.

TABLE 6-3

Portion Size of Starchy Vegetables and Fruit to Equal to One Carb Choice

Food	Amount to Equal One Serving
Baked beans	⅓ cup
Banana	1 small (6 inches long)
Corn	½ cup
Corn on the cob, medium	1 ear
Mixed vegetables with corn, peas, or pasta	1 cup
Peas, green (English peas)	½ cup
Plantain	½ cup
Potato, baked or boiled	1 small
Potato, mashed	½ cup
Squash, winter (acorn, butternut)	1 cup
Yam or sweet potato, plain	½ cup

Note: One carbohydrate choice equals 15g carbohydrates.

QUINOA: THE SUPER "GRAIN"

Quinoa (*keen*-wah) isn't exactly a grain, but this wonder food cooks like a grain, tastes like a grain, quacks like a grain. . .. You get the picture. Quinoa is actually a seed that is packed full of protein (including the all-important amino acid, lysine), calcium, and B-complex vitamins, including folic acid.

Quinoa is a wonder food with at least as complete a protein as whole milk and about as many carbs. Relatively new to North America, quinoa sustained the South American Incas, dating back at least 5,000 years. The seed itself closely resembles millet and comes in a variety of colors, ranging from red, orange, and yellow to white and black.

Before arriving at your grocery-store shelves, the seeds are processed to remove their bitter saponin coating. Unlike traditional refining, this process doesn't diminish the nutritional value of the quinoa; it simply makes it palatable.

You can find quinoa in most health-food stores and many larger grocery stores.

Dried beans, peas, and lentils

Dried beans and peas contain a fair amount of protein and are often counted as a meat substitute. They're low in glycemic load and can contain as many as 8 grams of dietary fiber per serving.

Table 6-4 lists some of these foods along with the portion size that counts as a carbohydrate choice.

TABLE 6-4 **Portion Size of Legumes to Equal to One Carb Choice**

Food	Amount to Equal One Serving
Beans and peas (garbanzo, pinto, kidney, white, split, black-eyed)	½ cup
Edamame (green soybeans)	½ cup
Lentils	½ cup
Lima beans	⅔ cup
Miso	3 tablespoons
Peanuts	3 ounces
Tofu, extra-firm	1 cup
Tofu, silken	1 cup

Note: One carbohydrate choice equals 15g carbohydrates.

Miso is a soybean paste that is a key ingredient in Japanese cuisine. Use it to quickly add the health benefits of soy to your meals, but watch how much you use if you're watching your blood pressure. This condiment is full of sodium. Speaking of soy, don't be afraid to try edamame (ed-ah-*mah*-may) or green soybeans. You can find these protein-packed pods in the produce department or in the freezer section of most grocery stores. Boiled in lightly salted water, they can satisfy a salty craving without adding much fat or sodium. A half cup has around 15 grams of dietary fiber, 70 mg of calcium, 10 grams of carbs, and 11 grams of protein. Munch away!

REMEMBER

If you don't eat animal products, but you want to follow a low-carb diet, use this group of Yellow Light foods as your Green Light proteins. If there is no meat, fish, or poultry at a meal, then the legumes and soy products count as protein, not starch. However, if there is an animal meat at the meal, you have to count these products as starch.

LEERY TO LOVE LEGUMES?

Maybe the word itself is a little intimidating. Legumes (*leh*-gooms) is a fancy word to describe the food family that includes black beans, black-eyed peas, garbanzo beans, Great Northern beans, kidney beans, lentils, navy beans, peanuts, pinto beans, soybeans, and practically any other kind of bean you can think of.

Once scorned as "the poor man's meat," legumes are a nutritional powerhouse. They're an inexpensive, health-promoting, land-sparing, nutritious food. They're full of fiber and protein, and some even contain decent amounts of calcium and very little fat. All legumes add essential vitamins and minerals to your diet.

Because they're relatively inexpensive, many countries and cultures have a long tradition of using them as the staple of their diet. In China and Japan, much of their cooking is related to soybean products, including sprouts, bean curd (tofu), and, of course, soy sauce. In India, lentils, beans, and chickpeas are the number-one protein source in everything from fritters to saucy curries. And what would Latin American cuisine be without black beans and pinto beans? Americans love their peanut butter, baked beans, Texas-style chili with beans, bean sprouts, garbanzo beans, and so on. What French farmhouse is complete without its homemade cassoulet? You get the picture.

Legumes are versatile and easy to prepare. You can find them dried, fresh, canned, or frozen. The canned variety are great for quick meals, but with a pressure cooker, you can have freshly cooked beans in minutes, compared to hours when cooked in the traditional method. Get a variety and find your favorites. Your stomach and intestines will thank you.

Some people do experience gas after eating legumes. Here are a couple of tips to alleviate the problem:

- Soak dried legumes overnight, then drain and rinse them before preparing them. This process seems to remove some of the gas-giving components. If using canned beans, just drain and rinse them.

- Use a commercially available food enzyme, like Beano. This enzyme helps your body break down the carbohydrate in the legumes so the bacteria in your intestines don't get the chance to break it down and create gas in the process.

Crackers and snacks

This is a category of food that has gotten completely out of hand in the American diet. Most of these foods in Table 6-5 are made from refined flour and are low in vitamins and minerals. Think about how frequently you choose these foods and try to substitute fresh fruit and veggies for your snack. When you do choose these foods, keep in mind that one serving equals approximately 15 grams of total carbohydrate.

TIP

To keep from overeating snack foods, take out the portion you need and then put the bag or box away. That way, you won't reach into a large bag of snacks and continue eating until the bag is empty. Try to include raw fruit, veggies, or low-fat cheese with your snack.

OH, SOY GOOD!

Soy is a unique food that's widely studied for its estrogenic and anti-estrogenic effects on the body. According to Harvard's Nutrition Source, results of recent population studies suggest that soy has either a beneficial or neutral effect on various health conditions. Soy is a nutrient-dense source of protein that can safely be consumed several times a week and is likely to provide health benefits.

Soy foods are packed full of great things including protein, carbs, calcium, vitamins, omega-3 fatty acids, and fiber. You name it, it's probably in there. The protein in soy is complete, meaning it has all eight essential amino acids.

Soy is packed full of antioxidants and isoflavones, which are powerful health-promoting compounds. Soy is believed to help reduce the risk of cardiovascular disease, by helping to lower LDL ("bad") cholesterol, and some kinds of cancer, including breast, prostate, and uterine cancer.

Soy estrogens are helping to alleviate menopausal symptoms for many women. Preliminary research indicates that soy foods are particularly good for diabetics at risk or experiencing symptoms of kidney disease.

If you haven't taken the plunge, try fitting soy products into your diet. Tofu may not sound appealing to you, but the best thing about it (besides the obvious nutrition) is that it takes on the flavor of whatever your cook it in or with. It's great in soups and sauce. Crumble a little in spaghetti sauce or chili.

Or you may prefer to try a type of soy that's completely different like edamame, miso, soy nuts, or soy milk. So rather than replace meat with tofu, just add soy products to your diet.

There is no official Recommended Daily Allowance (RDA) for soy protein; however, the U.S. Food and Drug Administration (FDA) established 25 grams of soy protein per day as the threshold intake required for cholesterol reduction. Many food producers are calling out soy protein grams separately on their food labels.

TABLE 6-5

Portion Size of Snacks to Equal to One Carb Choice

Food	Amount to Equal One Serving
Animal crackers	8
Graham crackers, 2½-inch square	3
Matzoh	¾ ounce
Melba toast	4 slices
Oyster crackers	24
Popcorn (popped, no fat added or low-fat microwave)	3 cups (½ bag)
Pretzels	¾ ounce
Rice cakes, 4 inches across	2
Saltine-type crackers	6
Snack chips (tortilla, potato, baked)	15 to 20 (1 ounce)
Soy nuts	1½ ounce
Vanilla wafers	5
Whole-wheat crackers, no fat added	2 to 5 (¾ ounce)

Note: One carbohydrate choice equals 15g carbohydrates.

Check out soy nuts if you haven't tried them. You get one and a half to two times the quantity compared to other snacks, plus you add calcium, protein, soy, and dietary fiber wrapped up in a snack-food package. Look for these in the snack-food aisle in many flavors — chile-lime, salt, teriyaki, and even barbecue.

Choosing the Best, Leaving the Rest

A general rule for making your carbohydrate selection each day is to stick to low-glycemic-load foods as often as possible. Choose whole grains for at least three of your carb choices and legumes for the other two for the healthiest diet. These foods will satisfy you longer, so you'll need to refuel less often. Occasionally, you can select more refined foods. Those foods will satisfy the occasional craving but typically have less fiber, vitamins, minerals, and overall nutrition. And always remember to count both with the appropriate number of carbohydrate choices.

Get a feel for high and low glycemic–load (GL) carbs and know how to strike a balance between the two. If your carb choices are all low glycemic load, then you shouldn't have any problems. But that isn't realistic. Those high glycemic load–carbs are just too tempting and sometimes they're the only food available. Of your five carb choices, you may tolerate three low GL choices and two high GL choices occasionally with no problems. However, if you edge over to two low GL foods and three high GL, you're getting in the danger zone of developing food cravings and overstimulating your appetite. Use the information in the following sections to find out where your limit of high glycemic load carbs is.

Low-glycemic-load carbs

Foods with a low–glycemic load affect your blood sugar slowly. Here are some examples of low–glycemic-load carbs and their serving sizes:

- » ½ cup of beans or peas (garbanzo, pinto, kidney, white, split, black-eyed)
- » ⅔ cup of lima beans
- » 1 slice of high-fiber bread (rye, whole-wheat, multigrain)
- » ¾ ounce (2 to 5) whole-wheat crackers
- » 3 cups of low-fat microwave popcorn

TIP

Whole-grain foods fall into the lower-glycemic-load category because they slow the digestion of starches into the bloodstream. These foods also have many other nutritional benefits, including the following:

- » They improve the health of the gastrointestinal tract by improving regularity.
- » They lower the risk of mouth, stomach, colon, gallbladder, and ovarian cancer.
- » They reduce LDL ("bad") cholesterol, while maintaining HDL ("good") cholesterol.
- » They may reduce some kinds of heart disease.
- » They contain valuable *phytochemicals* (naturally occurring plant-based chemicals that help fight disease).
- » They contain essential vitamins and minerals.

High-glycemic-load carbs

High-glycemic-load carbs quickly affect your blood sugar and may leave you hungrier more quickly than their low-glycemic-load counterparts. Starchy veggies with a high glycemic load like russet potatoes can be part of your diet and add to your daily fiber intake as long as you eat them in moderation. Other varieties of potatoes such as Yukon Gold or red potatoes tend to be lower in glycemic load. Stick to the portions outlined in the section, "Vegetables and fruit," earlier in this chapter to ensure you're staying within your daily allotment of carbohydrate choices.

Whenever possible, eat your starchy vegetables, like potatoes, with the skin intact. You're sure to get the most nutrients and an extra dose of dietary fiber. Better nutrition and a full tummy — what more can you ask for? Don't go crazy and start eating banana peels and spaghetti squash hulls, because that's just, well, silly — but eating a russet potato skin now and then won't hurt you.

Here are some examples of carbohydrate choices with a higher glycemic load:

>> 1 slice white bread

>> ½ cup of macaroni, spaghetti, or rice

>> ½ cup of potatoes

>> ¾ cup of unsweetened, ready-to-eat cereal

>> 6 saltine crackers

>> 5 vanilla wafers

For more on the glycemic load and glycemic index of foods, check out Appendix A.

Putting the Brakes on Refined Carbs

Refined carbs are foods that are highly processed and pre-packaged, like chips, cookies, cakes, candy, crackers, and bread. They may even have enticing packaging, claiming to be fat-free or cholesterol-free. But be very discriminating and read your nutrition labels so you know exactly what you're eating. (See Chapter 9 for more information on reading food labels the low-carb way.) You'll eat *some* refined carbs. You just don't want to eat them too frequently or in too great a quantity.

Refined carbs have a low nutrient density, meaning their nutrient value is low compared to the number of calories they pack. Many of these foods have become popular because they're low in fat. People see them as free foods because of their low fat grams, a big mistake.

When you do choose these foods, reduce your intake of the other carbohydrate foods to maintain balance and control in your eating. If you've spent your carbs for the day, remember you can still eat those Green Light foods in Chapter 5 —fruits, veggies, and lean proteins.

Trading off your carb choices for an occasional treat

Okay, so how do you handle a potato-chip craving that just can't be cured by microwave low-fat popcorn? Or what happens when the pop machine is out of no-calorie soda? Don't panic, just readjust your carbohydrate choices for the day with a trade-off. One snack-size (1-ounce) bag of potato chips has 16 grams of total carbohydrate, so you can trade one of your five carbohydrate choices for this puny bag.

One 12-ounce can of regular soda has 40 grams of total carbohydrate (and it's 100-percent sugar and 0-percent nutrients). If you choose a can of regular soda, count it as two and a half of your carb choices for the day. It's okay to make that kind of trade occasionally, but when you do, you can only have two and a half car-bohydrate choices for the rest of the day — not very many.

Say you're at a coworker's birthday party. You're handed a piece of birthday cake and you want to eat it. If it's a normal size serving of birthday cake, just count it as two carb choices and go on about your day. Now, if that unintended birthday cake means you've had your five carb choices by midafternoon, then no more carbs for you. *Remember:* On the Whole Foods Weight Loss Eating Plan, you can still eat your Green Light fruits, veggies, and lean proteins.

REMEMBER

These trade-offs may sound appealing, and you may be plotting your first trade-off as you read. But you can't underestimate the long-term detriment to your health of making these trade-offs too often. Without the critical fiber and nutri-tion you need daily, your general health and weight will suffer. Also, if you make those trade-offs too frequently, food cravings can return and get out of control. Then you have to conquer them all over again.

When evaluating the food labels of trade-off foods, here's a chart to help you work out your own trade-offs. (*Remember:* You can subtract the dietary fiber out of the total carb on the food label.) Check out Chapter 9 for more information on count-ing total carbohydrate.

Total Carbohydrates	Starch Count
6 to 10 grams	½ carb
11 to 19 grams	1 carb
20 to 25 grams	1½ carbs
26 to 35 grams	2 carbs

If your item has less than 5 grams of carbs per serving *and* you eat only one serving, don't count the carbs. Just keep in mind that a lot of 5-gram carb portions can add up in a day. So don't go crazy with this.

REMEMBER

The Nutrition Facts panel tells you how much *total* carbohydrate is in one serving. This includes the amount attributed to dietary fiber. You may subtract the dietary fiber from the total carbohydrate amount. Then calculate the number of carb choices per serving. For more on deciphering food labels, turn to Chapter 9.

Paying attention to sugar

You can eat sweets and sugar, if you count the carbohydrate they contain. The problem is that sugars and sweets don't have vitamins or minerals, and they do have a lot of calories, even in small servings. My best recommendation is to avoid hidden sugars in food, especially refined, pre-packaged, and processed foods. Make the sugar you eat count. Did you really enjoy that fat-free cookie? Probably not, but it likely contained 12 grams of carbs, which is equivalent to eating an entire *tablespoon* of sugar. You'd probably be more satisfied with ¾ cup of fresh strawberries, which contain the same number of carbs, have way more fiber and nutrients, and are pretty darn filling. And don't forget, strawberries are free to you — whereas the fat-free cookie will cost you one carb choice for the day.

Many foods contain both carbohydrate and fat, including sweets, such as cakes, pies, cookies, candy, ice cream, jelly, chocolate, and snack foods, such as chips and crackers.

Avoiding the urge to exceed your daily allowance

The best way to avoid exceeding the carb allowance is to build your meals around the Green Light foods. Always think of those free fruits and veggies first because the amounts are unlimited. Also, track your portion sizes of carb choice foods. Overeating a particular food is often a habit. It's surprising how satisfying a smaller portion can be, especially if you eat it with a variety of unlimited foods. If nothing seems to abate that sweet craving, then indulge it with a controlled amount. Eat it slowly, savor it, and then get back on track. You can compensate for what you've eaten by dropping a couple of carbs or increasing your exercise that day.

Evaluating Low-Calorie Sweeteners

Low-calorie sweeteners, sometimes referred to as *sugar substitutes* or *artificial sweeteners*, add to foods a taste that is similar to table sugar. These intense sweeteners are generally several hundred to several thousand times sweeter than sugar. Most don't contain calories, and they add essentially no calories to foods and beverages, but they aren't without concerns. All sweeteners are regulated by the FDA as food additives. Some research indicates that some of these sweeteners can stimulate insulin leading to fat storage, and some sweeteners can create a residual hunger leading to increased eating. In general, I classify natural sweeteners as "use in moderation" and artificial sweeteners as "use with caution."

Use in moderation

The following low-calorie sweeteners are considered natural sweeteners because they can be found in nature. They've been studied extensively and are considered safe to use:

>> **Allulose:** *Allulose* is a sweetener in the sugar family with a chemical structure similar to fructose. It's naturally found in figs, maple syrup, raisins, and kiwi. Even though it comes from the same family as other sugars, it doesn't substantially metabolize as sugar in the body. The FDA recognizes that allulose doesn't act like sugar, and as of 2019, no longer requires it to be listed with sugars on the U.S. nutrition labels. Allulose is about 70 percent as sweet as sugar, which is why it's sometimes combined with high-intensity sweeteners to make sugar substitutes. The conversion ratio for allulose is 1⅓ cups of allulose equals 1 cup of refined sugar.

>> **Erythritol:** Small amounts of *erythritol* occur naturally in some fruits. It's about 60 to 70 percent as sweet as table sugar and has at the most one-twentieth as many calories. Unlike the high-potency sweeteners (such as monk fruit and stevia leaf extract) erythritol provides the bulk and mouthfeel of sugar, making it a good substitute for sugar in baked goods. Erythritol is often combined with other sweeteners like monk fruit and stevia leaf extract to provide bulk and texture.

>> **Monk fruit:** *Monk fruit*, which is grown is Southeast Asia, was first used by Buddhist monks in the 13th century, giving the fruit its unusual name. Pure monk fruit extract has no sugar, which means that consuming it won't affect blood sugar levels. Even better, monk fruit has no harmful side effects. The FDA considers monk fruit sweeteners to be generally regarded as safe.

Monk fruit gets its sweetness from the antioxidant *mogrosides.* In fact, research found that the mogrosides in monk fruit extract may help reduce oxidative stress. Monk fruit extract is often mixed with erythritol to control its sweetness and to provide bulk in baked foods.

>> **Stevia leaf extract:** *Stevia leaf extract*, which comes from the stevia plant originating in South America, is made from the plant's leaves and is considered safe to consume. Stevia sweeteners are 200 to 350 times sweeter than sugar, which means you need only a very small amount to match the sweetness of sugar. Stevia leaf extract is also frequently mixed with erythritol to provide bulk and texture.

>> **Xylitol:** *Xylitol* is a naturally occurring sugar alcohol found in most plant material, including many fruits and vegetables. First extracted from birch wood to make medicine, xylitol now is widely used as a sugar substitute in sugar-free chewing gums, mints, and other candies. People also use xylitol to prevent cavities.

Xylitol tastes sweet, but unlike sugar, it isn't converted in the mouth to acids that cause tooth decay. It reduces levels of decay-causing bacteria in saliva and also acts against some bacteria that cause ear infections. Xylitol is better tolerated in the gastrointestinal tract than other sugar alcohols such as sorbitol or mannitol. That's why it's on this list and the other sugar alcohols aren't.

WARNING

Xylitol can be toxic to dogs, even when the relatively small amounts from candies are eaten, so keep it away from Spot. If your dog eats a product that contains xylitol, immediately take your fluffy friend to a veterinarian.

Use with caution

The following sweeteners are considered artificial sweeteners because they are manufactured and aren't naturally occurring in nature. They're synthetic sugar substitutes commonly added to foods such as soft drinks, powdered drink mixes, and other beverages, baked goods, candy, puddings, canned foods, jams and jellies, and dairy products. Artificial sweeteners are regulated by the FDA as food additives. According to the National Cancer Institute and other health agencies, there's no sound scientific evidence that any of the artificial sweeteners approved for use in the United States cause cancer or other serious health problems. Use the following with caution:

» **Acesulfame-potassium:** *Aceslfame potassium (Ace-K),* sold under the brand names of Sunett or Sweet One, keeps its sweetness at high temperatures, making it a good sweetener for baking. Some manufacturers refer to sweeteners in their products as "natural," even if the sweetener is processed or refined. Ace-K isn't natural. Although the FDA has deemed it as "generally safe," some researchers have noted it can have negative effects. More research is needed to see if these negative effects happen in humans.

» **Aspartame:** Known by trade names Nutrasweet, Equal, and Canderel, *aspartame* is an artificial non-saccharide sweetener 200 times sweeter than sugar. It's commonly used as a sugar substitute in foods and beverages, particularly diet drinks. Common side effects of consuming aspartame are headaches and migraine exacerbation.

TECHNICAL STUFF

Aspartame is a methyl ester of the aspartic acid/phenylalanine dipeptide. When subjected to heat, the methyl ester breaks down to free methanol, which if consumed regularly breaks down into formaldehyde, a known carcinogen and neurotoxin.

WARNING

In addition, aspartame is half phenylalanine, making it forbidden for people who have the genetic disease phenylketonuria (PKU). These individuals can't normally metabolize phenylalanine and need to avoid diet drinks and other products containing aspartame.

» **Sucralose:** *Sucralose* is a zero-calorie artificial sweetener, and the most common sucralose-based product is Splenda. Made from sugar in a multistep chemical process in which three hydrogen-oxygen groups are replaced with chlorine atoms, this alteration in its structure prevents enzymes in the digestive tract from breaking it down, which is an inherent part of its safety. About 85 percent of consumed sucralose isn't absorbed by the body and is excreted, unchanged in the feces.

REMEMBER

The FDA has determined sucralose to be safe by the FDA and can be an effective option to help control the amount of sugar and calories you eat. However, foods made highly palatable with sucralose activate brain regions of reward and pleasure. This positive association can enhance appetite, and, if left unchecked, the resulting increase in food intake can lead to overweight and obesity. Some researchers have expressed concern that activating reward pathways without delivering calories to the body may have unintended consequences.

» **Saccharin:** Known by trade name Sweet 'n Low, *saccharin* is an artificial sweetener with effectively no calories. It's about 300 to 400 times as sweet as sugar but can have a bitter or metallic aftertaste, especially at high concentrations. Saccharin is used to sweeten products such as drinks, candies, cookies, and medicines. It's heat-stable and stores well because it doesn't react chemically with other food ingredients.

» **Sugar alcohols:** Common *sugar alcohols* are *mannitol, sorbitol, and xylitol.* Sorbitol and xylitol can be found in nature. Mannitol is manufactured. Sugar alcohols aren't commonly used in home food preparation, but they're found in many processed foods. Food products labeled sugar-free, including hard candies, cookies, chewing gums, and soft drinks and even throat lozenges often consist of sugar alcohols. (They're also frequently used in toothpaste and mouthwash because they aren't converted in the mouth to acids causing tooth decay.)

Sugar alcohols and artificial sweeteners such as saccharin and aspartame have different caloric values. Although most artificial sweeteners contain zero calories, sugar alcohols contain about 2.6 calories per gram. The most common side effect of sugar alcohols is the possibility of bloating and diarrhea when sugar alcohols are eaten in excessive amounts. However, xylitol is better tolerated in the gastrointestinal tract than the other sugar alcohols. Be careful about offering any sugar alcohol or sugar-free food products to children.

Fitting in Your Daily Dietary Fiber

Fiber is an important contribution from many of the foods in this group. *Soluble fiber* is helpful in lowering your cholesterol and comes from whole grains like oats, barley, and rye and also from dried beans and peas. *Insoluble fiber* is helpful in lowering your risk of colon cancer and other cancers of the gastrointestinal tract. Whole grains on average provide 3 grams of dietary fiber per serving. Specialty cereals designed to provide more fiber (for example, Bran Flakes, All Bran, Fiber One) can provide 8 to 13 grams of dietary fiber per serving. Dried beans and peas can provide up to 8 grams of dietary fiber per serving. If you carefully select foods from this group, you can get the dietary fiber per day that your body needs.

The following sections explain the current dietary guidelines and how to incorporate them into your daily diet. Check out Appendix C for more on dietary fiber guidelines.

Current dietary fiber guidelines

Guidelines from the National Academy of Sciences recommend that women up to the age of 50 include 25 grams and men up to the age of 50 include 38 grams of fiber in their diet every day. Women over age 50 need 21 grams and men over age 50 need 30 grams of dietary fiber per day. Considering that the average person consumes 10 to 12 grams of fiber per day, this is quite an increase. Getting to the recommended level takes careful selection of the five carbohydrate servings. Don't forget to load up on the free fruits and veggies outlined in Chapter 5. They're chock-full of fiber and don't count as any (not one) of your daily carbohydrate choices.

Here are some examples of how to get the most fiber from your five carbohydrate choices:

½ cup cooked oatmeal = 3 grams dietary fiber

1 slice multigrain bread = 2 grams dietary fiber

¾ ounce (5) whole-wheat crackers = 2 grams fiber

3 cups low-fat microwave popcorn = 3 grams fiber

½ cup pinto beans = 8 grams dietary fiber

Total = 5 carb choices and 18 grams of dietary fiber

Add this to the 2 to 4 grams of dietary fiber that you get from each serving of the fruits and vegetables you eat, and you can easily meet the minimum recommendation of 25 grams of fiber for women up to age 50. Men may need a daily serving of the special high-fiber cereals to meet the higher recommendation of 38 grams of fiber for men up to age 50.

TIP

To estimate your dietary fiber intake, use Table 6-6 as your guide. For more specific information, check the food label or use a reliable reference.

TIP

Located at the Berkeley Nutrition Services website (www.nutritionquest.com) is a free Fruit/Veg/Fiber dietary screener that gives you a good estimate of the amount of fiber in your diet. It is quick and easy to use. If you aren't sure where you stand, visit the site to find out more.

TIP

If you can't get excited about ½ cup of All-Bran or Fiber One, mix them with ½ to ¾ cup Cheerios or Wheaties for two carb servings and 15 grams of fiber. Add 1 cup fresh strawberries and 1 cup of your choice of milk (refer to Chapter 8 for more about your dairy and dairy alternative options). You still have only used two carb choices and your fiber intake is 19 grams for one meal.

WARNING

If your usual diet is the typical 10 to 12 grams of dietary fiber, don't go to 25 to 38 grams of fiber overnight. Your intestinal tract will rebel and you'll experience gas, bloating, and discomfort. Instead, start gradually, adding about 3 extra grams of fiber per day, giving your system time to adjust. Also, when increasing fiber intake, remember to drink 6 to 8 glasses of fluid per day.

TABLE 6-6: **Your Dietary Fiber Intake**

Food	Amount	Grams of Fiber
Fruits and vegetables	½ cup cooked; 1 medium piece; or 1 to 2 cups raw	2 to 3
Starchy vegetables	½ cup	3
Legumes	½ cup	6 to 8
Cereals	½ to ¾ cup	2 to 4
Special high-fiber cereals	⅓ to ½ cup	8 to12
Breads and crackers, whole-grain	1 slice or 1 ounce	2 to 3
Nuts and seeds	½ ounce	1 to 2

Putting It on the Menu: The Daily Plan

As a rule, the best way to spend your five carb choices is to pick three of them from the whole-grains family (like whole-wheat crackers or whole-grain bread) and two of them from the legume group (like black beans or lentils) for the fiber. On occasion, you can definitely work in potatoes and bananas and so on. But really work on improving your intake of whole grains and legumes. You'll see results in both weight loss and general good health.

Here's a sample day to get you started. For more on menu planning see Chapter 10.

Breakfast:

½ cup Fiber One cereal (12 grams fiber) sprinkled with toasted almond (1 gram fiber)

1 cup your choice of milk

Fresh strawberries (4 grams fiber per cup) sweetened with stevia if needed

Carbohydrate choices: 1

Lunch:

Turkey sandwich:

    2 slices whole-wheat bread (4 grams fiber)

    Deli-style turkey breast

1 tablespoon reduced-fat mayonnaise

Mustard

Lettuce

Sliced tomatoes

½ sliced avocado

Orange sections (4 grams fiber per cup)

Iced tea, stevia optional

Carbohydrate choices: 2

Dinner:

Grilled salmon

Grilled mushrooms, bell peppers, and onions (2 grams fiber)

½ cup wild rice (2 grams fiber)

½ cup Pinto Bean Salad from Chapter 15 (6 grams fiber)

Watermelon chunks (1 gram fiber per cup)

Carbohydrate choices: 2

Snack:

6 ounces low-fat fruit-flavored yogurt

Total carbohydrate choices for the day: 5

Total fiber: 36 grams (24 grams from the carb choices, 12 from the fruits, veggies, and nuts)

Still hungry? Eat more strawberries, orange sections, or watermelon; veggies; or a little extra turkey meat or salmon. Or try any of the totally free, Green Light recipes in Chapters 13, 14, and 15, like Artichoke–Ham Bites, Eggplant Casserole, or Savory Carrots.

Chapter **7**

Shifting into Dairy Foods

Think only babies and young children need milk? Do you shun dairy foods when you're dieting because you think they're high in carbohydrate and fat? If you answered yes to either question, you're not alone — and you're also mistaken. The nutrients provided by dairy foods are as important when you're old as when you're young. Even though the jury is still out, some research indicates that calcium provided by dairy foods may help you lose weight.

In this chapter, I fill you in on the importance of dairy foods in your diet, focusing in particular on the benefits of calcium (and the risks you face if you aren't getting enough of it). I also let you know how to get calcium from other non-dairy sources. If you don't consume dairy products, I examine the wide array of dairy alternatives that are available.

Understanding the Benefits of Dairy Foods

Dairy foods such as milk, yogurt, cheese, and ice cream contain carbohydrate in the form of a milk sugar called *lactose*. Lactose is the principal carbohydrate of milk, making up about 5 percent of its weight. Lactose contributes 30 to 50 percent of milk's energy, depending on the milk's fat content. However, milk, yogurt, and other dairy products are low in glycemic load, so you can include them in your lower-carbohydrate meal plan. You're allowed two to three servings per day, and you don't count them as a carbohydrate choice on the Whole Foods Weight Loss

Eating Plan. Check out Chapter 2 for an overview of the eating plan. (For more information on glycemic load and its role in the foods you eat, turn to Chapter 3 and Appendix A.)

The fact that dairy products are low in glycemic load is a good thing because eating dairy foods has been demonstrated to reduce *hypertension* (high blood pressure) and the risk of osteoporosis, kidney stones, and colon cancer. The fat in dairy products is mostly saturated fat, which can increase the risk of heart disease; however, recent research has suggested that dairy products need not be stripped of its fat. Some studies have indicated full-fat sources may not play a role in cardiovascular disease (CVD)-related deaths and may even be protective in some cases. These dairy foods are also rich sources of vital nutrients that can prevent disease. In addition, grass-fed cows have more omega-3 fatty acids and up to 500 percent more conjugated linoleic acid (CLA). Studies suggest that CLA can have anti-cancer properties and help lower your body fat percentage. Also, some research is connecting the calcium from dairy products with weight loss (see the nearby sidebar for more information).

The following sections explore calcium's role in weight loss, the amount of calcium needed in the daily diet, the connection between vitamin D and calcium, and what you need to know to lower your risk of osteoporosis. Also, for those who can't tolerate dairy foods or those who prefer not to consume animal foods, there is a lengthy section on dairy alternatives from plant foods.

Got milk? Got nutrients

Dairy foods are excellent sources of calcium, phosphorous, riboflavin, protein, magnesium, vitamin A, vitamin B6, and vitamin B12. If fortified (and most milk *is* fortified), milk provides appreciable amounts of vitamin D as well. So what does this mean for your body? Take a look at just some of the benefits you stand to gain from the nutrients found in dairy products:

>> **Phosphorus:** This is an important mineral in bones and teeth and a part of every cell in the body.

>> **Riboflavin:** This vitamin supports normal vision and healthy skin. It's important to the production of energy in your body.

>> **Protein:** This nutrient builds and repairs body tissues.

>> **Magnesium:** This mineral is important in building healthy bones and teeth. It's also important in muscle contractions and nerve impulses.

>> **Vitamin A:** This is an important vitamin in maintaining healthy eyes and skin. It is also important in bone and tooth growth.

CALCIUM'S ROLE IN WEIGHT LOSS

The mineral calcium is a must for healthy bones, but a few studies show some kind of link between calcium and fat loss. Some studies exhibit that if you're deficient in calcium, you can lose more weight by adding more calcium from dairy foods to your weight-loss plan. Government studies show several groups of Americans don't meet the recommended daily intake for calcium, specifically boys and girls ages 9–18, women older than 50, and men older than 70. As dietary calcium intake increases, calcium levels within fat cells decrease. In turn, lower calcium levels within cells impact the metabolism of fat, in favor of weight loss. Fat synthesis decreases and fat breakdown increases. This shift in fat metabolism may result in less fat storage and a reduction in body weight.

In other words, getting enough calcium from dairy foods seems to trigger the body to burn more fat and make it harder for new fat cells to form. Of course, calcium can't work alone, but it's effective when combined with the rest of your weight-loss eating plan.

How much calcium do you need in order to lose weight? Even though a limited number of studies showed weight loss enhancement with calcium provided by dairy foods in the daily diet, the amount of calcium needed is still under investigation. Researchers continue to study the role of calcium in a reduced-calorie diet. Meanwhile, getting at least the recommended 1,000 mg of calcium per day from low-fat dairy products, calcium-fortified foods and beverages, and calcium-containing plant foods is a good idea.

>> **Vitamin B$_6$:** This vitamin helps make red blood cells and helps build proteins in your body.

>> **Vitamin B$_{12}$:** This vitamin prevents anemia and helps maintain healthy nerve cells.

>> **Vitamin D:** This vitamin helps maintain calcium and phosphorus for healthy bones.

If you were paying attention, you may have noticed calcium missing from that list. That's because the following section is devoted to the benefits of calcium (and what happens to your body if you don't get enough of it).

Calcium: It's everywhere!

Calcium is found in great abundance in the human body, and 99 percent of it is found in the bones and teeth. (That's why, when kids are growing, they need calcium to build strong bones and teeth.) But where is that remaining 1 percent of calcium found? In the blood. Calcium plays important roles in nerve conduction, muscle contraction, and blood clotting.

Knowing how much calcium you need

If calcium levels in the blood drop below normal, your body will pull calcium from your bones and put it into the blood in order to maintain the blood calcium levels it needs. If your blood borrows too much calcium from your bones, you're at risk for lots of conditions related to calcium deficiency, including osteoporosis. Consuming enough calcium throughout your lifetime, whether you're a man or a woman, is important in order to maintain adequate blood and bone calcium levels.

Check out Table 7-1 to see how much calcium and vitamin D you need every day (see the nearby sidebar, "Vitamin D and calcium: Their critical connection," for more information). These guidelines are the same for both men and women.

TABLE 7-1   **The Amount of Calcium and Vitamin D You Need**

Age	Calcium Amount (mg per day)	Vitamin D Amount (IU per day)
Infants 0 to 6 months	200 mg	400 IU
Infants 6 to 12 months	260 mg	400 IU
1 to 3	700 mg	600 IU
4 to 8	1,000 mg	600 IU
9 to 13	1,300 mg	600 IU
14 to 18	1,300 mg	600 IU
19 to 30	1,000 mg	600 IU
31 to 50	1,000 mg	600 IU
51- to 70-year-old males	1,000 mg	600 IU
51- to 70-year-old females	1,200 mg	600 IU
Older than 70	1,200 mg	800 IU
14 to 18, pregnant/lactating	1,200 mg	800 IU
19 to 50, pregnant/lactating	1,000 mg	800 IU

The National Institute of Health Consensus Conference and the National Osteoporosis Foundation recommend a higher calcium intake of 1,500 mg per day for postmenopausal women not taking estrogen and men and women 65 years or older. Talk to your healthcare provider or registered dietitian nutritionist about the amount of calcium that's right for you.

Although calcium offers many benefits, the old adage "If some is good, more is better" most definitely doesn't apply. If you take more than 2,500 mg of calcium per day, you may experience adverse side effects. High calcium intakes can lead to constipation and an increased chance of developing calcium kidney stones; it may also inhibit your absorption of iron and zinc, both of which are vital nutrients your body needs. Calcium supplements are better absorbed in divided doses. So, don't take 1,200 mg all at one time. Divide it into 600 mg in the morning and 600 mg at night.

If you're a nursing mother whose healthcare provider or lactation consultant has recommended that you cut back on your intake of dairy products because they're upsetting your baby's stomach, make sure you still get at least your minimum calcium requirement from nondairy sources and supplements. Sufficient calcium in your diet is essential in order to provide proper nutrition for you and your baby. For tips on nondairy calcium sources, check out the section, "Getting Enough Calcium," later in this chapter.

Recognizing what can happen if you don't get enough calcium

Calcium is a principal mineral provided by dairy foods. Everybody needs calcium, but as you age you need even more because your body naturally loses calcium *and* has a much tougher time absorbing it. Talk about a double whammy! Although dairy foods are a rich source of calcium, you can also get calcium from oranges, broccoli, dried beans, soy, spinach, and canned salmon with bones. Refer to the section, "Getting Enough Calcium," later in this chapter for more details.

Calcium can play a major role in disease prevention. Three good reasons to count on calcium are the prevention of osteoporosis, high blood pressure, and colon cancer.

OSTEOPOROSIS

Osteoporosis means "porous bone." It's a disease characterized by a decrease in bone mineral density and bone calcium content. What does osteoporosis mean in practical terms? It leads to an increased risk of fractures. One out of four women older than 65 and one out of eight men older than the age of 65 will develop osteoporosis. A diet high in calcium can help slow bone loss. Preserving bone mass helps reduce your risk of developing this bone-thinning and debilitating disease.

VITAMIN D AND CALCIUM: THEIR CRITICAL CONNECTION

Most foods that are fortified with calcium are also fortified with vitamin D. Vitamin D is a critical piece in the calcium-absorption puzzle. It enables your body to use the calcium you're taking in. Additionally, vitamin D helps your body reabsorb calcium in the kidneys rather than allow it to be removed from the body with waste. Vitamin D also helps your body maintain a proper balance of calcium and phosphorous in the bloodstream.

Current guidelines indicate that most people need between 200 and 800 IU (international units) of Vitamin D daily, depending on their age. Vitamin D supplements usually aren't necessary because vitamin D is available from fortified milk and foods such as fish and egg yolks.

Vitamin D is also known as the sunshine vitamin. You only need 15 minutes of sunlight exposure without sunscreen each day to maintain an adequate vitamin D level. The amount of skin exposed to the sun should be the equivalent of your face and arms. Sunscreens with a skin protection factor (SPF) of 8 or higher blocks vitamin D absorption. Persons living in climates with year-round cloudiness blocking the sun's rays will have less vitamin D absorption.

Vitamin D has been shown to produce adverse side effects such as *calcification* (hardening) of soft tissues (blood vessels, heart, lungs, kidneys, tissues around joints) at above 50 mcg or 2,000 IU a day. Examine Table 7-1 in this chapter to determine how much vitamin D you need.

To make sure you're getting enough vitamin D in your diet, take a look at some good sources of vitamin D:

Food	Serving Size	Vitamin D
Egg yolk	1 yolk	25 IU
Salmon	3 ounces	425 IU
Fortified milk	1 cup	100 IU
Fortified cereal	½ to 1 cup	40 IU
Sardines	3 ounces	255 IU

USING CALCIUM SUPPLEMENTS

As with any nutrient, food is always your best source of calcium because it's accompanied by additional essential nutrients that benefit your body. If your healthcare provider or registered dietitian nutritionist (RDN) recommends a calcium supplement, keep in mind that your body will absorb the calcium best if you take it with a meal.

Calcium in foods and in supplements occurs in a compound form. A *compound* is a substance that contains more than one ingredient. Calcium's most likely companions in a compound are carbonate and citrate.

The calcium in a compound is called *elemental calcium.* During digestion, the calcium compound dissolves and the elemental calcium becomes available to be absorbed into the blood. If a tablet contains 500 mg of calcium carbonate, it contains only 200 mg of elemental calcium. That's because only 40 percent of the calcium compound is elemental calcium; the other 60 percent, or 300 mg, is from the carbonate ingredient. Most calcium supplements list the elemental calcium content on the label. The elemental calcium is what counts toward your calcium total for the day.

Here are the main types of calcium supplements you'll find:

- **Calcium carbonate** is the most common type of calcium supplement on the market. It's found in products like Tums, Caltrate, and Os-Cal and usually requires extra stomach acid for digestion, so you should take it with a meal.

- **Calcium citrate** is another type of calcium supplement found in products like Citracal and most calcium-fortified juices. Calcium citrate contains 21 percent elemental calcium. Calcium citrate is the best absorbed supplemental form and does not require the presence of extra stomach acid to dissolve. It's much more expensive than calcium carbonate, so discuss the pros and cons of each type of calcium supplement with your healthcare provider.

Individuals at greater risk of developing osteoporosis include the following:

>> People with a low calcium and vitamin D intake (see the preceding section for recommendations on how much calcium and vitamin D you need)

>> Caucasian or Asian females

>> Females of any race who are thin and/or small-framed or who weigh less than 127 pounds

>> People older than 65

>> People with a family history of osteoporosis

>> Women who are postmenopausal or who have had a hysterectomy and who aren't on estrogen replacement therapy

>> People with a history of eating disorders

>> People who regularly follow a low-calorie diet of 1,200 calories or less

>> Women who are currently having or have had irregular periods or an absence of menstrual periods (lasting more than one year)

>> People with an inactive lifestyle

>> People who smoke cigarettes

>> People who drink more than two alcoholic drinks per day

>> Men with low testosterone levels

>> People who regularly use steroid or glucocorticoid medications (such as prednisone or cortisone) for treatment of asthma, arthritis, lupus, or another chronic disease

TIP

The more risk factors you have, the greater your risk of developing osteoporosis. Obviously, you can't do anything about some risk factors — like your age, your gender, your race, and your family history. However, you can and should consider the risk factors that are within your control. If you smoke, quit (not just because of osteoporosis, but for your overall health). If you drink heavily, cut back. If you lead an inactive lifestyle, become more active. And obviously, you can increase your intake of dairy products and calcium supplements. Making these kinds of lifestyle changes offers many health benefits, but lowering your risk of osteoporosis is a big one.

HIGH BLOOD PRESSURE

The prevalence of high blood pressure (also referred to as *hypertension*) among Americans is 33 percent for those older than 40 and the prevalence increases to 63 percent for those aged 60 and older. High blood pressure increases your risk of heart disease, stroke, and kidney disease. Calcium, potassium, and magnesium are three nutrients shown to reduce blood pressure. Research shows that increasing your calcium consumption to at least the recommended levels for your age (see "Knowing how much calcium you need," earlier in this chapter) is associated with a small but important reduction in blood pressure.

Potassium and magnesium help calcium lower blood pressure. Dairy foods contain ample amounts of all three of these nutrients. Getting all these nutrients in your diet can reduce your systolic blood pressure (the top number in a blood pressure measurement) by 8 to 14 points. Adding exercise will reduce it 4 to 9 points more.

COLON CANCER

Colon cancer is the second leading cause of cancer deaths in the United States. It has long been accepted that people who consume at least a moderate amount of calcium in their diet (700 to 800 mg per day) significantly reduce their risk of colon cancer by 40 to 50 percent. However, a recent study done at the University of North Carolina School of Medicine revealed that people with a history of pre-cancerous polyps that took a calcium supplement of 1,200 mg (with or without vitamin D) increased their risk of developing more cancerous polyps within six to ten years of starting the supplement. Within this group, women and smokers were the most at risk. Therefore, boosting your calcium intake through diet with dairy foods, along with consuming a high-fiber diet, may help reduce your risk of colon cancer. However, those people who have had at least one cancerous polyp should check with their healthcare provider or RDN before taking calcium supplements.

Getting Enough Calcium

The fat in dairy foods contains a high ratio of saturated fat, and high saturated fat intake has consistently been linked to high cholesterol levels and heart disease. Reducing your saturated fat intake as much as possible is a good idea.

TIP

Opt for low-fat or fat-free milk, yogurt, and cheese whenever possible. They contain fewer calories and little to no saturated fat but all the vitamins and minerals that the higher-fat versions contain.

REMEMBER

Children younger than 2 years of age need quite a bit of fat in their diet for adequate brain and nerve development, so they should drink whole milk instead of the low-fat or fat-free versions.

REMEMBER

Two to three servings per day of low-fat dairy foods are allowed on the Whole Foods Weight Loss Eating Plan. However, based on new evidence and a person's individual risk for osteoporosis, three to four servings may be more appropriate for some people. A serving is 1 cup of low-fat milk, 1 to 1½ ounces of cheese, or 6 to 8 ounces of yogurt.

No matter which number of servings is right for you, make sure your other food choices bring you in line with your minimum calcium requirements for your age.

Here's an example of how to fit your two to three servings in each day and add other foods to hit a 1,200 mg requirement:

>> **Breakfast:** Add 1 cup of skim milk to your whole-grain cereal (302 mg calcium).

>> **Lunch:** Toss a piece of low-fat string cheese into your lunchbox (183 mg calcium). Add a cup of raw broccoli (47 mg calcium).

>> **Afternoon snack:** Enjoy a container of nonfat or low-fat yogurt (400 mg calcium). Add some soy nuts for a quick salty treat (119 mg calcium).

>> **Dinner:** Try some braised kale as a side dish (180 mg calcium).

As you can tell from the preceding list, both dairy and nondairy foods can be good sources of calcium. Try to include calcium-rich foods from a variety of sources. To get you started, Table 7-2 lists appropriate serving sizes of some common dairy foods and their contribution to your daily calcium tally, and Table 7-3 lists non-dairy calcium-rich options. Many of the nondairy foods are Green Light foods on the Whole Foods Weight Loss Eating Plan.

TABLE 7-2   **Calcium-Rich Dairy Foods**

Dairy Food	Serving Size	Calcium
Buttermilk	1 cup	285 mg
Cheese, American	1 ounce	174 mg
Cheese, cheddar	1 ounce	204 mg
Cheese, mozzarella, part-skim	1 ounce	183 mg
Cheese, parmesan	1 tablespoon	69 mg
Cheese, ricotta	½ cup	257 mg
Cheese, Swiss	1½ ounces	408 mg
Cottage cheese, low-fat	1 cup	155 mg
Frozen yogurt, vanilla	1 cup	103 mg
Ice cream, vanilla	1 cup	168 mg
Milk, calcium-fortified	1 cup	500 mg
Milk, lactose-free, low-fat	1 cup	300 mg
Milk, skim	1 cup	302 mg
Milk, 2 percent	1 cup	297 mg
Yogurt, fruited, low-fat	1 cup	314 mg
Yogurt, plain, low-fat	1 cup	400 mg

TABLE 7-3

Calcium-Rich Nondairy Foods

Food Serving	Size	Calcium
Protein Foods		
Almonds	⅓ cup	120 mg
Almond milk	1 cup	450 mg
Pinto beans	½ cup	40 mg
Salmon (pink), canned, with bones	3 ounces	174 mg
Sardines, with bones	3 ounces	371 mg
Shrimp, canned	3 ounces	50 mg
Soy cheese, calcium-fortified	1 ounce	200 mg
Soy milk, calcium-fortified	1 cup	300 mg
Soy nuts, roasted, salted	½ cup	119 mg
Soy yogurt, calcium-fortified	⅔ cup	500 mg
Soybeans, boiled	1 cup	262 mg
Tempeh	½ cup	77 mg
Tofu, firm, calcium-fortified	½ cup	258 mg
Fruits and Vegetables		
Bok choy	1 cup	160 mg
Broccoli	½ cup	47 mg
Carrots	1 cup	48 mg
Collard greens, cooked	1 cup	358 mg
Kale, cooked	1 cup	180 mg
Mustard greens	1 cup	152 mg
Orange	1 medium	52 mg
Orange juice, calcium-fortified	½ cup	150 mg
Turnip greens	1 cup	250 mg

TIP

Calcium contents can vary, especially in calcium–fortified foods. Check the nutrition label. Good sources of calcium are those that provide 20 to 30 percent of the daily value (DV) for calcium.

MAKING OCCASIONAL SUBSTITUTIONS

The Whole Foods Weight Loss Eating Plan also allows for occasional substitutions of sugar-free ice cream or frozen yogurt for an occasional treat. Just make sure these treats don't exceed 90 to 130 calories per serving. Keep in mind that these are calorie-equivalent substitutions, and they don't include the same nutrients as a cup of skim milk, so you don't want to be making these substitutions frequently.

Many food manufacturers are capitalizing on the trend of increasing calcium in the diet and have fortified tons of food (literally!) with calcium, including ice cream and water. Although I don't consider them to be great sources of calcium, if you're going to splurge and eat it anyway, you may as well get a little calcium boost. Many of the Healthy Choice no-sugar-added ice creams contain as much as 200 mg of calcium per cup. Always double-check the nutrition label for the full "scoop" before you buy.

Considering Dairy Alternatives

Although some people like cow's milk, some people can't or choose not to drink milk due to personal preferences, dietary restrictions, allergies, or intolerances. Fortunately, plenty of nondairy alternatives are available. Look at the differences in the following popular types of milks to determine which best suits your needs. With all varieties, choose the unsweetened versions. Always check the nutrition facts label on these dairy alternatives especially the carbohydrate content. Milk contains 12 grams of carbohydrate per cup. Milk and milk alternatives can double their amount of carbohydrate (sugar) if they're sweetened with added sugars. Most dairy alternatives are lower in carbohydrate than cow's milk except for quinoa milk, which is similar to cow's milk in carb content. Oat milk and rice milk have double the carb content compared to cow's milk.

Here are nine nondairy substitutes for cow's milk in alphabetical order. Some will be familiar to you and some will be totally new.

Almond milk

Almond milk, made with either whole almonds or almond butter and water, has a light texture and a slightly sweet and nutty flavor. Compared to cow's milk, it contains less than a quarter of the calories and less than half the fat. It's also significantly lower in protein and carbohydrates. Of the nondairy milk alternatives, almond milk is one of the lowest-calorie choices available and is a great option for individuals wanting or needing to lower the number of calories they consume. In addition, almond milk is a natural source of vitamin E, a group of antioxidants that help protect the body from disease-causing substances known as free radicals.

Almond milk is a much less concentrated source of the beneficial nutrients found in whole almonds, including protein, fiber, and healthy fats. Almond milk consists of mostly water, and many brands contain only 2 percent almonds. Therefore, to make the most of almonds' nutrients and health benefits, choose brands of almond milk that contain a higher content of almonds, around 7 to 15 percent. Almonds also contain *phytic acid,* a substance that binds to iron, zinc, and calcium, reducing the absorption of these nutrients in the body.

Cashew milk

Cashew milk, made from a mixture of cashew nuts or cashew butter and water, is rich and creamy and has a sweet and subtle nutty flavor. It's great for thickening smoothies, as a cream in coffee, and as a substitute for cow's milk in desserts. As with most nut-based milks, the nut pulp is strained from the milk, which means the fiber, protein, vitamins, and minerals from the whole cashew are lost.

Cashew milk contains fewer that one-third of the calories of cow's milk, half the fat, and significantly less protein and carbohydrates. With only 23 to 50 calories per cup, unsweetened cashew milk is a great, low-calorie option for individuals looking to reduce their total daily calorie intake. Furthermore, the low carbohydrate and sugar content make cashew milk a suitable option for people who need to monitor their carb intakes.

Coconut milk

Coconut milk, made from water and the white flesh of brown coconuts, is sold in cartons alongside milk and is a more diluted version of the type of coconut milk commonly used in Southeast Asian and Indian cuisines, which is usually sold in cans. Coconut milk contains one-third the calories of cow's milk, half the fat, and significantly less protein and carbohydrates.

Coconut milk is a good choice for individuals looking to further reduce their carb intake. Ninety percent of the calories from coconut milk come from saturated fat, including a type of saturated fat known as *medium-chain triglycerides (MCTs)* (refer to Chapter 8 for more information about MCTs). Some research suggests that MCTs may help reduce appetite, assist with weight loss, and improve blood cholesterol levels; however, a review of 21 studies didn't support the improvement in blood cholesterol levels. Overall, very little quality research on the effects of coconut milk specifically has been conducted. Consuming a moderate amount of coconut milk as part of a healthy diet shouldn't be a cause for concern.

Hemp milk

Hemp milk is made from the seeds of the hemp plant, *Cannabis sativa*, the same species used to make the drug cannabis, also known as marijuana. Unlike marijuana, hemp seeds contain only trace amounts of tetrahydrocannabinol (THC), the chemical responsible for marijuana's mind-altering effects. Hemp milk has a slightly sweet, nutty taste and thin, watery texture. It works best as a substitute for lighter milks such as skim milk.

Hemp milk contains a similar amount of fat to cow's milk, but around half the calories and protein and significantly fewer carbohydrates. It's a good option for vegans and vegetarians because one glass provides 2 to 3 grams of high quality, complete protein with all the essential amino acids. In addition, hemp milk is a source of two essential fatty acids: the omega-3 fatty acid alpha-linolenic acid and the omega-6 fatty acid linoleic acid. Unsweetened hemp milk is very low in carbohydrates, making it a great option for people who want to reduce their carb intake.

Macadamia milk

Macadamia milk, made mostly of water and about 3 percent macadamia nuts, is fairly new to the market, and most brands are made in Australia using Australian macadamias. It has a richer, smoother, and creamier flavor than most nondairy milks and tastes great on its own or in coffee and smoothies.

Macadamia milk contains one-third the calories (about 50 to 55 calories per cup) and about half the fat of cow's milk. It's also somewhat lower in protein and carbohydrates, making it suitable for people with diabetes or those looking to reduce their carb intake. In addition, macadamia milk is a great source of healthy monounsaturated fats, helping to reduce blood cholesterol levels, blood pressure, and the risk of heart disease.

Oat milk

Oat milk is made from a mixture of oats and water to which manufacturers often add extra ingredients such as gum, oils, and salt to produce a desirable taste and texture. Hence, oat milk is naturally sweet and mild in favor. You can use it in cooking in the same way as cow's milk, and it tastes great with cereal or in smoothies. Oat milk contains a similar number of calories to cow's milk, but up to double the number of carbohydrates and about half the amount of protein and fat. Be sure to adjust your serving size of oat milk to a half cup if you want to keep the carb amount equivalent to cow's milk.

Oat milk is high in total fiber and *beta glucan,* a type of soluble fiber that forms a thick gel as it passes through the gut. Beta-glucan gel binds to cholesterol, reducing its absorption in the body thus lowering cholesterol, particularly LDL cholesterol, the type associated with increased risk of heart disease. Research has shown that beta-glucan may help increase feelings of fullness and lower blood sugar levels after a meal.

Quinoa milk

This dairy alternative is made from water and quinoa, an edible seed commonly prepared and consumed as a grain. The whole quinoa grain is very nutritious, gluten-free, and rich in high-quality protein. Even though quinoa has become a popular *superfood* (a nutrient-rich food considered to be especially beneficial to health) over recent years, quinoa milk is fairly new to the market. For this reason, it's slightly more expensive than other nondairy milks and can be a little harder to find.

Quinoa milk is slightly sweet and nutty and has a distinct quinoa flavor. It works best poured over cereal and in warm porridge. It contains a similar number of carbohydrates to cow's milk but fewer than half the calories and significantly less fat and protein. It consists mostly of water and contains 5 to 10 percent quinoa. It has a fairly well-balanced nutrition profile compared to other nondairy milks. Quinoa milk is a good plant-based source of complete protein for vegetarians and vegans.

Rice milk

Rice milk, which is made from milled white or brown rice and water, often contains thickeners to improve texture and taste (which is common with other nondairy milks). Rice milk is the least allergenic of the nondairy milks, making it a safe option for people with allergies or intolerances to dairy gluten, soy, or nuts. It's mild in taste and naturally sweet. It has a slightly watery consistency and is great to drink or use in smoothies, desserts, and with oatmeal.

Rice milk contains a similar number of calories to cow's milk but almost double the carbohydrates and considerably less protein and fat. Specifically rice milk contains about three times the carbohydrates of all the other nondairy milk alternatives. In addition, rice milk has a high glycemic index (GI) of 79 to 92, meaning the gut absorbs it quickly causing blood sugar levels to rapidly increase. Thus, rice milk may not be the best option for people with diabetes or for people who desire to lower their carb intake.

Rice milk has also been shown to contain high levels of inorganic arsenic, a toxic chemical found naturally in the environment. Long-term exposure to high levels of inorganic arsenic has been associated with an increased risk of certain cancers and heart problems. However, for most people, drinking rice milk shouldn't be a concern.

Soy milk

Soy milk, made with either soybeans or soy protein isolate, often contains thickeners and vegetable oils to improve taste consistency. It typically has a mild and creamy flavor, but the taste can vary between brands. It works best as a cow's milk substitute in savory dishes, with coffee, or on cereal. In terms of nutrition, soy milk is a close nondairy substitute for cow's milk. It contains a similar amount of protein, but around half the number of calories, fats, and carbohydrates. It's one of the few plant-based sources of high-quality complete protein providing all the essential amino acids. The human body can't produce these amino acids so they must be obtained from the diet.

Some people are concerned that soy contains large amounts of *isoflavones,* which can affect estrogen receptors in the body and affect the function of hormones. Although this topic is widely debated, currently no scientific evidence exists to suggest that moderate amounts of soy or soy milk will cause harm in otherwise healthy adults. Speak to your healthcare provider or registered dietitian nutritionist if you have any specific concerns.

Chapter **8**

Fueling Up with Fats: Good Fats, Bad Fats

Guess what? Fats are back, and some of them are even good for you — so good for you, in fact, that you should eat *more* of them. Eat more fat? Am I crazy? No, despite what you think, I'm not. The concept of eating less fat is so thoroughly ingrained in U.S. culture that anyone encouraging more fat is looked upon with suspicion. For the past 50 years, fat has been treated as public enemy number one. Some Americans got the message and successfully reduced their fat intake from 40 percent of calories to 34 percent of calories, but at the same time, others who reduced their fat intake increased their calorie intake (mainly by eating more carbohydrates). What did that do for their health? As a nation, Americans are fatter than ever. (For more on this phenomenon, check out Chapter 3.)

In this chapter, I tell you about two different (but very much related) concepts: fat, the nutrient, that functions in your body, and dietary fat that you eat, which may help or hurt your body. I show you how fats that naturally occur in some foods are actually very healthy for you *and* your heart. I introduce you to fats that are absolutely delicious and fun to eat — they not only satisfy your appetite, but also improve your health.

Recognizing How Fat Helps Your Body

Fat has negative connotations for many people, but in the body, fat is an essential nutrient. In fact, fat, in moderate amounts, is *necessary* for your health. In this section, I show you how fat helps your body.

Regulating body processes

All humans need fat in order to maintain healthy skin and regulate cholesterol metabolism. Fat is also necessary for the formation of hormone-like substances called *prostaglandins*, which regulate many body processes such as your body's inflammation response to injury and infection as well as blood vessel contractions and nerve impulses. The fat-soluble vitamins A, D, E, and K, stored in your body fat, play many specific roles in the growth and maintenance of your body.

Providing energy

Fat is a concentrated source of energy for the body by providing 9 calories per gram (compared with 4 calories per gram from either carbohydrates or protein). Fat is an important calorie source especially for infants and young children; 50 percent of the calories in human breast milk come from fat. Some storage of energy in your body in the form of fat is essential to your health.

Storing it up

The body uses whatever fat it needs for energy, and the rest is stored in various fatty tissues. Some fat is found in blood plasma and other body cells, but the largest amount is stored in the body's fat cells. These fat deposits not only act as storage for energy, but they're also important in insulating the body and supporting and cushioning organs.

Understanding the Different Kinds of Fat

Many people assume that dietary fat is directly connected with body fat and heart disease, but that isn't exactly true. Some studies show that women who eat the least amount of fat are the most overweight. As far as heart disease, some fats actually *protect* the heart, whereas others can certainly be harmful. So, just as not all carbohydrates are created equal, not all fats are created equal. Knowing the differences between the various kinds of fat and identifying where they're found in the foods you eat is key.

Fats are classified in three main categories: saturated, monounsaturated, and polyunsaturated (which I discuss in greater detail in the following sections). They differ primarily in the amount of hydrogen they contain. The degree of saturation determines whether the fat is a solid or a liquid at room temperature. The basic unit of a fat is called a *fatty acid.* Fats with lots of saturated fatty acids (like butter and lard) are more solid at room temperature; oils (like olive oil and canola oil) contain mostly unsaturated fatty acids and are liquid at room temperature.

Although the fat in food is often referred to as saturated, monounsaturated, and polyunsaturated, no dietary fat is 100 percent of any of those categories. Dietary fat is classified by the fatty acid that is present in the greatest quantity. For example, olive oil contains 13 percent saturated fat, 72 percent monounsaturated fat, and 8 percent polyunsaturated fat. Because it contains more monounsaturated fat than anything else, it's classified as a monounsaturated fat.

HDL is "good" cholesterol. It helps keep the arteries clear by picking up fatty fragments and taking them back to the liver where they are degraded. *LDL* is "bad" cholesterol. This type of cholesterol sticks to your arteries and forms plaque; the result can be reduced blood flow or the formation of a clot that totally blocks blood flow in an artery.

Having trouble remembering which is the "good" and which is the "bad" cholesterol? Try this:

>> **HDL cholesterol:** H = *H*ealthy, and you want it high (the higher the better, but at least above 40 mg/dl)

>> **LDL cholesterol:** L = *L*ousy, and you want it low (the lower the better, but at least below 130 mg/dl) ***Note:*** If you have diabetes or heart disease, your LDL cholesterol needs to be below 100 mg/dl.

Saturated fats

Saturated fatty acids are usually solid at room temperature, and they're more stable than other types of fats — that is, they don't turn rancid as quickly. Saturated fatty acids raise blood cholesterol, especially the LDL or "bad" cholesterol. Your risk of coronary heart disease rises as your blood cholesterol level increases.

The fat in meat is considered mostly saturated. You can see the visible fat of a piece of prime rib when it's served. You've probably noticed that when the juices that cook out of a roast start to cool, part of the fat starts to solidify and rise to the top. That fat that rises to the top is saturated fat. If you leave a stick of butter on the kitchen counter, it softens but doesn't become completely runny — that's because butter is saturated fat.

Trans fats are a subclass of saturated fat, but they started out as an unsaturated fat like vegetable oil. Food producers and snack makers *hydrogenated* (or added hydrogen to) the vegetable oils. Hydrogenated vegetable oils become more saturated and contain lots of trans fats. Hydrogenated vegetable oils are used in all kinds of common, everyday food products, such as fast food, french fries, stick margarine, and cookies.

In clinical studies, trans fatty acids, or hydrogenated fats, tend to raise total blood cholesterol levels more than unsaturated fats, but less than more saturated fatty acids. Trans fatty acids also tend to raise LDL cholesterol and lower HDL cholesterol. These changes in cholesterol levels may increase your risk of heart disease.

REMEMBER

Saturated fats and trans fatty acids are the two major culprits that have given fat its nasty reputation. These two troublemakers are associated with a whole host of medical conditions including heart disease, arteriosclerosis, cancer, high blood pressure, and diabetes. However, with a few changes to your diet, you can reduce the bad (saturated and trans fat), but still keep the good (and necessary!) mono- and polyunsaturated fats.

TIP

Limiting saturated fats in your diet basically means avoiding high-fat red meats and whole-fat dairy products. However, you don't need to eliminate all the saturated fat in your diet. Just eat saturated fats in the right proportion with unsaturated fats — at least 2 to 1 (unsaturated to saturated).

What that means for you is this:

>> Reduce the saturated fat in your diet as much as possible and always eat at least twice as much unsaturated fat as you eat saturated.

>> Eat only lean or extra-lean red meat.

>> Only eat low-fat dairy products or dairy alternatives. (Check out Chapter 7 for more on dairy alternatives.)

>> Eat more nuts and seeds.

>> Try to eat fish two times per week.

>> Use olive, canola, avocado, or peanut oils.

>> Eat more olives and avocados.

Also avoid *trans fat* whenever and wherever you can. All vegetable shortenings are packed with trans fats. So are most brands of stick margarines. Some margarine makers are now offering brands that are low in saturated fat and are virtually free of trans fats. Examine labels carefully and look for "Contains 0 grams of trans fatty acids" on the label. Also, check the ingredient panel on the food label. If you see the words *"hydrogenated"* or *"partially hydrogenated,"* then trans fats are in the food even if the label says *"no trans fat."* The Food and Drug Administration (FDA) allows a food to claim *"no trans fats"* if there is less than 0.50 grams of trans fat per serving. A *"trans fat–free"* food can have 0.49 grams of trans fat per serving. If you were to eat several servings of *"trans fat–free"* food, you can easily take in 1–2 grams of trans fat. The American Heart Association (AHA) recommends that trans fatty acids make up no more than <1 percent of calories. That means if you eat a 2,000-calorie diet, you should consume less than 2 grams of trans fat per day. That's about 20 calories.

Keep in mind that at least 50 percent of the trans fats you eat are hidden in commercially baked goods (like crackers, muffins, and cookies), in other prepared foods, and in fried foods prepared in restaurants.

COCONUT OIL: DON'T BE DECEIVED

Coconut oil has seen a surge in popularity in recent years due to many touted health benefits. The oil comes from a plant and is almost 100 percent fat, most of which is saturated fat. That's unusual because most saturated fats come from animals. However, the saturated fat in coconut oil is different from the saturated fat in animals. Most dietary fats are categorized as long-chain triglycerides (LCTs), whereas coconut oil contains some medium-chain triglycerides (MCTs), which are shorter fatty acid chains.

When you eat MCTs, they tend to go straight to your liver. Your body uses MCTs as a quick source of energy, and many people believe MCTs increase overall calorie burning. However, many of the health claims for coconut oil refer to research that used a special formulation of coconut oil made of 100 percent MCTs, not the commercial coconut oil most available on supermarket shelves. The coconut oil on the supermarket shelves actually contains 10 to 20 percent MCTs, so the health benefits reported from a specially constructed MCT coconut oil can't be applied directly to the coconut oil purchased in the supermarket.

Food sources of naturally occurring MCTs include dairy fat, coconut oil, goat milk, and palm kernel oil. Though the number of MCT foods is limited, if you drink milk, chances are you're getting some in your diet naturally. The use of MCT supplements to your diet is under investigation. In the meantime, check with your healthcare provider or registered dietitian nutritionist before supplementing your diet with MCTs.

Monounsaturated fats

Monounsaturated oils are liquid at room temperature but start to solidify at refrigerator temperatures. That's why salad dressing containing olive oil turns cloudy when refrigerated but is clear at room temperature — olive oil is a monounsaturated fat. Likewise, the fat in natural peanut butter is mostly unsaturated. If you let a jar of natural peanut butter sit for a while, you'll notice an oily layer forms on the top. That liquid is peanut oil, which is unsaturated fat and a liquid at room temperature.

Monounsaturated fatty acids lower blood cholesterol. They lower the LDL cholesterol and increase the HDL cholesterol (which is a good thing). They also seem to lower triglycerides in some people when substituted for carbohydrate in the diet.

REMEMBER

You can get your daily supply of monounsaturated fats from a variety of naturally occurring food sources including almonds, avocados, canola oil, cashews, olive oil, olives, peanut butter, peanut oil, peanuts, pecans, sesame seeds, and tahini paste made from sesame seeds.

Polyunsaturated fats

Polyunsaturated oils are liquid at room temperature and in the refrigerator. They easily combine with oxygen in the air to become rancid. Polyunsaturated fatty acids help lower total blood cholesterol — by lowering the LDL cholesterol but not the HDL cholesterol. The primary sources of polyunsaturated fat are margarine (the tub or squeeze kind, but not stick), English walnuts, corn oil, safflower oil, soybean oil, reduced-fat salad dressings, and mayonnaise.

Here are some classes of polyunsaturated fatty acids:

>> **Omega-3 fatty acids:** Found primarily in fish and fish oils they're also found in flaxseed, walnuts, and soy and canola oils. Studies suggest these fatty acids may help reduce your risk of heart disease, stroke, and cancer. Research shows that omega-3 fatty acids lower LDL cholesterol and triglycerides. Great sources of omega-3 fatty acids include salmon, albacore tuna, trout, herring, mackerel, flaxseeds, walnuts, canola oil, and non-hydrogenated soybean oil.

>> **Omega-6 fatty acids:** Linoleic acid comprises the majority of the polyunsaturated fat eaten in the United States and comes from a variety of commonly consumed animal and vegetable products, like corn, safflower, sunflower, and cottonseed oils.

FINDING TRANS FAT ON FOOD LABELS

To help foods stay fresh on the shelf or to get a solid fat product, such as margarine, food manufacturers *hydrogenate* (or add hydrogen to) polyunsaturated oils. These fats are trans fats, and you definitely want to avoid them. Trans fats increase LDL cholesterol and decrease HDL cholesterol, and raise triglycerides (another risk factor for heart disease). But how can you tell where they lurk? Products that list *partially hydrogenated vegetable oil* or *vegetable shortening* on the label are examples of trans fats.

Thanks to increased pressure from concerned consumers, dietitians, and other medical professionals, the Food and Drug Administration (FDA) now requires a listing of trans fats on the nutritional labels of all foods. Currently, the labels include total fat grams, saturated fat grams, and *trans* fat grams.

The FDA announced in 2003 it would require food manufacturers to list trans fatty acids on the Nutrition Facts label. This additional information gives consumers a more complete picture of the fat content of foods. Some food products already list trans fat on the food label, but food manufacturers were required to comply in January 2006. The Nutrition Facts Label was updated in 2016 to reflect updated scientific information. For example, "Calories from Fat" has been removed because research shows the type of fat consumed is more important than the amount. For more information, check out Chapter 9.

Watch out for promises on products like "97-percent fat-free." These messages may lead you to believe that if you eat a serving of this item, you'll only be getting 3 percent of the calories in fat grams. Not true! These types of statements reflect the percentage by weight, not by percentage of calories. The official FDA Nutrition Facts label is your best source for information on the true fat content of food.

Remember: Read the label! Products sold as healthy or cholesterol-free often contain vegetable oils that are so altered by processing that their inherent healthy properties have been stripped away.

In healthy populations that consume traditional diets, the ratio of omega-6 fat to omega-3 fat ranges from 5:1 to 10:1. In the American diet, the ratio is currently estimated to be 20:1. This imbalance is now potentially being linked to cancer, heart disease, and arthritis. Improving the ratio by substituting omega-3 fats for omega-6 fats in your diet can result in significant health benefits.

>> **Medium-chain triglycerides (MCTs):** MCTs are a class of saturated fat that contains fatty acids that have a chain length of 6–12 carbon atoms. Interest in MCTs has grown rapidly due to widely publicized benefits of coconut oil, which is a source of MCTs (see the nearby sidebar about coconut oil). MCT oil is available in supplement form. Be sure to check with your healthcare provider or registered dietitian nutritionist (RDN) before taking MCT supplements.

Knowing How Much Fat Is Enough

One serving of fat contains 45 calories and 5 grams of fat. For the average healthy adult, eight fat servings per day are appropriate. And most of those servings (at least six) should be unsaturated fat. That means more avocados but less mayonnaise; more nuts and olives but fewer full-fat dairy products; more fish and poultry; and only lean red meats.

So how do you keep your fat intake on track? Try the following suggestions:

>> Avoid saturated fat, which is animal fat found in red meat and full-fat dairy products, by eating lean meats, low-fat milk, and low-fat cheeses.

>> Eat more nuts, legumes, poultry, and fish.

>> Use nonstick cooking spray and liquid and spray margarine, soft tub plant butters, and margarine blends with yogurt.

>> Try the Olive Oil-Yogurt Spread recipe in Chapter 13 for an even better substitute for butter or margarine.

Check out Table 8-1 for guidelines on how much of the foods you eat constitutes a serving of fat.

TABLE 8-1   ## Fat Servings

Food	Amount for 1 Serving
Monounsaturated Fats	
Almonds	6
Avocado, medium	⅛ of an avocado
Canola oil	1 teaspoon
Cashews	6
Mixed nuts	(50 percent peanuts) 6
Olive oil	1 teaspoon
Olives, black	8 large
Olives, green, stuffed	10 large
Peanut butter	2 teaspoons
Peanut oil	1 teaspoon
Peanuts	10
Pecans	4 halves
Sesame seeds	1 tablespoon
Tahini paste	2 teaspoons
Polyunsaturated Fats	
Corn oil	2 tablespoons
Margarine	1 teaspoon
Margarine, lower fat (30-percent to 50-percent vegetable oil, the rest water)	1 tablespoon
Mayonnaise, reduced-fat	1 tablespoon
Miracle Whip Salad Dressing, reduced-fat	1 tablespoon
Pumpkin seeds	1 tablespoon
Safflower oil	2 tablespoons
Soybean oil	2 tablespoons
Sunflower seeds	1 tablespoon
Walnuts, English	4 halves

(continued)

TABLE 8-1 *(continued)*

Food	Amount for 1 Serving
Saturated Fat	
Bacon	1 slice
Butter, reduced-fat	1 tablespoon
Butter, stick	1 teaspoon
Butter, whipped	2 teaspoons
Cream, heavy, whipping	1 tablespoon
Cream, light or half-and-half	2 tablespoons
Cream cheese, reduced-fat	2 tablespoons
Cream cheese, regular	1 tablespoon
Neufchatel cheese	2 tablespoons
Salt pork	¼ ounce
Shortening or lard	1 teaspoon
Sour cream, reduced-fat	3 tablespoons
Sour cream, regular	2 tablespoons

Including More Healthy Fat in Your Diet

Replacing fats in your diet with refined carbohydrate creates new health problems; replacing saturated fat in the diet with unsaturated fat in the diet promotes better health. However, with a few simple changes, you can benefit from this proven diet plan.

TIP

Use liquid vegetable oils in cooking and at the table. Dipping bread in olive oil flavored with black pepper and coarse sea salt is a much better health choice than slathering it with butter. A little squeeze of liquid margarine is a better choice than pats of butter on steamed veggies.

Remember the calorie density of fat (9 calories per gram). Don't let fat dominate your food intake, but sneak good fats in. For example, when making a salad, add sliced olives instead of cheddar cheese. Toss in some sliced almonds instead of bacon with your green beans. Don't increase your total fat intake, but do change the type of fat you eat.

TIP

Use olive oil as a replacement for the saturated fat in your diet. Olive oil makes all food more flavorful, fresh-tasting, and delicious. Even better, it's a natural choice for good health. Olive oil contains no cholesterol, chemicals, or artificial additives. It's especially high in monounsaturated fat, which may reduce harmful LDL cholesterol and help maintain healthy HDL cholesterol levels when substituted for saturated fat. Check out the recipes for the healthy spreads in Chapter 13, and use them on salads, steamed veggies, fish and chicken, or that occasional bagel or cracker that's part of your carb count.

Improving Your Ratio of Good Fats to Bad Fats

Moderate, don't eliminate your fat intake. Mix up the kinds of fat you eat. Deliberately lower your saturated fat intake, but add more unsaturated fat, especially olive oil, peanut oil, canola oil, fish, olives, avocadoes, nuts, and nut oils. Eat two fish meals each week to increase your chances of getting omega-3 fatty acids in your diet.

TIP

Try to balance your intake of omega-3 and omega-6 fatty acids. Eat more fatty fish (salmon, albacore tuna, trout, herring, and mackerel), canola oil, flaxseed, and walnuts. Eat less corn, safflower, sunflower, and cottonseed oils.

Flaxseed contains high amounts of cancer fighters, as well as omega-3 fatty acids, which may help prevent heart disease. It also supplies iron, niacin, phosphorous, and vitamin E. To release the health benefits of flaxseed, the hard outer coating must be broken down. Place flaxseed in a small nonstick skillet; cook over low heat 5 minutes or until toasted, stirring constantly. Place the flaxseed in a blender; process just until chopped. Flaxseed keeps best when stored in the refrigerator. Toast and chop right before using.

Here are some other ways to improve your ratio of good fats to bad fats:

>> **Try a few almonds, Brazil nuts, cashews, macadamia, pecans, pistachios or English walnuts for a healthy snack.** But remember that 1 cup of nuts is about 800 calories, so don't eat too many!

>> **Use thin slices of avocado in place of mayonnaise.** This gives your sandwich a healthier spread.

- » **Always use the reduced-fat version of a high-fat food.** For example, try reduced-fat mayonnaise, reduced-fat salad dressing, reduced-fat Miracle Whip, and reduced-fat cheeses.

- » **Combine cheese with fruit to lower the fat percentage for the whole snack.** Doing so lowers the fat percentage of your snack rather than eating cheese alone.

- » **Avoid trans fats whenever possible.** Watch for ingredients like partially hydrogenated fat. Choose tub over stick margarine. Avoid shortening, commercially prepared breads, pastries, cookies, and french fries.

WHAT'S THE SKINNY ON NATURAL PEANUT BUTTER?

You'll recognize natural peanut butter by the oily layer that forms on the top. Don't pour this oil off. It's a monounsaturated fat and good for your heart. Also, pouring it off will leave a very thick peanut butter that not only sticks to the roof of your mouth but is impossible to spread on bread. You can handle the oil in two ways:

- Just turn the jar over until the oil seeps through to the other end. Periodically rotate the jar to keep the oil evenly dispersed in the peanut butter.

- Take a knife and carefully stir the oil back down into the peanut butter. When it's evenly mixed, store the peanut butter in the refrigerator to keep it from separating. When ready to use, take out the portion needed and soften it in the microwave for spreading.

3

Shopping and Cooking for a Low-Carb Lifestyle

Chapter 9

Navigating the Supermarket

You're headed home and you decide to run into the supermarket to pick up milk and bread; you leave 20 minutes later with four bags of groceries. But don't blame yourself. From the time you entered the store, your behavior was controlled. Supermarkets are carefully planned to see that you leave the store with more than you came in for.

Supermarket layout is an art and a science. They're creatively and scientifically designed to enhance your spending. From the music that you hear, to the aromas that you smell, you need to be aware of the environment you're entering — not only to keep your spending down, but to avoid those impulse items that are not part of your healthy eating plan.

Currently, supermarkets are undergoing exciting changes in both layout and operations. Today they're all about convenience: Picking up a healthy family meal at your local supermarket should be just as easy as picking up a less healthy fast-food meal; however, the control over your behavior when entering the store isn't any less than it was before all the updating changes. Having a firm awareness of navigating the store can help you avoid the impulse buying of less healthy items.

REMEMBER

If it goes in the grocery cart, it goes in the house and it goes in the mouth. Stop and think before you toss something into your cart. Try not to go to the supermarket hungry. When you're hungry, your resistance to temptation is lower.

Supermarket managers know you've already made the decision to spend money or you wouldn't be coming into their store. Without you realizing it, the store layout is set up to draw that money out of your pocket. The music, colors, aromas, and product arrangement are carefully designed to encourage more spending. This chapter guides you through the supermarket psychology and store layout to help you avoid that impulse buying that may deter your healthy eating plan.

Understanding Supermarket Psychology

Most shoppers don't give a second thought to where the cereal or green beans sit on the store's shelves. But, more than 50 percent of purchases are bought on impulse and supermarket managers know that shoppers' propensity to spend on impulse is highest in the supermarket. In many cases, representatives from food manufacturers work with supermarket managers to place their product lines on grocery store shelves. Depending on how well the products are arranged, they can boost profits or hurt sales.

Large supermarkets carry more than 50,000 items on their shelves with thousands of new products appearing every year. The competition for *shelf space*, or space for items to be placed on the shelves, is fierce. Products sitting on shelves too long and taking up space are quickly replaced by better-selling items. The objective is to keep the product line moving.

The layout of the supermarket is designed to keep you in the store longer than you planned because your time is critical. Every minute you spend browsing is another minute in which you're more likely to spend that extra dollar.

Even though products such as milk, bread, and meat are considered necessary commodities, you often find them at the back of the store, many times on opposite ends of the store. So, in your rush to pick up milk and bread, you'll likely travel the entire length (and maybe width) of the store.

TIP

Try out this scenario: When you enter the store, you first reach for the hand basket because you say to yourself, "It's only a couple of items. I can manage." But then you remember how heavy that gallon of milk is when you carry it in that small basket back up to the cashier at the front of the store. So, you choose the grocery cart instead. You pick up your gallon of milk and, on your way to the bread display, the wonderful aroma of baking bread gets your attention. So, you pick up the sandwich bread in the bread aisle you intended to buy and head for the bakery. Going back in front of the dairy case you notice crocks of butter. You think, "Now, that'd be good on warm bread." Picking up the butter you proceed to the bakery. Passing the meat counter, you catch a whiff of barbequed roast. You think, "Well, it's close to dinnertime, and I *am* feeling pretty hungry." That roast is fully prepared and ready to go. Placing it in your cart you head for the bakery. Slowing down for a minor traffic jam of grocery carts, you notice a bright display of canned baked beans marked "3 for $5." Picking up three cans, you head for the bakery. Arriving at the bakery, you're thinking, "Why am I here? Oh yeah, the bread."

Are you starting to get the picture? Store managers and food manufacturers got the picture a long time ago and have created ambience in grocery stores to encourage people to stay longer and longer. From the little café tables by the coffee vendor, to the familiar music they play, the longer you stay, the more you'll pay.

Knowing Supermarket Layout and Design

This sections shows you how your grocery store layout and design affects your purchases. Check out Figure 9-1 for an illustration of a typical grocery store layout.

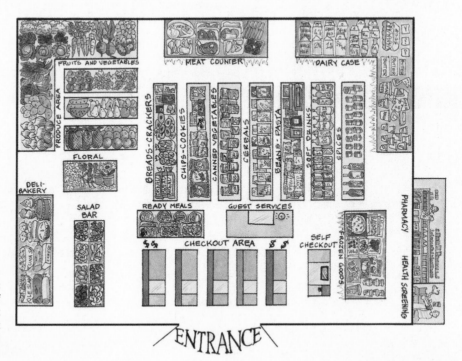

FIGURE 9-1:
The perimeter of the supermarket is your best bet for whole-food choices.

Illustration by Liz Kurtzman

Patrolling the perimeter

The most basic and nutritious foods are usually placed in areas around the perimeter of the store. That's where you find milk, bread, meat, and produce. At least one of these staple items is on every shopping list. Locating them around the edge and toward the back of the store provides more opportunity for bright-colored displays to catch your eye.

Eyeing the endcaps

Located at the end of the aisles, these eye-catching displays generally showcase items the store wants to sell quickly. These items may or may not be sale-priced.

Hitting at eye level

Costly items with the highest profit margins for the store are generally placed on shelves at shoppers' eye level. Check above or below for better deals.

Targeting your child

Cereals with cartoon characters and free toys are placed at a child's eye level. Larger bags of candy and specialty toys are at a kid's eye level as well.

Anticipating traffic jams

Some interruption of grocery-cart travel is allowed to occur in order to slow you down and cause you to browse.

Seducing you with signs

So-called "specials" may only be special to the store. When you see something labeled as a special, that doesn't guarantee the item will have a lower price.

When you see something marked with "as advertised," you may think that the item is on sale. But these signs don't necessarily translate into sale-priced or even regularly well-priced items.

Another trick to get you to buy more is advertising "3 for $5" or something similar. But if the management is playing fair, you can get the special price buying just one of the items — you don't have to pick up three.

Heading into the holidays

Supermarkets make purchasing items for holiday celebrations easy. But have you noticed how early it starts? Right after Labor Day you'll see Halloween candy in the store. How many trick-or-treaters do you see in September? The holiday is two months away! Buying candy too soon creates temptation for you, which candy makers hope will make you buy twice as much (some to eat now, some to give away later).

Luring you with free samples

Those nice workers encouraging you to sample their wares are demonstrating a highly successful selling technique. You wouldn't want to hurt their feelings by turning down their hospitality, would you? And if you're hungry when in the store, you may give in to tempting foods that end up in your cart.

Grooving to the music

Supermarket music is becoming synonymous with elevator music. The slow, lulling tempo encourages more browsing.

Steering Your Cart toward the Healthy Foods

Put the following locations on your radar screen as targets for healthy food:

>> **Perimeter:** The healthiest foods are around the perimeter of the store. This is where you'll find the most *whole foods* — foods free from processing and added sugar, salt, and fat.

>> **Dairy case:** Look for lower fat milk; low-fat and nonfat yogurt; reduced-fat cheeses; ricotta cheese; and liquid or tub margarines labeled with "no trans fatty acids" and plant butters. Some dairy alternatives may be in the dairy case, but not all dairy alternatives have to be refrigerated. You can also find dairy alternatives in the aisles; they'll need to be refrigerated after opening.

>> **Produce section:** People study years to memorize all the carotenoids, flavonoids, antioxidants, phytochemicals, and other wonderful stuff in fruits and vegetables. And face it, you're probably not that interested in the science behind it all. So, just concentrate on filling your cart with color. Get as many

colors in there as possible — red, yellow, orange, purple, blue, white, and especially green — and you'll cover all the bases. Buy fruit in season and in bags. Apples and oranges sold in bags are often cheaper than purchasing the same fruits individually.

Here are a few tips to help you select the best produce.

TIP

- Choose produce with a good color, not pale or browning.

- Select firm, not limp or soggy, produce. Hard pieces aren't yet ripe; soft pieces are too ripe. If you're making guacamole, select the mushiest avocados you can find — the riper the better.

- Avoid bruised or damaged items.

- Ask the produce manager if you can sample the food before buying. Nothing is more frustrating than getting home and discovering the grapes are sour.

REMEMBER

Supermarket salad bars offer a convenient variety of already prepared fruits and vegetables — no cutting, no mess. Also, try prepackaged salads, greens, veggies, and slaws. Containers of cut-up fruit (pineapple rings, sliced strawberries, melon balls, kiwi slices, mango, and papaya chunks) can be eaten as is or mixed into cereal or frozen yogurt. You may pay a little more, but sometimes paying for this convenience results in a healthier meal at home than a trip to a fast-food restaurant.

» **Meat counter:** Don't fear red meat, but look for the leanest cuts available. Red meat is an important source of zinc and iron. Check out those lean suggestions in Chapter 5 and on the grocery list in Appendix B.

» **Fish market:** Get acquainted with your store's fish market because fish is a heart-healthy food. The American Heart Association recommends two fish meals a week. Often the fishmonger will steam your fish for you ready to take home and eat. Or you can purchase prepared crab cakes ready to cook. Try the easy recipes located in Chapter 14.

TIP

Purchase fresh fish the same day you plan to prepare it. If you don't do that, store fresh fish sandwiched between layers of ice or in airtight plastic containers. Don't purchase fish with a "fishy" odor.

Making Good Use of New Features

New features in the supermarket are there to enhance shopper convenience, information, and pleasure. Look out for the following:

>> **Ready-made and heat-and-eat meals and dishes:** Even though most people want to cook a delicious and healthy meal for their family or for themselves every night, sometimes you just don't have the time, energy, or patience to do it. When that happens, go to the ready-meal section usually at the front of the store near the deli and salad bar and pick up an easy and delicious pre-made meal. Add a salad and a vegetable, and you're ready to go! Some may say "Why not eat out?" or "Call the pizza place?" These pre-made dinners are still healthier and cost way *less* than eating out. Not having to swing by the drive-thru will also *save you hundreds of dollars* over time.

>> **Senior shopping hours:** These special shopping hours are scheduled when the store is less crowded and when staff can give more attention and assistance to its older shoppers. Seniors or those with a disability can request help with bagging their groceries, transporting them to the car, and even loading them into the trunk. Ask at the customer service desk before you shop, and someone will be waiting to assist you. Check out the supermarket website or inquire at Guest Services for more information.

>> **Guest Services:** Sometimes referred to as Customer Service or Concierge Service, you go there to find that new product, get advice on how to cook a particular food, schedule a supermarket tour, plan catering for your special event, or ask any other question you may have.

>> **Floral arrangements:** Whether you're planning a party or even a wedding, your supermarket may be able to provide some stunning floral arrangements and much lower prices than your traditional florist. If you're simply picking up a bouquet, many floral departments will add ferns and wrap them beautifully at no extra charge.

>> **Pharmacy services:** Free health screenings such as blood pressure, blood sugar, or weight are often available in the area of the pharmacy. Also, flu, Covid, and shingles vaccinations are offered free or at a nominal fee.

>> **Medical nutrition counseling and special supermarket tours:** Many supermarkets offer shoppers a chance to meet with a registered dietitian nutritionist (RDN) to discover how to improve their diets and, ultimately, their health. Some will take shoppers on a guided store tour to introduce them to new foods they may not have tried or know how to cook.

Some of these tours may be disease specific such as diabetes, heart disease, hypertension, or weight control. A licensed RDN must legally perform individualized medical nutrition therapy. Often the supermarket can direct you to those professionals. Check out the supermarket website for more information, including how to schedule a tour.

>> **Self-checkout:** Customers hate waiting in line to pay for their purchases. Long lines can be a big deterrent, and customers often leave if they have to wait too long. That's where self-checkout can help you. In fact, many customers prefer

to pay for their purchases at the self-checkout. Doing so reduces the time spent waiting in line and minimizes contact with both staff and other shoppers. Less waiting means a better customer experience and increased customer satisfaction. Some companies are featuring apps that you activate when you enter the store and then every item you pick up and take out of the store is charged to your credit or debit card when you leave.

Focusing Only on the Healthy Foods in the Aisles

The middle aisles are where all the processed foods are (refer to Figure 9-1). The more ingredients a food has that you can't pronounce, the less it belongs in your shopping cart. But there are some good choices in the aisles if you know where to look.

Here are a few examples of healthy foods that are found in the aisles:

>> **Dried beans:** An inexpensive source of protein and fiber, dried beans and peas are a good way to spend one of your carbohydrate choices.

>> **Peanut butter:** Not all peanut butters are created equal. The healthiest choices are those that contain only peanuts and salt. Some have trace amounts (less than 1 percent) of hydrogenated vegetable oils (trans fatty acids that threaten heart health) or corn syrup. The small amount of hydrogenated oil keeps the peanut butter from separating and makes the peanut butter creamier. Read food labels carefully.

>> **Whole-grain bread:** Don't assume that breads with names like "wholegrain" are good sources of fiber. You must check the ingredient panel and look for the word *whole*. A *real* whole-grain bread will list "wholegrain wheat flour" as the first or second ingredient. Also, look for brands that contain at least 3 grams of fiber per serving.

>> **Canned fruits:** Look for fruits canned in a light syrup or in their own juice. They're great to keep in the pantry to add to a meal. Check out the recipes in Chapters 12 and 16 for ways to use canned fruit. Avoid canned fruit juice products that aren't 100-percent juice, and seek out those that have been fortified with vitamin C and calcium. Look for fruit prepackaged in individual serving containers for quick lunchbox additions.

>> **Canned vegetables:** Canned vegetables are better than no vegetables at all and in some cases may be better. Keep them in the pantry ready to add to a quick meal, salad, or soup.

Studies show that the phytochemicals known as carotenoids are better absorbed from many cooked, rather than raw, foods. *Carotenoids* are powerful antioxidants that are present in red, orange, and yellow vegetables and fruits. Lycopene, a phytochemical shown to fight cancer, becomes more available in tomato products that have been exposed to heat, such as canned or stewed tomatoes, pasta sauce, and ketchup. Carrots have higher levels of beta-carotene after cooking. Corn's antioxidant activity is increased the longer it is cooked. However, levels of folate (a B vitamin) and vitamin C can be decreased by cooking.

>> **Canned soups:** Canned soups are notorious for being high in sodium and fat. Don't assume that just because a soup claims to be low in fat that it is also low in sodium. Look for soups with less than 500 mg of sodium and less than 3 grams of fat per serving.

>> **Spaghetti sauce:** Spaghetti sauces differ in sodium content and fat content. Look for a sauce with fewer than 500 mg of sodium and 3 grams of fat per serving. Or try making your own spaghetti sauce using unseasoned canned tomato sauce and adding your own minced garlic and fresh basil. You can find brands of tomato sauce with as little as 0 grams of fat and 200 mg of sodium.

>> **Frozen foods:** Frozen dinners can be a healthy choice if you carefully select them. Look for dinners that contain about 1 cup of vegetables and about 350 to 400 calories. Plan to add a salad, a piece of fruit, or a glass of skim milk to improve the nutritional quality and to make the meal more satisfying. Many frozen dinners are high in sodium and fat so look for dinners with no more than 800 mg of sodium and no more than 30 percent of the daily value for total fat. Keep a few frozen dinners in the freezer. They're perfect for a quick dinner when time is limited or when you just don't feel like cooking.

Frozen vegetables (without sauces) are just as nutritious as fresh. Buy the large-sized bags. Take out what you need and save the rest for later. You can add bags or boxes of frozen veggies to already prepared soups, stews, and casseroles.

Deciphering Food Labels

When you're shopping, always read the labels. Get out of the habit of only looking at the fat content and look at the total carbohydrate content per serving. Determine how much is fiber and how much is sugar. Look at the ingredient list and determine the food sources of the fat, carbohydrate, and fiber. The more dietary fiber in the food the better it is.

REMEMBER

If the food you're evaluating has a high carb count and it's mainly high fructose corn syrup or table sugar, remember that 4 grams of sugar equal 1 teaspoon. Regular 12-ounce cans of soft drink contain 40 grams of carbohydrate — all sugar. That equals 10 teaspoons, or almost a quarter cup. It counts as three carbohydrate choices on your Whole Foods Weight Loss Eating Plan. That's a sobering thought.

Check out the serving sizes. All the nutrition information on the label applies to the stated serving size. Don't assume that a small box of any food or beverage is only one serving. Double-check the number of servings per container. Often a 16-ounce bottle contains 2 servings. But who only drinks half a bottle? You may be getting twice the sugar you thought.

The following sections help you better understand other aspects of the food label such as the ingredient panel and the Nutrition Facts label. These features provide valuable information that is important to identify when shopping.

Understanding the ingredient panel

Foods listed in the ingredient panel are required to be listed greatest in quantity (by weight) first and then on down the line. A breakfast cereal with sugar listed as first or second on the ingredient panel has more sugar than anything else.

WARNING

Look for the terms *hydrogenated* or *partially hydrogenated* oil on the ingredient panel. This indicates a source of trans fatty acids. Try to minimize your intake of this fat. You'll find it in many packaged goods, such as cakes, pastries, crackers, cookies, and cereals. For more on trans fats, see Chapter 8.

TIP

Fresh produce doesn't carry a nutrition label. However, the nutrition information should be available. Look for it on a flyer or poster in the produce department. Ask the produce manager if you can't find it.

Discovering the Nutrition Facts label

The Nutrition Facts label issued by the Food and Drug Administration (FDA) was updated in 2016, with the changes focused on recent scientific information, new nutrition research, and input from the public. This change was the first major update to the label in more than 20 years. The label's refreshed design and updated information simplify the shopping experience, allowing consumers to make more informed food choices that contribute to lifelong healthy eating habits.

Refer to Figure 9-2 to see the key changes to the updated Nutrition Facts label. They include the following:

>> **Servings:** The number of "Servings Per Container" and the "Serving Size" declaration have been increased and are now in larger and/or bolder type. Serving sizes have been updated to reflect what people actually eat and drink today. For example, the serving size for ice cream was previously ½ cup and now it's ⅔ cup.

>> **Calories:** "Calories" is now larger and bolder.

>> **Fats:** "Calories from Fat" has been removed because research shows the type of fat consumed is more important than the amount.

>> **Added Sugars:** "Added Sugars" in grams and as a percent Daily Value (%DV) are now required on the label. Added sugars include sugars that are either added during the processing of foods or are packaged as such (for example, a bag of table sugar); it also includes sugar from syrups and honey and sugars from concentrated fruit or vegetables juices. Scientific data shows that it's difficult to meet nutrient needs while staying within calorie limits if you consume more than 10 percent of your total daily calories from added sugars.

>> **Nutrients:** The lists of nutrients that are required or permitted on the label have been updated. Vitamin D and potassium are now required on the label because Americans don't always get the recommended amounts. Vitamins A and C are no longer required because deficiencies of these vitamins are rare today. The actual amount (in milligrams or micrograms) in addition to the %DV must be listed for vitamin D, calcium, iron, and potassium.

>> **Footnote: Percent (%) Daily Value:** The footnote at the bottom of the label has changed to better explain the meaning of %DV. The %DV helps you understand the nutrition information in the context of a total daily diet. A neat trick to use is to remember the 5 and 20 rule: If a food has 5 percent or less of a nutrient, it's considered low in that nutrient; if it has 20 percent or more, it's considered high.

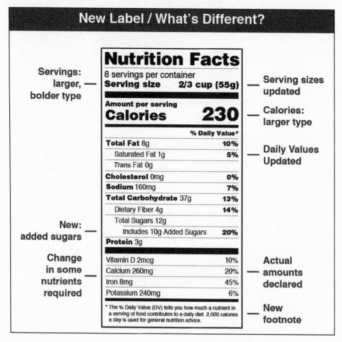

FIGURE 9-2:
The Nutrition
Facts Label.

U.S. Food and Drug Administration (FDA)

Considering labels on the Whole Foods Weight Loss Eating Plan

For the Whole Foods Weight Loss Eating Plan, you don't count the carbohydrate in fruits, vegetables, and milk. You only count the carbohydrate in the Yellow Light starchy foods. (See Chapter 6 for the full story.) Fruits, vegetables, and milk will show sugar as part of the total carbohydrate and total sugars on the food label, but this sugar is the naturally occurring simple sugar such as fructose, lactose, glucose, or galactose in the food. It isn't added sugar such as sucrose (table sugar). Added sugar will be listed separately under Total Sugars.

In the Yellow Light foods, 15 grams of total carbohydrate count as one carbohydrate choice. You may subtract the fiber from the total carbohydrate amount. For example, if one serving of a cereal contains 21 grams of total carbohydrate and 6 grams of dietary fiber, you may subtract the 6 grams of fiber from the total of 21 grams of carbohydrate. This gives you 15 grams of total carbohydrate for one serving, which equals one carb choice.

Chapter **10**

Planning Menus and Meals

Y ou're headed home from work, starting to relax, and then it hits you: What's for dinner? You picture hungry mouths meeting you at the door, and you hear your own stomach starting to rumble. Panic-time! Everyone is waiting for you, they're starving, and you don't have enough time to cook something. Then you see it, as if it were divinely placed in your view to answer your problem: golden arches gleaming in the setting sun. Your car turns as if drawn by a magnet. In no time, you've pulled into your driveway and opened the door laden with sustenance as if you're back from the hunt with the fattest beast. Cheers greet you and, for a brief moment, you are the family hero.

Sound familiar? Whatever fast-food restaurant it was that allowed you to be king or queen for a brief moment, that glory soon fades and the guilt sets in. You know you should be feeding your family healthier foods, but you just ran out of time, energy, and ideas. So, don't beat yourself up. Take some time to analyze this situation. How can this meal crisis be prevented? This chapter explains planning, shopping, and cooking in order to have healthy foods ready to go.

I have good news: Sensible lower-carb eating will make you and your family feel great and will give you the energy to enjoy busy days. But it doesn't come naturally in today's environment. It requires thoughtful planning. In this chapter, I give you all the information you need to plan low-carb meals and resist the fast-food temptation. Even though a low-carb diet isn't recommended for children, children will benefit from the reduction of refined and processed carbs and fast foods.

Planning Menus Ahead

Low-carb eating can quickly become a way of life. You'll be amazed at your heightened energy level that comes with reducing the amount and improving the quality of carbohydrate in your diet. Using complex carbs to help sustain you helps you avoid sugar highs and lows, keeping you fuller longer and keeping energy levels constant. With dedicated low-carb dieting, you'll also lose unwanted pounds. Notice I said *dedicated* dieting. One key ingredient in the recipe for low-carb dieting is planning. The better prepared you are to handle the unexpected obstacles that your busy life throws your way, the more successful you'll be and the sooner you'll achieve your desired results.

The following sections give you tips on planning and strategies to be prepared for unexpected events and special occasions. Don't be discouraged if you get off track. It takes practice for these strategies to become habits. Persevere and you and your family will enjoy the benefits of well-planned meals.

Failing to plan is planning to fail

A wise plan of food selection can be the key to many happy, healthy years. Do people like to plan their eating? No, not really. If you're like most people, you're used to eating as a natural response to hunger or tempting foods. It's a mindless activity. And no one knows that better than marketers of snacks, sodas, and fast food. They like to make your eating decisions for you. Reaching for a pre-packaged snack is always easier than creating your own healthy item when you're hungry. So plan your snacks *before* you're hungry.

Should you plan your eating? Most certainly, at least until choosing healthy foods becomes automatic. You plan other important aspects of your life. Just as you plan other important events in your life, plan your eating. Why plan? To ensure success.

Developing your food-plan strategy

If you know that you have ballet lessons, soccer practice, or Scouts on a particular night of the week, you can plan meals ahead of time rather than visit your local fast-food restaurant. If you know you'll be working late this week, make dinner ahead of time and freeze it for a healthy reheated meal. And you may consider just keeping a few things handy and ready in the freezer for those unexpected busy nights. Your strategy is as unique as your lifestyle. For more on examining your lifestyle with low-carb dieting in mind, check out Chapter 4.

TIP

Regardless of your lifestyle, these tips are helpful. Pick and choose your favorites.

>> **Go grocery shopping only once a week.** With supermarkets so handy (and many open 24 hours a day), limiting your shopping to once a week isn't always easy to do, but it certainly cuts down on impulse buying. In addition, it saves you time and will encourage you to at least roughly plan your daily menus instead of just grabbing whatever's handy.

>> **Cook in quantity.** Instead of one entree, make two. Enjoy one right away and freeze the other one to use later. Soups, spaghetti sauce, meat, and poultry dishes freeze well, so keep one of these in your freezer for when you don't feel like cooking. You can even freeze leftovers in individual serving containers. These containers are particularly handy for quick healthy frozen lunches.

>> **Prepare larger cuts of meat like a roast, whole chicken, or a turkey breast.** Doing so is a great way to provide several family meals but cook only once. Talk about tasty sandwiches and delicious lunchbox foods!

>> **Have a marathon cooking session during the weekend.** If you're chopping onions for soup, you may as well keep chopping for spaghetti sauce. And since you're cooking in volume, you can definitely justify the cleanup of time-saving equipment like food processors. Cook and freeze for the week. This not only helps control the foods you consume, but cooking for the rest of the week is a breeze — and think of the cleanup saving! What a great stress relief!

>> **Write it down!** Keep a food journal, especially keeping track of your carb choices. You can review it at the end of every day to make sure you're getting enough whole grains and legumes and not exceeding your daily carbohydrate choices. Refer to Chapter 4 for more specifics on keeping a food journal.

TIP

Work on your own food strategy and spend some time with the Whole Foods Weight Loss Eating Plan:

>> **Review the Green Light Foods in Chapter 5.** Mark the ones you really like and the ones you're willing to try. Add a new food to your grocery list every week.

>> **Check out the Yellow Light list of starchy carbs in Chapter 6.** Select the ones to use and get to know the appropriate portion sizes.

>> **Stock up on low-fat 1 percent milk instead of whole milk and 2 percent.** Chapter 8 discusses dairy and dairy alternatives in greater detail.

>> **Start replacing saturated fats with unsaturated fats.** Switch to soft tub margarine olive oil–based, yogurt-based, or vegetable oil–based (no trans fatty acids) rather than butter or stick margarine. Try the new plant butters on the market. Replace full-fat cheeses with crunchy nuts in your salads.

Linoleic acid, an omega-6 fatty acid, comprises the majority of the polyunsaturated fat eaten in the world. It's found in corn, safflower, sunflower, and cottonseed oils. Replacing these oils with omega-3 fatty acids is better for our health and weight management. Omega-3 fatty acids are found in fish, flaxseed oil, soybean oil, canola oil, nuts and seeds such as chia seeds and walnuts, and dietary supplements such as fish oil. See Chapter 8 for more information.

>> **Keep lean meats on hand for quick entrees and snacks.** A rolled-up piece of lean deli turkey is a great snack, right out of the package.

Scheduling for special occasions

Like most people, you're probably conditioned to celebrate with food. Baby showers, birthday parties, wedding receptions, and many other occasions call for special and often carb-heavy foods. If you know you have a special occasion on a particular day, compensate by adjusting your carbohydrate intake the rest of the day. That doesn't mean you should starve yourself all day because you're going to indulge in a big dinner.

Take advantage of the Green Light list in Chapter 5 and continue to eat through the day. Save your carb choices for a glass of wine or piece of cake.

Look for Green Light foods on the buffet. Veggie trays are a great place to find free foods. Be sure to watch the dips and count milk and carb choices as needed. Cocktail shrimp are definite Green Light foods. Meat and cheese trays can be a lifesaver if you're looking for a quick bite.

TIP

If you must turn your meat and cheese into a sandwich, choose the darkest, grainiest bread available. Without a food label handy, you won't be able to ensure that you have a whole-grain choice, but it's the most likely candidate. Also, choose mustard or vinegar rather than mayo.

Avoid the fried items like chicken wings or egg rolls. One egg-roll wrapper has 12 to 13 grams of carbs, and that doesn't even count the filling or dipping sauce! If they're just too tempting to avoid, make sure you count them with the appropriate carb choice.

The bottom line: Save your carb choices for the occasion, and make them count. Don't consume unwanted carbs in sugary marinades, like barbecue sauce or pre-packaged chips and dips. Go for the most unrefined, natural food choices available at your event. And make sure you count your carb choices.

REMEMBER

You have five carb choices to use every day — at least three of them should be whole-grain choices. Each carb serving is made up of around 15 grams of carbs. Check out Chapter 6 for serving sizes of your favorite foods.

Getting Organized

Any plan is only as good as its execution, and executing your plan is much easier if you're organized and ready. Here are a few easy tips that will get you ready to go in no time:

» **Arrange your pantry and freezer with foods sorted by their Whole Foods Weight Loss Eating Plan color, like Green Light on one shelf, Yellow Light on another, and so on.** This strategy makes it easy to grab ingredients that fit your needs. You can also take a quick visual inventory of what you have and don't have on grocery-shopping day.

» **Stock your pantry, refrigerator, and freezer with easy-to-fix, low-carb friendly foods, such as canned and frozen vegetables, lean meats, fish fillets, and chicken.** Look for individually quick-frozen proteins, so you can thaw only what you need. You can find large bags of these individual chicken breasts at grocery stores and warehouse stores, so you can still save money and make small portions. Also, there's little to no waste with these trimmed prepared proteins. The fish portions are usually ready to use right out of the bag — no messy bones or skin to mess with. You can find frozen shrimp in a variety of forms: cooked, raw, or with or without shells. You can find individual beef burgers and chicken burgers for easy weeknight dinners.

» **Enlist family members to help with the planning.** Make the planning process a game using your recipe cards. Spread a few low-carb–friendly recipes out, face down on the table. Take turns picking up cards to create the weekly menu. Post the menu on the fridge, bulletin board, or chalkboard — wherever everyone is likely to see it. That way, whoever is home first knows what's for dinner and can start cooking.

>> **Make friends with your microwave.** Microwave ovens are great for vegetables. They usually save time, retain nutrients, and maximize the natural flavor of vegetables. To get started, try Microwave Zucchini in Chapter 15. Or cook an entire ear of corn (husk and all) in the microwave, three minutes per ear. Remove the husk before eating, though, because no one needs that much fiber. Microwaving is also great for heating leftover vegetables. Try microwave or quick stovetop versions of dishes you usually bake.

TIP

Always pay attention to standing times in microwave recipes. Because microwave ovens can heat unevenly, these standing times give your dish a chance to even out temperature-wise. Also, know the power of your microwave because some recipes specify a certain microwave power.

>> **Use other labor-saving devices, such as a food processor, convection oven, pressure cooker, slow cooker, or indoor grill.** Any cut of meat becomes tastier when stewed in a slow cooker. Dried beans, peas, and lentils are a snap to prepare quickly with a pressure cooker. The more you use a food processor, the more you'll wonder how you ever got along without it — especially if you cook in volume. You can dice 10 pounds of onions without shedding a single tear.

Maintaining grocery lists

Keep a running shopping list on your phone so you can jot down needed items as you think of them. Post your paper list in a conspicuous place, like on the fridge, and keep a pencil handy. Invite all family members to add to the list letting them know there may be substitutions for high-calorie, high-carbohydrate foods. To get started, take a look at the form in Appendix B. It lists all the foods in the book and puts them in their appropriate categories. I've given you some extra spaces to fill in other items I've left off. Make copies of this great list and take one with you to the market — you'll always have a reminder of the best choices for your low-carb lifestyle.

Use your weekly menu to finish up your grocery list. It doesn't do much good to create a menu and advertise it for the family to see, only to find you don't have the items in the house to create your low-carb delights. Make sure that if you're going to have Jim's Sausage Soup (see Chapter 12 for details), you have Healthy Choice small link sausages on your list. An extra trip to the grocery store means more opportunity for impulse buying. Also, note any unusual quantities that you may need, so if you're making a double batch of Marilyn's Orange Pineapple Delight from Chapter 13, you'll have the necessary two 11-ounce cans of mandarin oranges.

REMEMBER

Make sure you have your grocery list with you on your weekly visit. If you like to write it, take a picture with your phone. All your hard work and planning is out the window if your list stays stuck to the fridge. Better yet, keep your list on your phone. Add to it every time you think of something you need. Even though you may be able to avoid impulse buys, you're likely to make it home without that one secret ingredient for your Aunt Bunny's beef stew that you've painstakingly converted to a new low-carb entrée. For details on converting your own recipes, see Chapter 14.

TIP

If you're a budget-conscious shopper, take time to cross-reference your grocery list with the weekly grocery sales circular from the newspaper or online. You can make a notation by each of your items regarding which store has the best deals, saving you time and money. Many supermarkets send out digital deals by email. You automatically get credit for the special when you check out.

Creating a snack list

Snacks are a necessary (and delicious!) part of healthy, low-carb dieting. Gone are the days of the nutrition advice, "Three square meals a day, and no in-between meal snacks." Instead, I recommend *preventive eating*, meaning eating healthy foods before you're hungry, to stave off hunger and eliminate the urge to overeat high-carb, prepackaged snacks.

REMEMBER

Preventive eating is eating in order *not* to eat. In other words, use your Green Light foods to strategically place snacks in your day to help control your appetite at meals. Strategic times are mid-morning, mid-afternoon, arrival at home before dinner, or at bedtime. Other critical times include before a party or restaurant meal when you know you'll be tempted by high-calorie foods. Use only your Green Light foods for this purpose. Look for suggestions in the section, "Snacking the Good-Carb Way," later in this chapter. Any recipe in this book marked with a Green Light is a great snacking choice. Check out Chapters 13 and 14 for lots of great recipes.

Be sure to include room in your weekly menu and grocery list for preplanned snacks. Here are a few suggestions for your own snack list to get you started:

>> An orange

>> A bunch of grapes

>> An 8-ounce container of low-fat yogurt

>> A can of unsweetened applesauce, diced peaches, or mixed fruit

>> A glass of skim, ½-percent, or 1-percent milk

- >> Dried apricots

- >> A handful of raisins

- >> A big green (or red) apple

- >> Raw vegetables (baby carrots, cherry tomatoes, green beans, pepper strips, radishes, celery, cucumber) with a low-fat salad dressing

- >> Sliced turkey rolled up in a lettuce leaf

- >> Boiled shrimp with zesty cocktail sauce

- >> Skim-milk mozzarella string cheese

REMEMBER

Yellow Light foods make appropriate snacks on occasion, but you must plan for them and count them in your daily carbohydrate totals. Here are a few one-carb choice examples:

- >> 3 cups of low-fat microwave popcorn

- >> 1½ ounces of barbecued soy nuts

- >> Yogurt smoothie (see Chapter 16 for my Four-Fruit Shake)

TIP

Keep a whiteboard or notepad on the fridge listing the snacks you have on hand. Kids think it's fun because it feels like a snack-bar menu, and it's handy because you don't have to hunt through the produce drawer. They can choose from fresh grapes, homemade granola, jicama chips, or sliced oranges. Just advertise the healthy choices that are your family's daily specials and reinforce good habits for the whole family. When you run out of one snack, just erase it or replace it with another.

Ensuring Breakfast Is Quick and Easy

Breakfast is a meal that is often neglected and surrounded with excuses. Like, "I don't like bacon and eggs, and cereal makes me gag in the morning!", "I'm way too rushed in the morning, so I don't have enough time to eat," "I'm really not hungry when I first wake up," or, "I'm trying to lose weight, so I'll just save those calories." None of those excuses are valid.

But analyze those excuses for a minute:

- >> **"I don't like traditional breakfast foods."** Your breakfast meal can be any combination of Green Light foods. Check out Chapter 5 for some ideas and

Chapter 11 for some easy breakfast recipes. Your breakfast can even be leftovers from dinner the night before. Breakfast is also a good place to add in Yellow Light carbs such as whole grain toast or muffin, oatmeal, or whole grain cereal (see Chapter 6). Carbs are necessary to provide energy. Be sure to add a lean protein or a low-fat dairy food with it to provide additional energy and to keep you feeling "full." Fiber-rich whole-grain foods can also add to the feeling of fullness.

>> **"My mornings are too hectic. There's just not enough time."** Plan ahead and stock the fridge with grab-and-go breakfasts. Whether you eat your breakfast in your kitchen, take it with you, or keep breakfast on hand at the office, it's faster than the drive-thru and a lot healthier. You can get a quick metabolism boost, by following a few easy tips:

- Try setting out your breakfast the night before or getting ingredients together in the refrigerator. If you want a breakfast omelet, do your prep the night before. Chop veggies, grate cheese, cook your bacon, and store it in the fridge. In the morning, you can break an egg or two and get going.

- Stock your desk with nonperishable foods, such as packages of instant oatmeal, snack packs of raisins or other dried fruit, snack packs of nuts, small cans of 100-percent fruit juice or fruit canned in light syrup, jars of dried beef, or small tubs of applesauce or beef jerky.

- Bring resealable plastic bags with premeasured portions of granola or other high-fiber cereal. Some vending machines in offices now carry both cereal and milk, and occasionally there are some whole-grain choices available. But don't count on it. Bring your own to ensure you can stay on your plan and hit your goals.

- Keep packages of cheese and crackers or peanut butter and crackers to combine with a small can of fruit.

- If you have a refrigerator at work, keep yogurt, low-fat cheese, skim milk, or fresh fruit. Be sure to count your carbs appropriately.

- Buy a bigger lunchbox. Pack your breakfast — and your lunch — the night before.

>> **"I just can't eat in the morning"** An early work schedule or just concentrating on getting ready for the day make it difficult for some people to get in the mood to eat breakfast. But inevitably, hunger appears later in the morning. Don't be tempted by the pastry cart, lunch wagon, or vending machine. Before you leave the house, try starting off with something small like cheese or peanut butter and six crackers or cottage cheese and fruit. At least drink some milk or juice before heading out. Then later in the morning, eat something more substantial like a whole-wheat muffin and a handful of grapes.

> >> **"I'm trying to lose weight, so I want to save my breakfast calories."** So
> you think skipping breakfast translates into automatic weight loss? Missing an
> entire meal would seem to eliminate a great deal of calories; however, when
> that meal is in the morning it can lead to bad habits like eating more high-
> calorie snacks and meals later on. Skipping breakfast leads to intense hunger,
> which makes it more difficult to make wise food choices. Eating breakfast
> jump-starts your metabolism and gets you started burning more calories,
> earlier in the day. Even just a quick container of low-fat or nonfat yogurt, a
> piece of fruit, or an ounce of low-fat cheese can get your calorie clock started.

Breakfast can energize you, maximize your mental potential, and keep your dietary intake on track. Start today developing your personal breakfast strategy.

Waking up fresh and healthy

Choose your main dish — whether it's cereal and milk, an egg, or a lean meat
dish. If the dish is hearty, like hot cereal for example, you may want to serve a
refreshing fruit juice with it. On the other hand, if it's less filling, a fruit combination or spiced fruit may lend an exciting contrast.

Check out a few ideas for easy breakfast menus. Flip to Chapter 11 for other breakfast recipes.

Wake-up #1

Here's an easy family breakfast to get your day started right:

>> Sparkling Fresh Fruit Cups (see Chapter 16)

>> Scrambled Eggs (check out Chapter 11)

>> Multigrain toast (counts as one carb choice)

>> Soft tub plant butter or avocado spread

>> 1 cup skim milk, coffee, or tea

Wake-up #2

The beauty of this menu is that it can all be done ahead of time — great for families that start their morning on different time schedules. If you think brie isn't the
best choice for a morning cheese, consider substituting your family's favorite, like
low-fat Monterey Jack, Colby, or cheddar. Try the following;

- » Fruit and Brie Kabobs (flip to Chapter 13)

- » Hearty Whole Wheat Muffin (see Chapter 11)

- » 1 slice broiled Canadian bacon

- » 1 cup skim milk, coffee, or tea

REMEMBER

Make sure you count your muffin as one carbohydrate choice.

Wake-up #3

Perfect on a cold morning! This is the breakfast childhood was based on. I recommend that you use quick-cooking oats for a fast and easy weekday breakfast. Instant oatmeal can be a good choice — just watch how much sugar is added. Compare the nutrition labels of several varieties and watch the fiber stay constant while the overall carb count varies. That variation has to do with the amount of refined sugar the manufacturer adds. Consider the following:

- » ¾ cup 100-percent orange juice

- » Hot instant, high fiber oatmeal

- » Raisins or other dried fruit for topping, small handful

- » 1 tablespoon soft yogurt-based tub margarine (such as Brummel and Brown)

- » Honey, brown sugar, or non-calorie sweeteners (optional)

- » 1 broiled reduced-fat sausage patty

- » 1 cup skim milk, coffee, or tea

REMEMBER

Drink only 100-percent fruit juice. Juice drinks and punch are loaded with extra sugar and calories.

Grab-and-go breakfasts

Grab-and-go breakfasts are easy breakfasts that require little to no cooking and boast very easy cleanup, like yogurt topped with granola or berries or toast topped with eggs prepared in any fashion.

Try keeping a few things on this list handy in your fridge or pantry so you can grab and go in a hurry:

- » Hard-boiled eggs or deviled eggs (see Chapter 11)

- » Small containers of 100-percent fruit juice

- » Small containers of fruit packed in light syrup

- » String cheese and whole-wheat crackers

- » Veggies and low-fat dip

- » Peanut butter and celery sticks

Here are some great grab–and–go breakfast options.

Grab-and-go breakfast #1

I like to sprinkle some of the granola into my yogurt to add a little crunch. You can portion out the granola in a resealable plastic bag the night before for extra speed:

- » 1 container of low-fat fruit-flavored yogurt

- » ½ cup Homemade Granola (see Chapter 11 for recipe)

- » 1 small can of 100-percent fruit juice

Grab-and-go breakfast #2

String cheese is great to keep on hand. It stars in this delicious breakfast suggestion:

- » 1 small can of 100-percent fruit juice

- » 1 Fiber-Friendly Muffin (see Chapter 11 for recipe)

- » 1 package of low-fat string cheese

Making Power Lunches

Lunch is the midday break for refueling, relaxing, and refreshing. Wherever you are — at home, the office, school, or a restaurant — take time to sit down and enjoy the food you're eating. Take a breather from whatever occupied the morning and restore your mental and physical energies for the afternoon's activities. Avoid heavy, high-carb meals. They will only leave you lethargic and sleepy at that after–lunch conference. The recipes in Chapter 12 can help you start. These sections give you some great power lunch options.

Noontime fuel

Use your lunchtime as a pit stop to power-up with Green Light foods and carbs low in glycemic load. For more on Green Light foods, see Chapter 5.

Because lunchtime is a time to refuel for the day, it's another good place to use one or two of your carbohydrate choices. Here are a couple of tasty power lunches to get you through your day. As always, count your carb choices appropriately and if you find yourself still a bit hungrier, choose a food from the Green Light list.

Noontime fuel #1

This lunch requires a little work ahead of time, but it's well worth the effort. Share this lunch with special friends:

>> Artichoke-Ham Bites (see Chapter 13)

>> Tasty Chicken Roll-Ups, 7 (see Chapter 13)

>> 1 cup steamy tomato soup

>> 14 stone-ground whole-wheat thin crackers

>> Frosty Fruit Cup (check out Chapter 17)

>> Tea or coffee

REMEMBER

If you eat one serving of each item on this menu, count it as a total of two carb choices. Seven roll-ups equal one carb choice and 14 crackers equal one carb choice.

Noontime fuel #2

This filling salad makes the meal! You won't believe you're dieting. If you're making it for a group, try using several different kinds of beans, like pinto, black beans, and cannellini beans:

>> South of the Border Salad (see Chapter 12)

>> Lo-Cal Salad Dressing (check out Chapter 12)

>> Blue Corn Crackers (refer to Chapter 16 for recipe)

>> Light vanilla ice cream, ½ cup with fresh strawberries

>> Tea or coffee

This salad has lots of Green Light foods, but make sure you count your carb choices. Seven crackers and the equivalent of ½ cup of beans in the salad count as one carb choice each for a total of two. If you also indulge in dessert, count your ½ cup scoop of ice cream as one dairy choice.

Noontime fuel #3

This lunch is almost too decadent to fall into the simple "fuel" category. It's a great choice for a leisurely weekend lunch when you have some extra time to linger over your cupcake and coffee:

- » Tossed green salad ready-mix
- » Lo-Cal Salad Dressing (see Chapter 12)
- » Onion-Lemon Fish with Quick Dill Sauce (refer to Chapter 14)
- » Summer Squash Medley (check out Chapter 15)
- » 1 slice Oat-Bran Bread (see Chapter 11)
- » 1 Peanutty Cupcake (refer to Chapter 16)
- » Tea or coffee

You won't even mind counting these carbohydrate choices. For each 1½-inch slice of Oat-Bran Bread, count one carb choice. One cupcake will cost you one carb choice — and you won't even ask for change.

Brown-bag bounty or working at home

Whether you're taking it with you or preparing it at home, start viewing your lunch as a positive thing. It keeps you from standing in the fast-food line (or sitting in the drive-thru), eating out of the vending machine (at astronomical prices), or going out for a heavier lunch than you planned. It also gives you complete control over portion sizes. Be creative when making that sandwich, and vary the menu by taking a salad or left-over foods from home. Choose foods ahead of time that fit your individual meal plan. Realize how much better you feel and how energized you are for the afternoon when you eat a healthy lunch.

Be wary when shopping for lunch items at the grocery store. Use processed foods and prepackaged products, like frozen entrées, sparingly. They tend to be overloaded with carbs, fat, preservatives, sugar, and sodium.

As with most rules, there are always exceptions, so look for these individually portioned foods to make brown–bagging a breeze *and* low–carb friendly:

>> Unsweetened applesauce

>> Canned fruits in their own juice

>> Cans of tomato or vegetable juice

>> Carrot and hummus packets

>> Cottage cheese

>> Fresh berries — strawberries, raspberries, blackberries, blueberries

>> Beef jerky, no sugar added

>> Sugar-free and fat-free pudding and gelatin

>> Greek yogurt

>> Low-fat or fat-free yogurt

>> Mini snacking peppers

>> Mini guacamole pack

>> Mixed nuts

>> String cheese, low-fat mozzarella

>> Tuna salad

>> Peanut butter and cheese crackers

>> Fruit-filled cereal bars

Brown-bag bounty #1

This is a basic sack lunch, but it's a welcome treat when the clock strikes 12! Try the following:

>> Baby carrots with low-fat dip

>> Ham-and-cheese sandwich made with

- 2 slices whole-wheat, 40-calorie bread

- Thin-sliced Swiss cheese

- Thin-sliced lean honey ham

- Lettuce leaves and sliced tomatoes

- Light mayonnaise and spicy mustard (optional)

>> Dill pickle

>> Apple wedges with Apple-Cheese Spread (see Chapter 13)

>> Bottle of sparkling water

TIP

Package the lettuce and sliced tomatoes separately and add them to your sandwich before eating — this keeps your bread from getting soggy and keeps your lettuce crisp!

REMEMBER

If you're using the 40-calorie-per-slice whole-wheat bread, count two slices as one carb choice. Two pieces of any other bread will likely cost you two carb choices — check your food labels to be sure. Go whole grains!

Brown-bag bounty #2

Make this chicken salad the night before to save time in the morning. Sometimes I skip the crackers and eat my chicken salad with a fork. That way, I can enjoy another carb choice, like low-fat microwave popcorn, for a midafternoon snack. That's the great thing about this plan: You choose what's right for you on any given day. Include the following:

>> 1 small bunch of seedless grapes

>> Chicken-Vegetable Salad (see Chapter 12)

>> 6 saltine crackers (1 carb choice)

>> Cherry tomatoes

>> Bottle of sparkling water

TIP

To take a salad for lunch, place the salad in a large resealable plastic bag with the dressing sealed in a separate sandwich-sized bag. Place the small bag in the larger one. At lunchtime, pour the dressing over the salad in the larger bag, seal tightly, and shake. No soggy salad, no messy cleanup, and no containers to tote back and forth between home and work. Assemble it the night before for even greater efficiency!

Putting Together Satisfying Suppers

Unless your family has the luxury of similar departing times in the morning, dinner is probably the only meal at which every member is present and accounted for. Dinner deserves careful planning to ensure the right foods, but also to ensure pleasure and enjoyment. It's worth the extra effort because healthful food and pleasant feelings create a warm family atmosphere.

Evening nourishment

This is the winding down of your day and not the time to fuel up as breakfast and lunch are. Here you should be catching up on lean meats and green veggies. Keep your carb choices low at this time of day because you won't be burning them. Concentrate on building your meals around lean protein, fruit, and veggies.

Evening nourishment #1

This is a great way to enjoy a delicious variety of foods, with fairly easy preparation. Try the following:

>> Broiled Cinnamon Peaches (check out Chapter 15)

>> Grilled boneless, skinless chicken breast with teriyaki sauce

>> ½ cup wild rice with mushrooms

>> Steamed broccoli

>> Pineapple Sundaes (see Chapter 17)

TIP

Count ½ cup wild rice as one carb choice. And count your pineapple sundae as one milk serving for the day because each sundae has ½ cup of light ice cream.

REMEMBER

You can enjoy two to three servings of milk each day. For more information about dairy foods and low-carb dieting, take a peek at Chapter 7.

Evening nourishment #2

Roll up the leftover roast in butter lettuce leaves for a quick Green Light lunch the day after. Here is another great way to end your day:

>> Tossed green salad with cherry or grape tomatoes and red onion

>> 2 tablespoons reduced-fat salad dressing

>> Betty's Busy Day Roast (refer to Chapter 14)

>> Corn Medley (see Chapter 16)

>> Green Beans with Onions (see Chapter 15)

>> Iced tea with lemon wedges

>> Thumbprint Cookies (see Chapter 17)

TIP

Count ½ cup Corn Medley as one carb choice and two Thumbprint Cookies as one carb choice.

Evening nourishment #3

This is a great way to start working seafood into your diet if you're not a fan of it. If you're running low on carbohydrate choices for the day, skip the French bread and add another Green Light food.

>> Baked Catfish Delight (refer to Chapter 14)

>> Zucchini-Tomato Bake (check out Chapter 15)

>> 1 slice sliced French bread with garlic butter

>> Peach Salad Cups (see Chapter 15)

>> Chocolate-Almond Crisps (flip to Chapter 17)

TIP

Count each ½-inch slice of bread as one carb choice and three Chocolate-Almond Crisps as one carb choice. Indulge in each as your daily food plan permits.

Company's coming

Don't think your food-related social life is over just because you're low-carb dieting. Invite people to your place so you can control the menu. Your guests will love these dishes and may not even notice that they're low in carbs.

Company's coming #1

This is a great menu if you're looking for a change from the everyday surf and turf, starting with the mushroom cocktail instead of shrimp cocktail. The most common version of Wellington is Beef Wellington, typically made with beef tenderloin stuffed with mushroom duxelles (minced mushrooms sautéed in butter and garlic) then wrapped in puff pastry or phyllo dough. This version is rich and delicious in its own right. Bon appetit! Consider the following:

>> Mushroom Cocktail (refer to Chapter 13)

>> Bertie Jo's Salmon Wellington (check out Chapter 14)

>> Savory Carrots (see Chapter 15)

>> Microwave Zucchini (refer to Chapter 15)

>> Peach-Yogurt Freeze (see Chapter 17)

>> Iced tea

TIP

Count one carb for the puff pastry in Bertie Jo's Salmon Wellington.

Company's coming #2

This menu is a tasty one for breezy summer nights. The Key Lime Pudding Cakes are tart and refreshing, and you make them in the microwave. Try these foods:

>> Avocado-Orange Salad (refer to Chapter 12)

>> Cajun Shrimp (check out Chapter 14)

>> Baked-Stuffed Potatoes (see Chapter 16)

>> Harold's Stir-Fry (flip to Chapter 14)

>> Key Lime Pudding Cakes (see Chapter 17)

>> Ice tea or lemonade

TIP

Count one serving of Key Lime Pudding Cakes as ½ carb choice. You may want to double the portion size to one carb choice, for ease of counting — and because it's just plain good! Each serving of Baked Stuffed Potatoes is one carb choice.

Snacking the Good-Carb Way

Wholesome snacks, chosen from nutritious foods, give a necessary lift. Also, when strategically placed in your day, they allow for good appetite control. Snacking can be a healthy part of your life. In fact, it's not at all unnatural to want to eat between meals. If you don't eat something about every four hours, your blood sugar dips, which can make you feel tired, cranky, and mentally sluggish.

Although many people believe that snacking causes weight gain, the reverse is often true. People who force themselves to resist snacks are more likely to be ravenous at mealtime and will probably overeat. Of course, the key to that is what you choose to snack on. Instead of pigging out on chips, approach snacking as you would any other meal. Be selective about what you eat and watch your portions of everything except for the Green Light foods. (For a list of the Green Light foods, check out Chapter 5.) Think of those between–meal bites as a chance to add vital nutrients to your diet and an opportunity to keep excess hunger in check.

TIP

Here are a few tips to get you going:

>> **Develop a taste for fresh fruit and crunchy vegetables.** Buy fruit at peak ripeness for sweetness and keep veggies sliced and seeded and ready to go.

>> **For a satisfying snack, make a smoothie with low-fat yogurt, skim milk, and a soft fruit like strawberries, cantaloupe, or banana.** Remember to count the banana as a carb choice.

>> **Buy resealable plastic bags.** The snack-size ones are great for more carb-intense choices. For easy snacking, you can make pre-portioned servings of Homemade Granola (see Chapter 11). You can make your own trail mix with peanuts, raisins, dried apricots, or whatever appeals to you and portion them out so they're easy to grab. It's great to keep the quart- or sandwich-size bags on hand for portioning out prepped Green Light veggies, like broccoli, pepper strips, and carrot sticks. These are quick snacks and easy salad fixings.

I often choose toothpicks as my snack–delivery system. Here are some of my favorite choices for snack kabobs:

>> Pineapple chunks with a cube of ham

>> Cooked chicken cubes with cucumber twists

>> Roast beef cubes with chunks of dill pickle

>> Cheese and ham cubes

>> Luncheon meat cubes with cherry tomatoes

Use Green Light foods stuffed with Green Light snacks to create edible bowls. They're pretty, filling, and you can eat the bowl when you're done! Consider the following:

>> Tomato shell stuffed with cottage cheese

>> Tomato shell stuffed with tuna salad

>> Bell pepper shell with fillers

>> Roll-ups:

- Spread a slice of lunch meat with cream cheese or pimento cheese. Sprinkle with chopped pecans. Roll and secure with toothpick.

- Stuff celery with egg salad, pimento cheese, cream cheese, or peanut butter. Chapter 13 is chock-full of recipes for snacks (and appetizers you can turn into snacks). The Orange-Pineapple Delight recipe in Chapter 12 is another great recipe for snacks.

Chapter 11

Starting the Day with Breakfast

The word breakfast comes from the phrase "break the fast." Your time of sleep isn't only a time for rest and restoration, it's also the longest time most of you go in a 24-hour period without eating. The overnight fast from dinner until you wake up depletes the glucose stores necessary to keep your brain alert. During sleep, your metabolism drops to a maintenance level. A well-balanced morning meal ignites your mind and muscles for the day.

Many folks say, "I'm just not hungry in the morning." On the Whole Foods Weight Loss Eating Plan, you don't have to eat a large breakfast, and you don't have to eat first thing in the morning. A slice of whole grain toast with an avocado spread and piece of fruit or sliced tomatoes will do the trick. It's like stoking the furnace or adding fresh wood to the dwindling campfire. Research demonstrates that skipping breakfast lowers mental performance especially in youth and young adults. You may not be hungry in the morning because you ate so much the night before. And if you can't or don't eat first thing in the morning, you may find yourself hungry a couple of hours after awakening. That's when a grab-and-go breakfast as I suggest in Chapter 10 can hit the spot.

If you're used to eating cereal and milk, toaster pastries, or cinnamon rolls for breakfast, then breakfast may be difficult for you when you switch to a low-carb diet. But breakfast is a very important meal, so you should choose your foods wisely. Proteins like the ones I list in Chapter 5 are especially important at breakfast or any time of day.

Who says breakfast has to be bacon and eggs, cereal and milk, or pancakes and syrup? Even left-over veggie or cheese pizza or a peanut butter sandwich with orange juice can make a good breakfast. Just about any food can be a breakfast food with some exceptions. Avoid breakfasts high in refined carbohydrates or sugars. Sugary cereals, doughnuts, pastries, or pancakes and syrup may provide an immediate energy boost, but later in the morning you're likely to be hungrier and sleepy.

This chapter provides some tasty and low-carb recipes to help you get your day started off right.

Creating Some Egg-cellent Choices

Eggs are a nutritional powerhouse containing a large number of nutrients. They contain minerals, proteins, vitamins, and some fat, but the fat they contain is mainly the healthy unsaturated kind. A single egg contains vitamins A, B_2 (riboflavin), B_5 (pantothenic acid), B_{12}, and the mineral, *selenium*. In fact, eggs contain a small amount of almost every mineral and vitamin that the human body requires, including iron, calcium, zinc, potassium, folate, vitamin E, choline, and manganese. Eggs also contain two antioxidants, *lutein* and *zeaxanthin*, that are extremely important for protection of the eyes.

Eggs have a higher than average cholesterol content. Fifty years ago when heart disease was shown to be related to cholesterol plague in people's arteries, the scientific community immediately came down hard on eggs. Later scientists discovered that cholesterol in the human diet has little to do with cholesterol in the arteries. The human liver manufactures cholesterol every day. If a large amount comes in through the diet, the liver makes less; if little cholesterol comes in through the diet, the liver makes more. Interestingly, more recent research shows that plague in arteries is more related to the intake of refined carbohydrates than to dietary cholesterol intake. All that to say, this low carb diet is good for your heart!

TIP

A QUICK, LOW-CARB BREAKFAST: HARD-BOILED EGGS

Hard-boiled eggs are a great high-protein, low-carb food. I hard-boil several eggs at once, usually six or so, to save time. Then they're always available to chop up into salad, make into deviled eggs, or just eat as a snack. Everyone can boil an egg, right? Well, maybe. Believe it or not, there are many ways to boil eggs.

Here's my favorite method:

1. **Place a few eggs in a small saucepan.**

2. **Cover the eggs with water.**

   Make sure there's at least a ½ inch of water over the eggs.

3. **Bring the water to a rolling boil and continue to boil for approximately 7 minutes.**

4. **Turn the water off, and allow the eggs to sit in the hot water for 10 minutes or so.**

5. **Run cool water over the eggs.**

6. **Peel and eat, or store unpeeled eggs in the fridge for up to one week.**

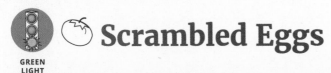

Scrambled Eggs

GREEN LIGHT

PREP TIME: 5 MIN	COOK TIME: 5 MIN	YIELD: 3 SERVINGS

INGREDIENTS

4 eggs

¼ cup low-fat milk

¼ teaspoon salt

Dash of pepper

Nonstick cooking spray

DIRECTIONS

1 In a small bowl, combine the eggs, milk, and seasonings. Heat a skillet over medium or medium–high heat.

2 Spray the heated skillet with nonstick cooking spray. Immediately, pour the eggs into a frying pan and stir from the outside edge toward the center, allowing the uncooked egg in the center to flow to the outside. Continue stirring until all the egg has cooked solid and has a creamy golden yellow appearance.

TIP: If you like super-fluffy scrambled eggs, try substituting water for the milk in this recipe. The water steams the eggs from the inside causing them to be lighter and fluffier.

PER SERVING: *Calories 107 (From Fat 61); Fat 7 g (Saturated 2 g); Cholesterol 284 mg; Sodium 288 mg; Carbohydrate 2 g (Dietary Fiber 0 g); Protein 9 g.*

SOME EXTRA FLAVOR FOR YOUR EGGS

Scrambled eggs are easy to make. You can eat them any time of day, not just breakfast. Occasionally, they need some Green Light pizzazz to keep them from being boring. Be creative and consider the following to mix them up:

- Add chopped lean ham, chopped bell peppers and onions, or chopped mushrooms. Serve with picante sauce for a spicy flair.

- Add goat cheese, blistered tomatoes, and garlic. Heat 1 tablespoon olive oil to a high heat and add a pint of grape tomatoes. Cook 2 minutes without stirring. Then stir them around and add one sliced garlic glove. Cook 2 more minutes, stirring often. Remove from the pan and set aside. Prepare the scrambled eggs in the same skillet. Stir goat cheese into the hot eggs. Top with blistered tomatoes and garnish with fresh herbs, such as thyme, basil, oregano, or parsley.

GREEN LIGHT

Zucchini Frittata

PREP TIME: 20 MIN	COOK TIME: 30 MIN	YIELD: 4 SERVINGS

INGREDIENTS

1 large onion, minced

2 cloves garlic, minced

3 tablespoons olive oil

2 tablespoons parsley

2 tablespoons Italian seasoning

1 tablespoon Maggi seasoning

1 teaspoon salt, optional

1 teaspoon pepper

10 small zucchini

8 eggs

¾ cup grated Parmesan cheese

1 tomato, peeled and chopped for garnish

DIRECTIONS

1 Preheat oven to 350 degrees.

2 Sauté onion and garlic in oil until onion is limp. Add herbs and seasonings. Slice zucchini very thin. Add to onion mixture and sauté 5 minutes.

3 Mix eggs and cheese, pour zucchini, and mix thoroughly. Pour mixture into baking dish. Bake for 30 minutes at 350 degrees or until eggs are set.

4 Garnish with chopped tomatoes.

NOTE: Maggi seasoning is a product used all over the world. You can use up to nine different formulations that differ among nations and regions. The Swiss version, which has a savory flavor, is the original flavor and the version used in this recipe. Some people claim that it tastes like soy sauce and Worcestershire sauce mixed together. You can purchase it in grocery stores, gourmet stores, and online.

PER SERVING: *Calories 307 (From Fat 193); Fat 21 g (Saturated 5 g); Cholesterol 332 mg; Sodium 1033 mg; Carbohydrate 16 g (Dietary Fiber 5 g); Protein 18 g.*

Ham & Feta Omelet

PREP TIME: 20 MIN | COOK TIME: 10 MIN | YIELD: 2 SERVINGS

INGREDIENTS

4 eggs

1 green onion chopped

1 tablespoon low-fat milk

¼ teaspoon dried basil

¼ teaspoon dried oregano

Dash garlic powder

Dash salt

Dash pepper

1 tablespoon plant butter

½ cup crumbled feta cheese

3 slices deli ham, chopped

1 plum tomato, chopped

2 teaspoons balsamic vinaigrette

DIRECTIONS

1 In a small bowl, whisk the eggs, green onion, milk, and seasonings until blended. In a large nonstick skillet, heat plant butter over medium-high heat. Pour in egg mixture. Mixture should set immediately at edge.

2 As eggs set, push cooked portions toward the center, letting uncooked eggs flow underneath. When eggs are thickened and no liquid egg remains, top 1 side with cheese and ham.

3 Fold omelet in half; cut into two portions. Slide onto plates; top with tomato. Drizzle with vinaigrette before serving.

NOTE: Refer to the color insert for a photo of the Ham & Feta Omelet recipe.

PER SERVING: *Calories 414 (From Fat 265); Fat 30 g (Saturated 14 g); Cholesterol 445 mg; Sodium 1286 mg; Carbohydrate 11 g (Dietary Fiber 3 g); Protein 27 g.*

Eggs Benedict

| PREP TIME: 10 MIN | COOK TIME: 4 MIN | YIELD: 4 SERVINGS (*1 CARB CHOICE PER SERVING) |

INGREDIENTS

2 whole English muffins*

Four 1-ounce slices lean cooked ham

1 medium tomato, cut into 4 slices

4 eggs, poached and kept warm

¼ cup plus 2 tablespoons plain low-fat yogurt

1 tablespoon lemon juice

1 teaspoon prepared mustard

DIRECTIONS

1 Slice the muffins in half and toast. Place one ham slice and one tomato slice on each muffin half. Broil 4 minutes.

2 Top each muffin half with one poached egg. Combine lemon juice and mustard; blend with a wire whip, then add to the room-temperature yogurt, blending with a wire whip. Spoon 2 tablespoons yogurt mixture over each egg and serve immediately.

NOTE: Refer to the color insert for a photo of Eggs Benedict.

PER SERVING: *Calories 181 (From Fat 54); Fat 6 g (Saturated 2 g); Cholesterol 178 mg; Sodium 512 mg; Carbohydrate 16 g (Dietary Fiber 1 g); Protein 15 g.*

MAKING POACHED EGGS

Poached eggs are essentially eggs that are boiled without their shell. They're not difficult to make, but they do take a little practice. To make a perfectly poached egg, do the following:

1. **Choose a nonstick saucepan or skillet filled with 1 inch of water; heat the water.**

2. **Add 1 teaspoon kosher salt and 2 teaspoons white vinegar; bring to a simmer over medium heat.** Meanwhile, crack 1 very fresh cold large egg into a custard cup or small ramekin. Use the handle of a spatula or spoon to quickly stir the water in one direction until it's all smoothly spinning around.

3. **Add the egg.**

   Tip: Use this whirlpool method when poaching a single serving (one or two eggs). For bigger batches, heat the water, salt, and vinegar in a 12-inch nonstick skillet and don't stir. Carefully drop the egg into the center of the whirlpool. The swirling water helps prevent the white from *feathering* or spreading out in the pan.

4. **Let the egg poach by turning off the heat and covering the pan.** Set your timer for 5 minutes. Don't peek, poke, or accost the egg in any way.

5. **Remove the egg with a slotted spoon and serve immediately.**

Using a Carb Choice for Breakfast

Because grains are a carbohydrate source, they're often off limits on many low-carb diets. However, several types of grains are high in fiber, offsetting part of the carbohydrate value. Whole grains such as whole wheat, oats, barley, and rye are healthy for your heart and provide fiber to your diet. Your Whole Foods Weight Loss Eating Plan allows you to have up to five carbohydrate choices per day, and breakfast is a good place to spend one or two carb choices.

The following recipes count as one carb choice per serving. They're made from healthy grains, are high in fiber, and are good for your heart. Enjoy one or two servings of them with your Green Light eggs, ham, cheese, or yogurt breakfast along with a variety of fruit such as watermelon, fresh orange slices, strawberries, and blueberries.

Hearty Breakfast Muffins

PREP TIME: 20 MIN	COOK TIME: 20 TO 25 MIN	YIELD: 12 SERVINGS (*1 CARBOHYDRATE CHOICE PER SERVING)

INGREDIENTS

½ cup whole-wheat flour*

½ cup all-purpose flour*

½ cup cornmeal*

2 teaspoons baking powder

⅛ teaspoon salt

½ cup chopped lean cooked ham

½ cup reduced-fat sharp cheddar cheese, cut into small cubes

1 cup skim milk

½ cup instant grits*

3 tablespoons canola oil

2 eggs, beaten

Vegetable cooking spray

DIRECTIONS

1 Preheat oven to 375 degrees. Combine the flours, cornmeal, baking powder, salt, ham, and cheese in a large bowl; make a well in the center of the mixture. Set aside.

2 Place the milk in a small saucepan; cook over low heat, stirring constantly, until the mixture reaches 120 to 130 degrees. Cool to 105 to 115 degrees. (Use a candy thermometer to check the temperature.) Combine the grits and the milk, stirring well. Combine the canola oil and eggs in a small bowl. Add the grits mixture and egg mixture to the dry ingredients, stirring just until moistened.

3 Spoon the batter into the muffin pans lined with muffin cup liners, filling each three-fourths full. Bake for 20 to 25 minutes, or until the muffins are lightly browned.

PER SERVING: *Calories 154 (From Fat 53); Fat 6 g (Saturated 1 g); Cholesterol 41 mg; Sodium 313 mg; Carbohydrate 19 g (Dietary Fiber 1 g); Protein 6 g.*

Friendly Fiber Muffins

PREP TIME: 20 MIN	COOK TIME: 15–20 MIN	YIELD: 12 SERVINGS (*1 CARBOHYDRATE CHOICE PER SERVING)

INGREDIENTS

Nonstick cooking spray

1 cup whole-wheat flour*

2 teaspoons baking powder

½ teaspoon salt

1¾ cups Kashi Good Friends Original cereal*

¾ cup skim milk

1 egg

¼ cup honey*

6-ounce jar baby food bananas*

2½-ounce jar baby food applesauce

DIRECTIONS

1 Preheat oven to 375 degrees. Spray 12-cup muffin pan with cooking spray; set aside. In a small bowl, stir together the flour, baking powder, and salt. Set aside.

2 In a large mixing bowl, combine the cereal and milk; let stand for 2 to 3 minutes. Add the egg and beat well. Stir in the honey, bananas, and applesauce. Add the flour mixture and mix only until the dry ingredients are moistened.

3 Divide the batter between the prepared muffin cups. Bake 15 to 20 minutes or until lightly brown.

TIP: If you're trying to find ways to add more fiber to your diet, here's a great place to start. Eat these muffins for breakfast or anytime you need a filling snack.

NOTE: Refer to the color insert for a photo of Friendly Fiber Muffins.

PER SERVING: Calories 97 (From Fat 8); Fat 1 g (Saturated 0 g); Cholesterol 18 mg; Sodium 189 mg; Carbohydrate 22 g (Dietary Fiber 3 g); Protein 3 g.

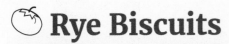 # Rye Biscuits

PREP TIME: 15 MIN	COOK TIME: 12 MIN	YIELD: 12 SERVINGS (*1 CARBOHYDRATE CHOICE PER SERVING)

INGREDIENTS

1½ cups all-purpose flour*

½ cup medium rye flour*

1 tablespoon baking powder

¼ teaspoon salt

1 teaspoon caraway seeds, crushed

3 tablespoon plant butter, softened

¾ cup low-fat buttermilk

Vegetable cooking spray

DIRECTIONS

1 Preheat oven to 450 degrees. Sift together the flours, baking powder, and salt; stir in the caraway seeds. Cut in the plant butter with a pastry blender until the mixture resembles coarse meal. Add the buttermilk, stirring just until the dry ingredients are moistened.

2 Turn the dough out onto a lightly floured surface; knead three to four times. Roll to ¾-inch thickness; cut into rounds with a 2-inch biscuit cutter. Place on a baking sheet coated with cooking spray.

3 Bake for 12 minutes or until golden brown.

TIP: You can find rye flour at any natural food store and at some larger supermarkets.

VARY IT: If you have trouble finding it, you can substitute any whole-grain flour for the rye flour.

PER SERVING: *Calories 104 (From Fat 29); Fat 3 g (Saturated 1 g); Cholesterol 1 mg; Sodium 193 mg; Carbohydrate 16 g (Dietary Fiber 1 g); Protein 3 g.*

🍅 Oat Bran Bread

PREP TIME: 45 MIN (PLUS APPROXIMATELY 1 HOUR 10 MIN RESTING TIME)	COOK TIME: 30–45 MIN	YIELD: 2 LOAVES, 16 SLICES PER LOAF (*1 CARBOHYDRATE CHOICE PER SLICE)

INGREDIENTS

2 cups whole-wheat flour*

1 package (.04 ounce) dry yeast

½ teaspoon salt

2 cups skim milk

¼ cup molasses*

2 tablespoons plant butter

½ cup plus 1 tablespoon unprocessed oat bran, uncooked, divided*

3 cups all-purpose flour*

Vegetable cooking spray

1 egg white, lightly beaten

2 teaspoons unprocessed oat bran, uncooked*

DIRECTIONS

1 Combine the whole-wheat flour, yeast, and salt in a large mixing bowl; stir well. Set aside. Combine the milk, molasses, and plant butter in a small saucepan; cook over medium heat until very warm, but not boiling (120 to 130 degrees). Remove from heat.

2 Gradually add the milk mixture to the flour mixture, beating at medium speed with an electric mixer for three minutes. Stir in the oat bran and enough all-purpose flour to make a soft dough. Turn the dough out onto a lightly floured surface; knead until smooth and elastic, about 8 to 10 minutes. Place in a bowl that has been coated with cooking spray, turning to grease the entire loaf. Cover and let rise in a warm place (about 85 degrees), free from drafts, 35 minutes or until doubled in bulk. (A laundry room with the dryer going works great for this purpose.)

3 Preheat oven to 375 degrees. Punch the dough down; divide into two portions. Cover and let the dough rest 10 minutes. Shape each portion into a loaf. Place in two 8½-x-4½-x-3-inch loaf pans that have been coated with cooking spray. Brush the loaves with egg white; sprinkle 1½ teaspoons oat bran over each loaf. Cover and let rise in a warm place, free from drafts, 30 to 60 minutes or until doubled in bulk. Bake for 30 to 45 minutes or until loaves sound hollow when tapped. Remove from the pans, and let cool on wire racks.

NOTE: The Whole Foods Weight Loss Eating Plan lets you indulge in this high fiber bread. Toast a slice with a little cheese or spread it with one of the new plant butters for a filling breakfast start to your day. Give it a shot and make those Yellow Light carbohydrate choices count.

PER SERVING: *Calories 92 (From Fat 10); Fat 1 g (Saturated 0 g); Cholesterol 0 mg; Sodium 48 mg; Carbohydrate 18 g; Dietary Fiber 2 g; Protein 3 g.*

🍅 Mildred's Cheesy Grits

PREP TIME: 5 MIN	COOK TIME: 20 MIN	YIELD: 4 SERVINGS (*1 CARBOHYDRATE CHOICE PER SERVING)

INGREDIENTS

2 cups water

½ cup quick grits, uncooked*

4 ounces processed cheese spread, cubed

Dash of garlic powder (optional)

Paprika to sprinkle

DIRECTIONS

1 Bring the water to a boil; slowly stir in the grits. Reduce the heat; simmer 3 to 4 minutes or until thick, stirring occasionally.

2 Add the cheese and garlic powder; continue cooking until the cheese is melted, about 2 to 3 minutes. Sprinkle with paprika.

PER SERVING: *Calories 179 (From Fat 66); Fat 7 g (Saturated 5 g); Cholesterol 24 mg; Sodium 394 mg; Carbohydrate 19 g (Dietary Fiber 0 g); Protein 8 g.*

Homemade Granola

| PREP TIME: 20 MIN | COOK TIME: 40 MIN | YIELD: ABOUT 9 CUPS (*1 CARBOHYDRATE CHOICE PER ½ CUP SERVING) |

INGREDIENTS

3 cups rolled oats*

½ cup honey*

½ cup canola oil

1½ cups wheat germ*

½ cup dry milk

1 cup coarsely chopped almonds

½ cup rye flakes*

½ cup sesame seeds

1 cup hulled sunflower seeds

1 cup raisins or other dried fruit

DIRECTIONS

1 Preheat the oven to 300 degrees. Toast the oats in a 13-x-9-inch pan for about 15 minutes, stirring frequently.

2 In a separate saucepan, combine the honey and the canola oil. Heat slowly. Stir in the wheat germ, dry milk, almonds, rye flakes, sesame seeds, and sunflower seeds.

3 Combine the honey mixture with the toasted oats and spread thinly in the pan, continuing to toast and to stir frequently another 15 minutes or until the ingredients are all toasted. Remove from the oven and mix in the raisins or dried fruit. Cool thoroughly and store tightly covered in the refrigerator. Eat dry or with skim milk or yogurt.

TIP: Visit your local whole-foods or natural foods market to find the ingredients for this awesome granola. You may even find that you can find the ingredients in bulk and pre-measure buying just the amount you need. That way, when you get home, you can just dump in your bulk bags and munch.

PER SERVING (½ CUP): *Calories 281 (From Fat 132); Fat 15 g (Saturated 1 g); Cholesterol 0 mg; Sodium 14 mg; Carbohydrate 32 g (Dietary Fiber 5 g); Protein 8 g.*

Chapter **12**

Perfect for Lunch: Soups and Salads

Lunch, an abbreviation for the word luncheon, is generally considered a light meal eaten in the middle of the day. Lunch is an important meal for everyone, providing energy and nutrients to keep the body and brain working efficiently through the afternoon. Keeping your lunch lower in carbs helps to avoid the sluggishness and drowsiness that follows a high carb meal.

A soup and salad are a light and healthy way to have your meals during your lunch break whether you're at home, at work or school, or on the go. Soups and salads are not only perfect for lunch, but they also can be eaten any time of day. Lunch is also a great way to incorporate more fruits and veggies in your daily diet. Many of the recipes in this chapter are made completely with Green Light foods, which makes them free on the Whole Foods Weight Loss Eating Plan. Everyone needs to eat more fruits and veggies (especially dark green and orange) and legumes, and soups and salads are a great way to eat them because they're popular soup and salad ingredients. The key is to make them ahead and have them ready to go. See Chapter 10 for hints on providing your noontime fuel.

Making Hearty Soups

Nothing spells comfort to your family more than a hearty soup, which is a flavorful and nutritious liquid food. Spend a carbohydrate choice here and add a fruity dessert from Chapter 16 to complete the meal. If possible, start your soup at least a couple hours before serving. You can also make your soups the night or day before and refrigerate overnight. Any excess fat solidifies on top for easy removal. For an added bonus, the soup thickens in the fridge making it extra delicious the next day.

The Hearty Vegetable Soup is a filling Green Light food and is great any time, especially on a cold day. The other soups use convenient canned veggies or dried beans for the carbohydrate choice. (See the nearby sidebar on canned fruits and veggies.) Have a small cup of soup with your meal or as your meal, and experience the full and satisfying effect of your soup.

INCORPORATING CANNED FRUITS AND VEGGIES

You may consider canned fruits and veggies as gross, thinking canned foods are nutritionally inferior. However, canned veggies are better than no veggies at all. The nutritional hierarchy is considered to be fresh is best, then frozen, and then canned. But you may be surprised to know that the nutritional value varies little among the three. The primary difference is sodium content. By draining and rinsing canned vegetables with water prior to cooking, you can reduce the sodium content by as much as 41 percent. Canned fruits and vegetables are budget-friendly and should be pantry staples for a quick meal or soup. Everyone should eat more fruits and vegetables for better health, and canned fruits and veggies can help.

GREEN LIGHT

Hearty Vegetable Soup

| PREP TIME: 15 MIN | COOK TIME: 40 MIN | YIELD: NINE 1½-CUPS |

INGREDIENTS

16-ounce can tomato juice

14.5-ounce can fat-free chicken broth

Two 28-ounce cans diced tomatoes, not drained

6 medium carrots, sliced

1 medium onion, sliced

2 cups frozen sliced okra

2 cups frozen sliced green beans

3 tablespoons Worcestershire sauce

2 teaspoons Mrs. Dash Table Blend

DIRECTIONS

1 Mix the juice, broth, and canned tomatoes in a 3-quart saucepan.

2 Simmer the carrots and onions for 10 minutes before adding the frozen vegetables.

3 Stir in the seasonings.

4 Cook over medium–high heat for 10 minutes. Reduce the heat and simmer for 30 minutes until vegetables are tender.

5 Store in the refrigerator for up to one week or freeze to enjoy any time.

VARY IT! To make a hearty meal, add leftover chicken. Try other vegetable combinations like tomatoes, okra, and squash; or cabbage, bell pepper, and mushroom. Anything on the Green Light list is fair game.

PER SERVING: *Calories 95 (From Fat 0); Fat 0g (Saturated 0g); Cholesterol 0mg; Sodium 580mg; Carbohydrate 22g (Dietary Fiber 6g); Protein 4g.*

Jim's Sausage Soup

| PREP TIME: 10 MIN | COOK TIME: 45 MIN | YIELD: 8 (*1 CARB CHOICE PER SERVING) |

INGREDIENTS

Vegetable cooking spray

16-ounce package Healthy Choice small link sausages, cut-in pieces

1 medium to large onion, quartered

Two 14.5-ounce cans sliced potatoes, drained*

Two 10-ounce cans diced tomatoes and green chilies

14.5-ounce can stewed Mexican-style tomatoes

16-ounce can tomato juice

Two 4-ounce cans mushroom stems and pieces, drained

16 ounces water, if needed

DIRECTIONS

1 Spray the bottom of a 4-quart saucepan with cooking spray. Brown the sausages and onion.

2 Add all the other ingredients to the saucepan. Simmer for 30 minutes.

NOTE: This soup is a breeze to prepare. You can easily make a hearty weeknight meal in under an hour. Of course, the longer it simmers, the better the flavor — but either way this soup's a winner!

VARY IT: To lower the sodium in this soup: Drain and rinse the sliced potatoes and use low sodium or "No Salt Added" tomatoes and tomato juice.

PER SERVING: *Calories 160 (From Fat 15); Fat 2g (Saturated 1g); Cholesterol 20mg; Sodium 1,426mg; Carbohydrate 26g (Dietary Fiber 3g); Protein 9g.*

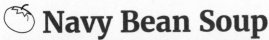 Navy Bean Soup

PREP TIME: 30 MIN PLUS OVERNIGHT	COOK TIME: APPROXIMATELY 2 HRS	YIELD: 6 (*1 CARB CHOICE PER SERVING)

INGREDIENTS

1½ cups dried navy beans*

Vegetable cooking spray

1 medium onion, chopped

½ cup chopped carrots

½ cup chopped celery

4 cups water

1 tablespoons plus 1 teaspoon chicken-flavored bouillon granules

⅛ teaspoon pepper

1 bay leaf

DIRECTIONS

1 Sort and wash the beans; place them in a large bowl. Cover with water 2 inches above the beans; soak overnight. Drain and rinse the beans, and set aside.

2 Coat a large Dutch oven with cooking spray. Place over medium heat until hot. Add the onion, carrots, and celery. Sauté until the vegetables are crisp-tender.

3 Add the reserved beans to the vegetable mixture. Stir in the water and the remaining ingredients. Bring to a boil. Cover; reduce heat, and simmer 1 hour.

4 Remove and discard the bay leaf. Pour half of the mixture into an electric blender or food processor; process until smooth. Return to the Dutch oven; stir well. Cook over low heat until thoroughly heated.

TIP: A stick mixer is a handy tool for this recipe. You can find them at many discount stores that sell small kitchen appliances. You'll save the time on pouring soup back and forth from the blender and have less cleanup.

PER SERVING: *Calories 185 (From Fat 8); Fat 1g (Saturated 0g); Cholesterol 1mg; Sodium 635mg; Carbohydrate 35g (Dietary Fiber 8g); Protein 11g.*

Beefy Chili

PREP TIME: 10 MIN	COOK TIME: 30 MIN	YIELD: 4 SERVINGS (*1 CARB CHOICE PER SERVING)

INGREDIENTS

1 pound lean ground beef

½ cup chopped onion

1 tablespoon chili powder

2 tablespoons ground cumin

1 tablespoon taco seasoning

1 teaspoon salt

One 16-ounce can crushed tomatoes, undrained

One 15-ounce can kidney beans, undrained*

3 cups water

DIRECTIONS

1 Brown ground meat and onion over medium heat in a nonstick skillet; drain. Add chili powder, cumin, taco seasoning, and salt to meat mixture. Stir until evenly mixed.

2 Combine tomato and beans in a saucepan. Add water,

3 Add meat mixture to saucepan. Bring to a boil; reduce heat, and simmer uncovered, 30 to 40 minutes.

TIP: For extra flavor, prepare recipe ahead of time. Refrigerate overnight, allowing flavors to blend and intensify. Reheat before serving.

PER SERVING: Calories 406 (From Fat 165); Fat 18g (Saturated 7g); Cholesterol 102mg; Sodium 1394mg; Carbohydrate 23g (Dietary Fiber 7g); Protein 37g.

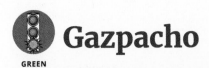

Gazpacho

GREEN LIGHT

PREP TIME: 20 MIN (PLUS 8 HRS CHILLING TIME)	COOK TIME: NONE	YIELD: 6 CUPS

INGREDIENTS

3 medium tomatoes, peeled, seeded, and diced

3 cups tomato juice

¼ cup diced onion

¼ cup diced celery

1 medium green pepper, seeded and diced

¼ cup sliced green onions

1 medium cucumber, peeled and chopped

3 cloves garlic, minced

2 tablespoons chopped fresh parsley

1 teaspoon chopped fresh cilantro

3 tablespoons red wine vinegar

Dash of hot sauce

⅛ teaspoon freshly ground pepper

DIRECTIONS

1 Combine all ingredients in a large non-metallic bowl. Stir well.

2 Cover and chill at least 8 hours or overnight.

3 Stir well and ladle into soup bowls. Garnish with additional ground pepper and chopped fresh parsley or cilantro, if desired. Store in refrigerator for four or five days.

TIP: Make sure you leave plenty of time for the flavors of this soup to meld or come together. The longer the soup sits, the more flavorful it becomes.

NOTE: This chilled soup is a staple of the Spanish diet, and it can be part of your low-carb eating plan as well. The best thing about this soup is that you don't ever have to cook it, you can make it ahead of time, and you can eat as much as you want. It's made from Green Light, free foods.

PER SERVING (1 CUP): *Calories 61 (From Fat 3); Fat 0g (Saturated 0g); Cholesterol 0mg; Sodium 445mg; Carbohydrate 13g (Dietary Fiber 3g); Protein 3g.*

Tossing Together Healthy Salads and Easy Dressings

Eating salads is a super-convenient way to work in a few servings of the fruits and veggies in the Green Light category of foods. You can make a green salad at home in 5 minutes, armed with a bag of prewashed salad greens, a few carrots or other veggies, and a bottle of light salad dressing. Salads are cool, crunchy, and fun to eat (lots of textures, colors, and flavors), and most people enjoy eating salads — even kids! You can customize them to include the fruits and vegetables that appeal to you the most, and whichever ones you have on hand. Add your favorite protein such as tuna, chicken, ham, and cheese, and you have a satisfying meal.

Eating a little good fat (like monounsaturated fat found in olive oil, avocado, and nuts) with your vegetables helps your body absorb protective *phytochemicals* (bio-active compounds found in plants), like lycopene from tomatoes and lutein from dark green vegetables. A study from Ohio State University measured how well phytochemicals were absorbed by the body after people ate a salad of lettuce, carrot, and spinach, with or without 2½ tablespoons of avocado. The avocado-eaters absorbed eight times more alpha-carotene and more than 13 times more beta-carotene (both of which are thought to help protect against cancer and heart disease) than the group eating salads without avocado. See Chapter 8 for more on healthy fats.

Following are some tasty and healthy salad recipes you can toss together for lunch or a light dinner.

South-of-the-Border Salad

PREP TIME: 20 MIN	COOK TIME: 5 TO 10 MIN	YIELD: 4 SERVINGS (*1 CARB CHOICE PER SERVING)

INGREDIENTS

1 pound extra-lean ground beef

1 small onion, chopped

2 tablespoons canola oil

3 cloves garlic, minced

2 teaspoons chili powder

½ teaspoon ground cumin

1 head of lettuce

2 small tomatoes, chopped

1 avocado, peeled and diced

4-ounce can sliced ripe olives, drained

16-ounce can pinto beans, drained*

2 cups grated reduced-fat sharp cheddar cheese

DIRECTIONS

1 Brown the meat and onion in the oil until the onion is translucent. Drain off the excess liquid. Stir in the garlic, chili powder, and cumin. Continue to cook 5 to 10 minutes. Set aside and let cool.

2 Tear up the leaves of lettuce. Add the tomato, avocado, olives, beans, cheese, and the meat mixture. Toss gently to mix.

TIP: Try this great salad with different types of beans, like black beans, kidney beans, or garbanzo beans — whatever you have handy and in your pantry for a quick weeknight meal. Serve it with your favorite salad dressing and Blue Corn Crackers (see Chapter 16).

VARY IT: If you leave the beans out of this salad, it turns it into a Green Light food.

NOTE: Refer to the color insert for a photo of this salad.

PER SERVING: *Calories 509 (From Fat 316); Fat 35g (Saturated 13g); Cholesterol 71mg; Sodium 696mg; Carbohydrate 14g (Dietary Fiber 7g); Protein 35g.*

Green Wonder Salad

PREP TIME: 15 MIN	COOK TIME: 0 MIN PLUS REFRIGERATION TIME	YIELD: 8 CUPS

INGREDIENTS

One 14.5-ounce can French-style green beans

One 14.5-ounce can small English peas

One 15-ounce can fancy Chinese vegetables w/o meat

One 8-ounce can water chestnuts, sliced

1½ cups celery, sliced very thin

3 medium sweet onions, thinly sliced

⅓ cup apple cider vinegar

1 tablespoon plus 2 teaspoons Truvia Spoonable

1 teaspoon salt

Pepper or Greek seasoning to taste

DIRECTIONS

1 Drain all vegetables and then mix in a large bowl.

2 Mix vinegar, sweetener, and seasoning and pour over vegetables.

3 Cover and refrigerate for several hours or overnight. Keeps well for several days refrigerated.

NOTE: This salad is a popular dish to take to a potluck dinner. It's easy to prepare and offers a sweet and sour flavor and a crunchy texture. It's a nice contrast to other foods.

PER SERVING (6 SERVINGS): *Calories 83 (From Fat 3); Fat 0g (Saturated 0g); Cholesterol 0mg; Sodium 551mg; Carbohydrate 17g (Dietary Fiber 5g); Protein 4g.*

**GREEN
LIGHT**

Avocado-Orange Salad

| PREP TIME: 15 MIN | COOK TIME: NONE | YIELD: 4 SERVINGS |

INGREDIENTS

3 tablespoons orange juice

1½ tablespoons olive oil

1 tablespoon lemon juice

Sugar substitute equivalent to 1½ teaspoons sugar

1 teaspoon Dijon mustard

½ teaspoon salt

½ teaspoon pepper

10-ounce bag mixed salad greens

1 ripe avocado, peeled, seeded, and diced

11-ounce can mandarin oranges, drained

3 green onions, thinly sliced

DIRECTIONS

1 Combine the orange juice, olive oil, lemon juice, sugar substitute, mustard, salt, and pepper together in a medium bowl. Whisk in to blend and make the dressing.

2 Combine the salad greens, avocado, mandarin oranges, and onions in a large bowl. Toss gently with the dressing to coat.

PER SERVING: *Calories 161 (From Fat 105); Fat 12g (Saturated 2g); Cholesterol 0mg; Sodium 345mg; Carbohydrate 15g (Dietary Fiber 6g); Protein 3g.*

GREEN LIGHT

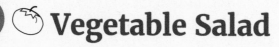 # Vegetable Salad

PREP TIME: 10 MIN	COOK TIME: NONE	YIELD: 5 SERVINGS

INGREDIENTS

5 cups Romaine lettuce, torn in pieces

1 pint cherry tomatoes, sweet grape size, cut in half

2¼-ounce can sliced black olives

14-ounce can artichoke hearts, drained well, cut in quarters

4 ounces sliced mushrooms

1 small bell pepper, chopped

¼ cup low-fat Italian dressing

4 ounces feta cheese crumbles

DIRECTIONS

1 Toss together all the ingredients except for the feta cheese.

2 Sprinkle with the cheese.

VARY IT! Try different combinations of veggies and cheeses. Or add 1 cup cooked, diced, skinless chicken meat.

TIP: To reduce the sodium, use a lite feta.

PER SERVING: Calories 149 (From Fat 70); Fat 8g (Saturated 4g); Cholesterol 20mg; Sodium 755mg; Carbohydrate 14g (Dietary Fiber 5g); Protein 8g.

Chicken–Vegetable Salad

GREEN LIGHT

PREP TIME: 10 MIN PLUS 2 HRS TO CHILL	COOK TIME: NONE	YIELD: 4 SERVINGS

INGREDIENTS

2 tablespoons lemon juice

¼ cup reduced-fat mayo

1 tablespoon minced parsley or parsley flakes

¼ teaspoon salt

3 cups cooked chicken, cubed

1 cup thinly sliced celery

½ cup frozen green peas, thawed

5-ounce can (½ cup) sliced mushrooms, drained

Paprika (optional)

Pimento (optional)

DIRECTIONS

1 In a medium mixing bowl, combine lemon juice, mayo, parsley, and salt. Add the chicken and the celery. Mix well.

2 Gently fold in the peas and mushrooms. Chill before serving. Garnish with pimento or paprika, if desired.

NOTE: The small amount of green peas per serving is negligible for your carb count.

TIP: The chicken in this recipe is delicious by itself or can be used on salads, in soups, or in other recipes. Paired with fresh fruits and veggies, it makes a great kid-friendly meal. And there are no hidden sugars or marinades that you find in the precooked, grilled chicken in the freezer section of your grocery store.

PER SERVING: *Calories 238 (From Fat 91); Fat 10g (Saturated 2g); Cholesterol 83mg; Sodium 485mg; Carbohydrate 8g (Dietary Fiber 2g); Protein 28g.*

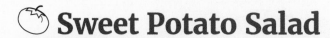 Sweet Potato Salad

PREP TIME: 10 MIN	COOK TIME: 6 TO 7 MIN PLUS 2 MIN STANDING TIME	YIELD: 4 SERVINGS (*1 CARB CHOICE PER SERVING)

INGREDIENTS

¾ pound sweet potatoes, peeled and cubed*

3 tablespoons water

1 tablespoon vegetable oil

1 tablespoon lemon juice

Sugar substitute to equal ½ teaspoon sugar

Curly lettuce leaves

DIRECTIONS

1 Place the sweet potatoes and water in a 1-quart casserole dish. Cover and microwave on high for 6 to 7 minutes, stirring after 3 minutes. Let stand 2 minutes in the microwave. Drain the potatoes well, and set aside.

2 Combine the vegetable oil, lemon juice, and sugar substitute; pour over the reserved potatoes. Toss gently to coat. Serve at room temperature on curly lettuce leaves.

NOTE: Sweet potatoes are a nutrition powerhouse with their excellent source of beta-carotene, vitamin C, and potassium; they're also a decent source of many other vitamins and minerals. Sweet potatoes rank low in glycemic load. One-half cup counts as a carb choice.

NOTE: This is a great side salad. Choose a cup of soup from the section, "Making Hearty Soups," earlier in this chapter.

PER SERVING: *Calories 104 (From Fat 33); Fat 4g (Saturated 0g); Cholesterol 0mg; Sodium 9mg; Carbohydrate 17g (Dietary Fiber 1g); Protein 1g.*

Lo-Cal Salad Dressing

GREEN
LIGHT

PREP TIME: 5 MIN	COOK TIME: NONE	YIELD: 12 OUNCES

INGREDIENTS

6 ounces white vinegar

6 ounces water

1 heaping teaspoon garlic salt

Sugar substitute to equal
½ teaspoon sugar

DIRECTIONS

1 Combine all the ingredients in a dressing bottle. Shake vigorously. Store in the refrigerator, shaking well before each use.

TIP: Add a tablespoon of a healthy monounsaturated olive, avocado, or peanut oil if desired.

PER SERVING (1 TABLESPOON): *Calories 0 (From Fat 0); Fat 0g (Saturated 0g); Cholesterol 0mg; Sodium 76mg; Carbohydrate 0g (Dietary Fiber 0g); Protein 0g.*

GREEN LIGHT

Honey–Lime Dressing

| PREP TIME: 5 MIN | COOK TIME: NONE | YIELD: 1 CUP |

INGREDIENTS

⅔ cup honey

⅓ cup lime juice

DIRECTIONS

1 Combine the honey and lime juice in a clean glass bottle. Shake vigorously to mix.

TIP: Keep this delicious dressing in the refrigerator to pour over fresh fruit any time.

PER SERVING (1 TABLESPOON): *Calories 45 (From Fat 0); Fat 0g (Saturated 0g); Cholesterol 0mg; Sodium 1mg; Carbohydrate 12g (Dietary Fiber 0g); Protein 0g.*

Chapter **13**

Fixing Low-Carb Finger Food: Appetizers and Snacks

Appetizers are great to add to a meal. Traditionally, appetizers are finger foods usually served before a meal with their main function being to increase your hunger and prepare you for the main course to come. But appetizers are much more versatile than that. Just as you can increase your hunger for the meal with light appetizers, you can also use them to satisfy your need for a meal. So, eat your appetizers strategically; the sky is your limit with the wide variety in appetizers. The only requirement is that you keep everything small enough to be picked up with your fingers and eaten with little mess.

TIP

You can combine two to three appetizers in this chapter to make a meal for lunch or dinner. Try the Spicy Meatballs, Fruit and Brie Kabobs, and the Bell Pepper Nachos for a healthy meal and explosion of flavors and textures. You can also make several appetizers at a time and use them as snacks throughout the day. That means spotting those Green Light foods — fruit, veggies, and lean protein — to add to your snack list.

Perhaps the simplest appetizer/snack is an arrangement of fresh fruits or vegetables. Choose a variety of items that are complementary in color and then cut them in attractive shapes. For example, you can serve a platter of thinly sliced cucumbers, chunks of red bell pepper, and baby carrots. For a fruit tray, consider serving red and green grapes as well as chunks of mango with toothpicks. Health-conscious guests will be grateful for a tasty selection of fresh fare.

Starting with Some Tasty Low-Carb Appetizers

Appetizers are often the bane of healthy eating. Making frequent appearances on cocktail-party buffets, appetizers are often rich in fat or combined with an oil or butter base to buffer the impact of alcohol on the system. If guests fill up on these fat-laden goodies, they have no room to enjoy the main courses.

The following easy appetizer recipes are light and healthy. They work for you and not against you in your quest for good health. Appetizers and snacks made from fruits and veggies can add up to an adequate amount of fiber before the main course is ever served.

REMEMBER

You don't always have to eat appetizers right before a meal. If you do, you can easily make them ahead of time and eat them as a mid-afternoon or bedtime snack, or as something to grab when you have the munchies, guilt-free. Eat the Green Light ones freely.

GREEN LIGHT

Marinated Mushrooms

PREP TIME: 10 MIN (PLUS 24 HRS STANDING TIME)	COOK TIME: NONE	YIELD: 2 CUPS

INGREDIENTS

1 pound small white button-type mushrooms, cleaned

⅓ cup bottled vinaigrette dressing

2 tablespoons chopped fresh parsley

¼ teaspoon crushed red pepper

DIRECTIONS

1 Combine all ingredients in a nonmetallic bowl.

2 Marinate at least 1 hour, preferably overnight in the refrigerator.

3 Spear onto toothpicks and arrange on a platter.

NOTE: These mushrooms are great as a party appetizer, speared on colorful toothpicks. But they're so delicious you can serve them as the main ingredient in a hearty salad. They're complete in their own dressing.

PER SERVING (¼ CUP): *Calories 35 (From Fat 17); Fat 2g (Saturated 0g); Cholesterol 0mg; Sodium 85mg; Carbohydrate 4g (Dietary Fiber 1g); Protein 2g.*

SAVE TIME WITH MARINATED MUSHROOMS

If you're in a time crunch and need the mushrooms to marinate fast, you can try these quick marinating tips:

- **Quarter the mushrooms.** You create more surface area on the porous mushrooms to quickly soak up the marinade. The chunky quarters should be big enough for your guests to spear.

- **Steam the mushrooms briefly in the microwave.** Place the mushrooms in a microwave-safe bowl. Cover with plastic wrap. Cut a few vent holes in the plastic, and then microwave on high for 2 minutes. Allow the mushrooms to stand in the microwave for 3 minutes, before preparing as directed in the recipe.

GREEN LIGHT

Crunchy Stuffed Mushrooms

PREP TIME: 20 MIN	COOK TIME: 4 MIN	YIELD: 12 APPETIZERS

INGREDIENTS

12 large fresh mushrooms

2 tablespoons chopped onions

2 tablespoons plant butter

½ cup pecans, chopped

½ cup fine breadcrumbs

1 teaspoon lemon juice

½ teaspoon salt

DIRECTIONS

1 Wash mushrooms gently in cold water. Remove stems and chop. Sauté onion in butter.

2 Combine onion, chopped mushrooms stems, pecans, breadcrumbs, lemon juice, and salt. Mix well.

3 Mound mushrooms caps with stuffing.

4 Broil for 4 minutes, about 4 inches from heat, or microwave on 100 percent power for 2 to 3 minutes until cooked throughout.

PER SERVING (3 MUSHROOMS): Calories 150 (From Fat 90); Fat 10g (Saturated 4g); Cholesterol 15mg; Sodium 437mg; Carbohydrate 13g (Dietary Fiber 2g); Protein 5g.

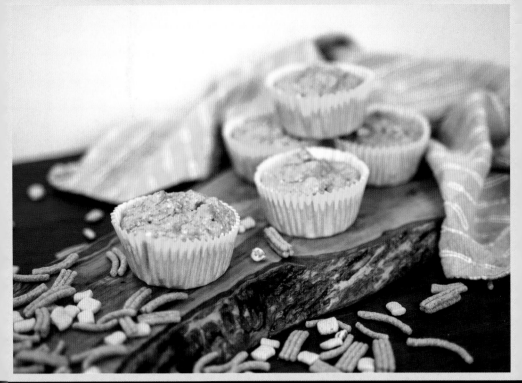

The Friendly Fiber Muffins in Chapter 11 are great for a tasty breakfast or lunch.

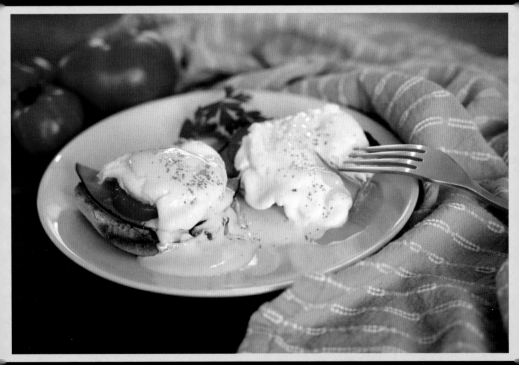

The Eggs Benedict in Chapter 11 are a perfectly delicious breakfast tradition.

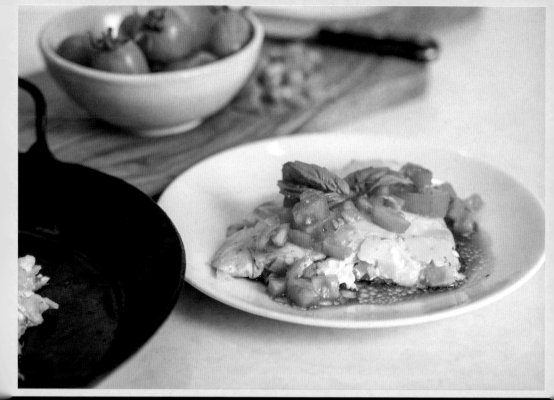

Start your day off with the hearty Ham and Feta Omelet in Chapter 11.

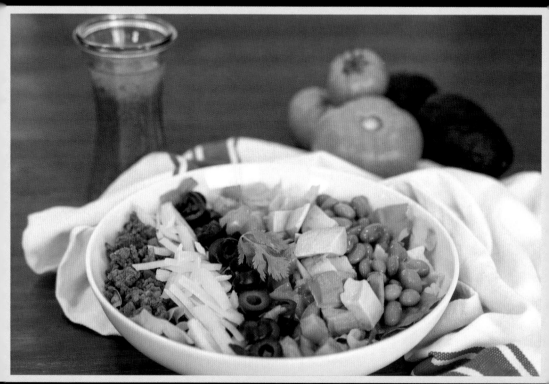

You can serve the South-of-the-Border Salad in Chapter 12 any time anywhere for a filling

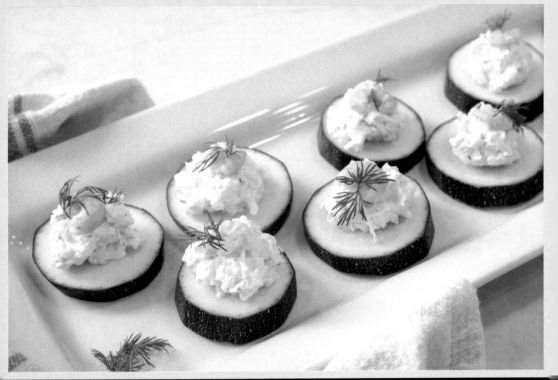

The Zucchini-Shrimp Canapés in Chapter 13 are an elegant appetizer to feel a little pampered.

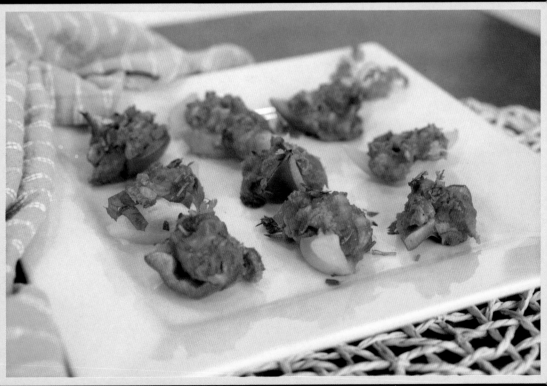

The Bell Pepper Nachos in Chapter 13 are perfect for low-carb eating before the big game.

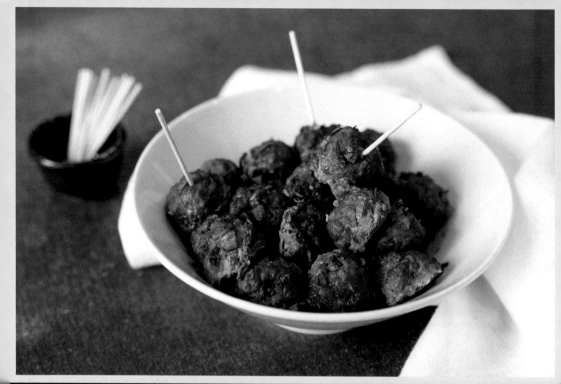

Serve the Spicy Meatballs in Chapter 13 as a tasty appetizer at your next party or family gathering.

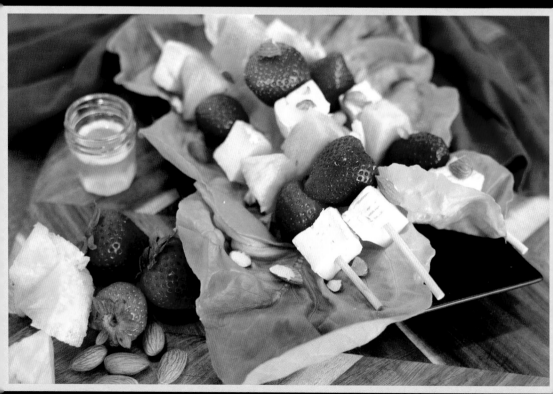

The Fruit and Brie Kabobs (refer to Chapter 13) are tasty and irresistible.

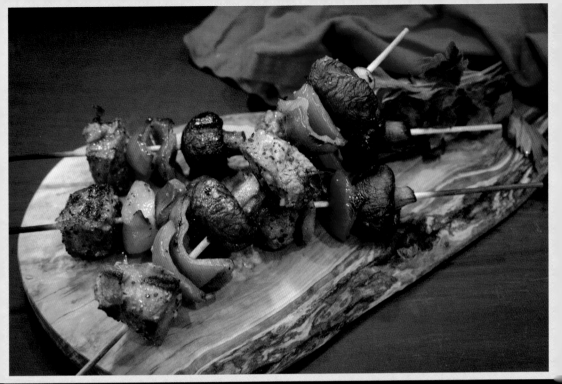

The Spicy Beef and Mushroom Brochettes (refer to Chapter 14) can serve as an impressive entree or as a featured appetizer.

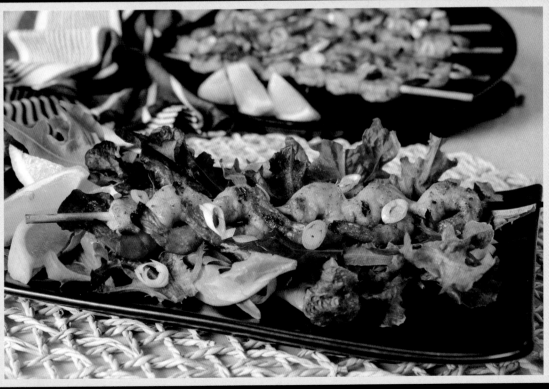

You can eat the Cajun Shrimp in Chapter 14 as an entree or as a salad topper.

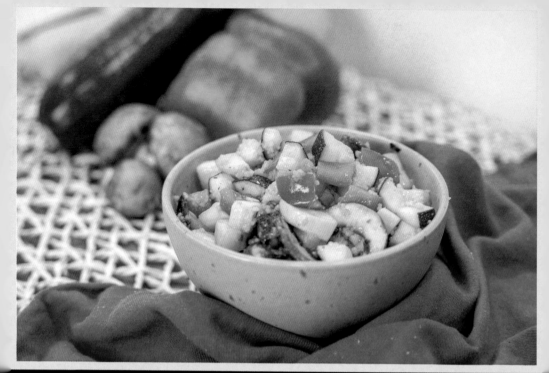

The Vegetable Couscous in Chapter 14 can boost the nutrients in any meal.

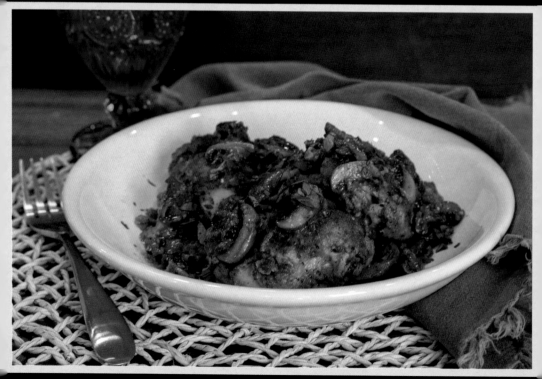

The Wine-Braised Chicken with Mushrooms in Chapter 14 will please your dinner guests.

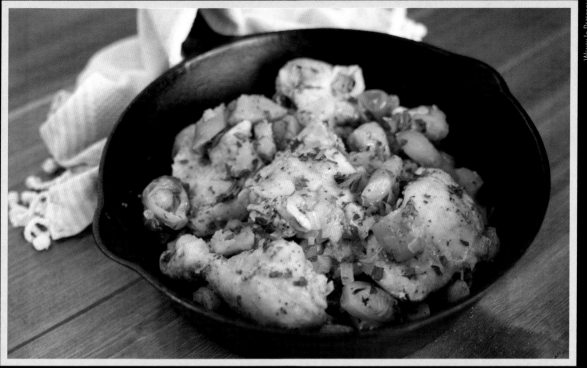

The Baked Chicken with Winter Vegetables in Chapter 14 is a welcome meal on a cold wintry night.

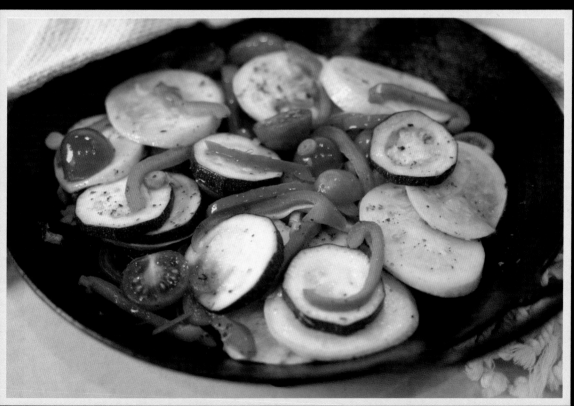

The Summer Squash Medley in Chapter 15 is a year-round flavorful and nutritious side dish for any meal.

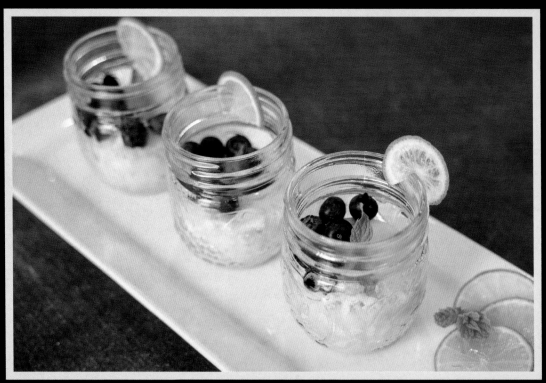

The Key Lime Pudding Cakes in Chapter 16) are always a tasty and tart treat.

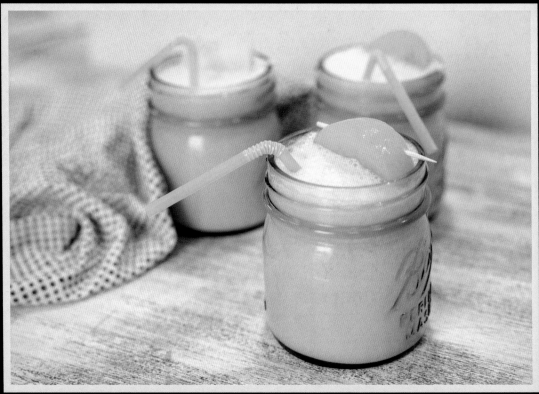

You can enjoy the Pineapple-Peach Smoothie in Chapter 16 for breakfast or as a refreshing treat.

Fruit and Brie Kabobs

| PREP TIME: 20 MIN | COOK TIME: NONE | YIELD: 30 APPETIZERS |

INGREDIENTS

One 3-pound cored, fresh pineapple (or pineapple chunks, canned in own juice)

8 ounces round brie cheese, cut into ¾-inch cubes

4 cups fresh strawberries

Leaf lettuce

2 tablespoons honey

1 tablespoon lemon juice

1 tablespoon plus 1½ teaspoons chopped almonds, toasted

DIRECTIONS

1 Cut the pineapple into 1-inch pieces or drain the canned pineapple chunks.

2 Thread the cheese cubes, pineapple, and strawberries onto 30 6-inch bamboo skewers.

3 Line a serving platter with the leaf lettuce. Arrange the kabobs over the lettuce.

4 Combine the honey and lemon juice; drizzle over the fruit kabobs. Sprinkle with the almonds.

TIP: Check with the produce manager at your supermarket to see if they can core a fresh pineapple for you. They usually have a handy machine that peels and cores this tasty fruit in one easy step, saving you some prep time.

VARY IT: If you aren't a fan of brie cheese try cubes of mozzarella, white cheddar, or pepper jack.

NOTE: Refer to the color insert for a photo of this recipe.

PER SERVING (PER KABOB): *Calories 50 (From Fat 22); Fat 3g (Saturated 1g); Cholesterol 8mg; Sodium 48mg; Carbohydrate 6g (Dietary Fiber 1g); Protein 2g.*

Zucchini-Shrimp Canapés

PREP TIME: 20 MIN (PLUS 4 HRS CHILLING TIME)	COOK TIME: NONE	YIELD: 2 DOZEN

INGREDIENTS

4 ounces (½ of an 8-ounce package) Neufchatel cheese, softened

½ cup reduced-calorie mayonnaise

¼ cup yellow or white onion, minced

¼ teaspoon dried dill

2 large zucchini, cut crosswise into 24 ⅛-inch-thick slices

4½-ounce can tiny shrimp, rinsed and drained

Fresh dill sprigs (optional)

DIRECTIONS

1 Combine the cheese, mayo, onion, and dill in a small bowl; mix well. Cover and chill thoroughly, at least 4 hours.

2 Arrange the zucchini slices on a serving platter. Top each slice with 1 teaspoon of the chilled mixture. Top each canapé with 1 shrimp.

3 Garnish with dill sprigs, if desired.

TIP: Using zucchini slices in place of the bread rounds or crackers found in traditional canapés makes this elegant appetizer a Green Light food.

VARY IT! Toss the shrimp in a little lemon juice and pepper for a zesty variation.

NOTE: Refer to the color insert for a photo of Zucchini-Shrimp Canapés.

PER SERVING: *Calories 40 (From Fat 26); Fat 3g (Saturated 1g); Cholesterol 15mg; Sodium 69mg; Carbohydrate 2g (Dietary Fiber 0g); Protein 2g.*

Bell-Pepper Nachos

PREP TIME: 30 MIN	COOK TIME: 8 TO 10 MIN	YIELD: 8 SERVINGS (*1 CARBOHYDRATE CHOICE)

INGREDIENTS

Nonstick vegetable cooking spray

1 medium green bell pepper

1 medium yellow or red bell pepper

2 Roma tomatoes, seeded and chopped

¼ cup finely chopped onion

2 teaspoons chili powder

16-ounce can fat-free refried beans*

½ cup shredded reduced-fat Monterey Jack cheese

2 tablespoons chopped fresh cilantro

¼ teaspoon hot pepper sauce

½ cup shredded reduced-fat sharp cheddar cheese

DIRECTIONS

1 Preheat oven to 400 degrees. Spray large nonstick baking sheet with nonstick cooking spray; set aside.

2 Cut bell peppers in half; seed. Cut peppers into 2-x-1½-inch strips; cut strips into bite-sized triangles. Set aside.

3 Spray nonstick skillet with nonstick cooking spray. Add tomatoes, onion, and chili powder. Cook over medium heat 3 minutes or until onion is tender, stirring occasionally. Remove from the heat. Stir in refried beans, Monterey Jack cheese, cilantro, and pepper sauce.

4 Assemble the nachos. Top each pepper triangle with approximately 2 tablespoons of the bean mixture; sprinkle with cheddar cheese. Place the nachos on prepared baking sheets; cover with plastic wrap. Refrigerate up to 8 hours before serving. When ready to serve, remove the plastic wrap. Bake for 8 to 10 minutes, or until the cheese melts and the bean mixture is warmed through.

VARY IT! Mix it up a little and try different colored sweet peppers. Create a nacho rainbow: Add orange and purple sweet peppers.

NOTE: Refer to the color insert for a photo of Bell-Pepper Nachos.

PER SERVING (4 PIECES): *Calories 101 (From Fat 29); Fat 3g (Saturated 2g); Cholesterol 10mg; Sodium 292mg; Carbohydrate 12g (Dietary Fiber 4g); Protein 7g.*

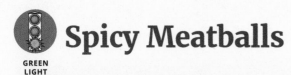

Spicy Meatballs

GREEN LIGHT

PREP TIME: 10 MIN	COOK TIME: 12 TO 15 MIN	YIELD: 60 MEATBALLS

INGREDIENTS

1 pound extra-lean ground beef

1 tablespoon sugar or sugar-substitute equivalent

¼ teaspoon ground cloves

¼ teaspoon cinnamon

1 teaspoon salt

½ cup chopped raisins

4-ounce can diced green chilies

1 egg, beaten

1 tablespoon dry sherry

DIRECTIONS

1 Preheat oven to 500 degrees.

2 Combine all ingredients. Shape into tiny balls. Arrange balls on ungreased, rimmed baking sheet.

3 Bake for 12 to 15 minutes, turning occasionally. Serve with wooden toothpicks.

TIP: A rimmed baking sheet helps you keep control of these tiny, round, tasty treats. As you pull out the tray to turn them, you'll see them roll around the cookie sheet a bit and will quickly appreciate the edge that saves them from the fiery depths of your oven. Also, consider lining your baking sheet with foil to avoid messy cleanup later.

NOTE: Refer to the color insert for a photo of Spicy Meatballs.

PER SERVING (PER MEATBALL): *Calories 17 (From Fat 5); Fat 1g (Saturated 0g); Cholesterol 5mg; Sodium 7mg; Carbohydrate 2g (Dietary Fiber 0g); Protein 1g.*

Artichoke-Ham Bites

PREP TIME: 10 MIN (PLUS MARINATING TIME)	COOK TIME: 10 MIN	YIELD: 24 BITES

INGREDIENTS

14-ounce can artichoke hearts

½ cup low-calorie Italian salad dressing

⅛ teaspoon garlic powder

6 slices boiled ham

DIRECTIONS

1 Preheat oven to 300 degrees.

2 Drain artichoke hearts; cut in half. Combine the dressing and garlic powder; add the artichokes. Marinate several hours, or overnight; drain.

3 Cut the ham into 1-x-4-inch strips. Wrap one strip around each artichoke-heart half. Secure with a wooden toothpick.

PER SERVING: *Calories 19 (From Fat 11); Fat 1g (Saturated 0g); Cholesterol 2mg; Sodium 126mg; Carbohydrate 2g (Dietary Fiber 0g); Protein 1g.*

Mushroom Cocktail

PREP TIME: 10 MIN (PLUS CHILLING TIME)	COOK TIME: NONE	YIELD: 6 SERVINGS

INGREDIENTS

⅓ cup ketchup

1 tablespoon vinegar

¼ teaspoon prepared horseradish

Lettuce leaves

1½ cups lettuce, shredded

12 fresh medium mushrooms, sliced

DIRECTIONS

1 In a small bowl, blend the ketchup, vinegar, and horseradish. Chill for at least 1 hour. Line six sherbet cups with lettuce leaves; layer with shredded lettuce.

2 Arrange about ¼ cup sliced mushrooms atop each. Chill at least 30 minutes. Just before serving, drizzle each with 1 tablespoon of the ketchup mixture.

PER SERVING: *Calories 25 (From Fat 2); Fat 0g (Saturated 0g); Cholesterol 0mg; Sodium 164mg; Carbohydrate 6g (Dietary Fiber 1g); Protein 1g.*

Tasty Chicken Roll-Ups

PREP TIME: 10 MIN (PLUS 2 HOURS CHILLING TIME)	COOK TIME: NONE	YIELD: 35 ROLL-UPS (*1 CARBOHYDRATE CHOICE PER SERVING)

INGREDIENTS

¼ cup light cream cheese, softened

3 tablespoons canned chopped green chiles

2 teaspoons tomato sauce

½ teaspoon chili powder

Five 7-inch flour tortillas*

Two 2½-ounce packages very thinly sliced chicken

2 tablespoons chopped ripe olives

DIRECTIONS

1 Beat cream cheese in a bowl at medium speed with an electric mixer until smooth. Add chiles, tomato sauce, and chili powder; stir well. Spread over tortillas.

2 Top with chicken and olives. Roll up the tortillas jellyroll fashion, as shown in Figure 13-1. Cover with plastic wrap; chill 2 hours. Cut into 1-inch pieces.

TIP: Keep the uncut roll-ups in the fridge for a quick snack. These also make a delicious quick lunch for kids.

PER SERVING (7 ROLL-UPS): *Calories 171 (From Fat 46); Fat 5g (Saturated 2g); Cholesterol 33mg; Sodium 173mg; Carbohydrate 17g (Dietary Fiber 1g); Protein 14g.*

ROLLING UP A TORTILLA FOR ROLL-UPS

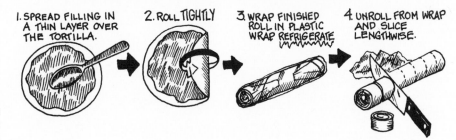

1. SPREAD FILLING IN A THIN LAYER OVER THE TORTILLA.

2. ROLL TIGHTLY

3. WRAP FINISHED ROLL IN PLASTIC WRAP REFRIGERATE

4. UNROLL FROM WRAP AND SLICE LENGTHWISE.

FIGURE 13-1: Rolling up tortillas jellyroll-style.

Illustration by Liz Kurtzman

GREEN LIGHT

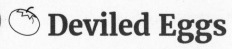 Deviled Eggs

PREP TIME: AT LEAST ONE HR CHILLING TIME	COOK TIME: NONE	YIELD: 4 SERVINGS

INGREDIENTS

4 hard-cooked eggs, halved

2 teaspoons lite mayo

1 teaspoon vinegar

½ teaspoon dry mustard

¼ teaspoon salt

Dash of onion powder

Dash of pepper

Paprika

DIRECTIONS

1 Remove egg yolks from the egg whites and mash. Set egg white halves aside.

2 Combine yolks, mayonnaise, vinegar, dry mustard, salt, onion powder, and pepper, stirring well.

3 Pipe or spoon yolk mixture into egg white halves. Sprinkle with paprika.

PER SERVING: *Calories 80 (From Fat 50); Fat 6g (Saturated 2g); Cholesterol 187mg; Sodium 238mg; Carbohydrate 1g (Dietary Fiber 0g); Protein 6g.*

Feeling the Snack Itch? Feed It with These Low-Carb Snacks

Snacks can be an important part of your eating plan. Just be sure you're eating snacks and not treats. A snack is a light meal containing two food groups like the snacks in the next paragraph. Snacks satisfy your hunger until mealtime. A treat is a cookie, candy bar, chips, cake, or other refined carb that temporarily tastes good, but does nothing to satisfy your hunger and often increases it. Always choose Green Light foods for your snacks and carefully plan them in your day. The following recipes are a great place to start.

REMEMBER

Raw fruits and veggies make great snacks and satisfy your appetite on their own. However, I've found that the protein foods taste better with a fruit or veggie partner. Here are some examples:

>> String cheese and seedless grapes

>> Chicken salad with light mayonnaise and Granny Smith apples

>> Lettuce-wrapped Chihuahua cheese and salsa

>> Boiled shrimp and zingy tomato cocktail sauce

>> Prosciutto and melon

Here are some of my favorite choices for snack kabobs:

>> Pineapple chunks with a cube of ham

>> Cooked chicken cubes with cucumber twists

>> Roast beef cubes with chunks of dill pickle

>> Cheese and ham cubes

>> Luncheon meat cubes with cherry tomatoes

Use Green Light foods stuffed with Green Light snacks to create edible bowls. They're pretty and filling, and you can eat the bowl when you're done:

» Tomato shell stuffed with cottage cheese

» Tomato shell stuffed with tuna salad

» Bell pepper shells stuffed with fillers

» Roll-ups:

- A slice of lunch meat with cream cheese or pimento cheese

- Celery with egg salad, pimento cheese, or peanut butter

**GREEN
LIGHT**

🍅 **Jicama Chips**

PREP TIME: 10 MIN	COOK TIME: NONE	YIELD: 32 CHIPS

INGREDIENTS

1 jicama, peeled and cut into
¼-inch slices

DIRECTIONS

1 Cut jicama slices with assorted 1–inch cookie cutters. Store in an airtight container in the refrigerator.

NOTE: Jicama (see Figure 13-2) is a root vegetable that resembles a cross between a turnip and a potato. It has a fresh, slightly sweet flavor and a crisp texture similar to an apple or water chestnut. It's delicious raw or cooked.

VARY IT! If you'd like a bit more flavor, try sprinkling these chips with lime juice and a touch of chili powder.

PER SERVING (8 CHIPS): *Calories 40 (From Fat 0); Fat 0g (Saturated 0g); Cholesterol 0mg; Sodium 4mg; Carbohydrate 9g (Dietary Fiber 5g); Protein 1g.*

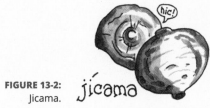

FIGURE 13-2:
Jicama.

Illustration by Liz Kurtzman

Sharon's Zesty Cottage Cheese

PREP TIME: 10 MIN	COOK TIME: NONE	YIELD: 6 SERVINGS

INGREDIENTS

24-ounce container cottage cheese

2 Roma tomatoes, seeded and diced

6 medium green onions, thinly sliced

1 medium cucumber, peeled, seeded, and diced

1 teaspoon seasoning salt

DIRECTIONS

1 In a small mixing bowl, combine the cottage cheese, tomatoes, onion, cucumber, and seasoning salt; mix well.

2 Arrange ½ cup cottage cheese on the lettuce leaves for individual salads, if desired.

TIP: Feel free to substitute whatever veggies you have on hand for a quick snack with no shopping. Any blend of spices that you like works well.

PER SERVING: *Calories 130 (From Fat 48); Fat 5g (Saturated 3g); Cholesterol 17mg; Sodium 617mg; Carbohydrate 6g (Dietary Fiber 1g); Protein 15g.*

GREEN LIGHT

🍅 Apple Treats

PREP TIME: 10 MIN	COOK TIME: NONE	YIELD: 24 SLICES

INGREDIENTS

2 tablespoons chopped dates

1 ounce Neufchatel cheese, softened

1 tablespoon peanut butter

½ teaspoon grated orange rind

4 medium Red Delicious apples, cored

DIRECTIONS

1 Combine the dates, cheese, peanut butter, and orange rind, stirring well.

2 Stuff 1 tablespoon of the mixture into the cavity of each apple. Cut each stuffed apple into 6 slices. Serve immediately.

PER SLICE: *Calories 23 (From Fat 6); Fat 1g (Saturated 0g); Cholesterol 1mg; Sodium 8mg; Carbohydrate 4g; (Dietary Fiber 1g); Protein 0g.*

GREEN LIGHT

Pimiento Cheese–Apple Wedges

PREP TIME: 10 MIN	COOK TIME: NONE	YIELD: 24 PIECES (6 SERVINGS)

INGREDIENTS

2 tablespoons shredded reduced-fat sharp cheddar cheese

1 tablespoon chopped pecans, toasted

1 tablespoon diced pimiento

2 ounces Neufchatel cheese, softened

2 drops hot sauce

4 medium Red Delicious apples, cored

DIRECTIONS

1 Combine the cheddar cheese, pecans, pimiento, Neufchatel cheese, and hot sauce in a small bowl; spoon evenly into the cavity of each apple.

2 Cut each apple into 6 wedges or slice crosswise into 6 slices. Serve immediately.

PER PIECE: *Calories 24 (From Fat 9); Fat 1g (Saturated 1g); Cholesterol 2mg; Sodium 10mg; Carbohydrate 4g (Dietary Fiber 1g); Protein 1g.*

220   PART 3 Shopping and Cooking for a Low-Carb Lifestyle

GREEN LIGHT

 # Marilyn's Orange-Pineapple Delight

PREP TIME: 10 MIN	COOK TIME: NONE	YIELD: 8 SERVINGS

INGREDIENTS

1 large package of sugar-free orange gelatin

24-ounce container cottage cheese

11-ounce can mandarin oranges, drained well

14.5-ounce can pineapple tidbits in pineapple juice, drained well

½ cup Cool Whip

DIRECTIONS

1 Mix the gelatin powder with the cottage cheese until dissolved.

2 Stir in the drained fruits.

3 Add just enough Cool Whip to smooth out the texture. Store in the refrigerator for up to one week.

VARY IT! Make up your own combination of cottage cheese, sugar-free gelatin, and fruit.

PER SERVING: *Calories 139 (From Fat 42); Fat 5g (Saturated 3g); Cholesterol 13mg; Sodium 411mg; Carbohydrate 11g (Dietary Fiber 1g); Protein 12g.*

Blue Corn Crackers

PREP TIME: 10 MIN	COOK TIME: 8 TO 10 MIN	YIELD: 5 DOZEN (*1 CARBOHYDRATE CHOICE PER SERVING)

INGREDIENTS

¾ cup plus 2 teaspoons blue cornmeal*

½ cup all-purpose flour*

¼ teaspoon salt

⅓ cup plant butter

¼ cup skim milk

DIRECTIONS

1 Preheat the oven to 375 degrees. Combine ¾ cup of the blue cornmeal, the flour, and the salt in a medium bowl. Cut in the softened margarine with a pastry blender until the mixture resembles coarse meal. Sprinkle the skim milk over the cornmeal mixture, stirring just until the dry ingredients are moistened.

2 Turn the dough out onto a lightly floured surface; knead five to six times. Roll the dough to ⅛-inch thickness on a lightly floured surface; cut into rounds with a 2-inch biscuit cutter.

3 Place the rounds on an ungreased baking sheet. Sprinkle evenly with the remaining 2 teaspoons of cornmeal. Bake for 8 to 10 minutes or until lightly browned.

4 Remove from the baking sheet immediately, and cool on wire racks. Store in an airtight container.

VARY IT! Brush the crackers lightly with water and sprinkle on Mrs. Dash Table Blend instead of cornmeal before baking. It's delicious and doesn't add any sodium, fat, or sugar.

NOTE: These crunchy crackers are a great accompaniment to the South-of-the-Border Salad in Chapter 12. They're a great alternative to the store-bought hydrogenated variety. They add crunch without the guilt.

PER SERVING (7 CRACKERS): *Calories 139 (From Fat 66); Fat 7g (Saturated 2g); Cholesterol 0mg; Sodium 155mg; Carbohydrate 16g (Dietary Fiber 1g); Protein 2g.*

Whipping Up Low-Carb Spreads and Salsas for Snacking

Check out these recipes for healthy spreads and use them on salads, steamed veggies, fish, and chicken, or as a snack on that occasional bagel or cracker that's part of your carb count. Olive oil makes them smooth and flavorful. They can be refrigerated for three or four days or frozen. Prepare them in advance for parties, special occasions, or use them as a dip for those raw veggie and fruit snack trays.

The following salsa recipes make a great snack because they're loaded with healthy fruits and vegetables. You can also use them as a dip for other pieces of food or incorporate the salsa into meals as a condiment or topping to add more flavor.

TIP

Spread a thin slice of cucumber, zucchini, or yellow squash with the Mushroom and Sun-Dried Tomato Spread, and top with a spoonful of the Avocado Salsa. Or, spend a carb choice of (seven reduced-fat round crackers), and spread with Herb-Parmesan Spread or top with a spoonful of Mango Salsa.

CHOLESTEROL-REDUCING SPREADS

If you glance at the butter/margarine section in the dairy case at your local supermarket, you'll view a wide selection of plant butters and margarines. All these products are designed to lower cholesterol and improve health. Take Control, Benecol, and Benecol Lights are brand names of margarines that have been designed to lower cholesterol.

Some of these products are made from plant sterol esters from canola or soybean oil. This food ingredient can help reduce LDL cholesterol by blocking the absorption of cholesterol from the digestive tract. However, you need to eat two to three servings per day to reap the cholesterol lowering benefits. For people with high cholesterol, these products can complement the effectiveness of their cholesterol-lowering medication The newer category of plant butters make it clear to consumers there is absolutely no animal produce in their products. Although margarines are made up of vegetable fats, some include milk products. One of the main differences between plant-based alternatives and butter and margarine are the social and environmental values that come with the former. These vegan spreads are based on various ingredients, including nut oils and avocado oils.

Yogurt–Olive Oil Spread or Base

PREP TIME: 15 MIN (PLUS 24 HRS STANDING TIME)	COOK TIME: NONE	YIELD: 12 OUNCES OR ABOUT 1½ CUPS

INGREDIENTS

32-ounce container nonfat plain yogurt

3 tablespoons olive oil

½ teaspoon salt (optional)

DIRECTIONS

1 Line a medium–size strainer with a coffee filter or a double layer of cheese cloth hanging over the rim. Suspend over a bowl to catch the whey (watery, liquid drippings that form). Spoon the yogurt into the prepared strainer and let stand, covered, for 24 hours in the refrigerator. It should yield about 20 ounces (1½ cups) drained yogurt. Reserve the whey for another use or discard it.

2 Place the drained yogurt in a mixing bowl. Slowly drizzle in the olive oil while stirring constantly until all the oil is incorporated. Add salt, if desired. Serve as is, or proceed with your recipe of choice. Store in the refrigerator for up to 1 week.

NOTE: You can use this recipe as a spread or salad dressing; as a topping for steamed vegetables, grilled chicken, fish, or lamb; as a marinade for chicken, fish, or lamb; or as a dip for raw vegetables or fruit. Use the remaining liquid in soups, stews, sauces, and so on.

PER SERVING (1 TABLESPOON): *Calories 32 (From Fat 15); Fat 2g (Saturated 0g); Cholesterol 1mg; Sodium 23mg; Carbohydrate 3g (Dietary Fiber 0g); Protein 2g.*

GREEN LIGHT

Herb-Parmesan Spread

PREP TIME: 15 MIN (PLUS 1 HR STANDING TIME)	COOK TIME: NONE	YIELD: ABOUT 3 CUPS

INGREDIENTS

Yogurt–Olive Oil Spread or Base (see previous recipe)

¾ cup finely chopped green onion, white and green parts

½ cup grated Parmesan cheese

¼ teaspoon ground pepper

⅓ cup chopped flat-leaf parsley

DIRECTIONS

1 Place the Yogurt–Olive Oil Spread or Base in a mixing bowl. Add the other ingredients, mix well, and let stand for 1 hour, allowing the flavors to marry.

2 Serve as a spread on allowed crackers or melba toast, as a dip for raw vegetables, or as a topping for steamed vegetables.

PER SERVING (1 TABLESPOON): *Calories 20 (From Fat 10); Fat 1g (Saturated 0g); Cholesterol 1mg; Sodium 27mg; Carbohydrate 2g (Dietary Fiber 0g); Protein 1g.*

🍅 **Mushroom and Sun-Dried Tomato Spread**

PREP TIME: 15 MIN (PLUS 1 HR STANDING TIME)	COOK TIME: NONE	YIELD: 1 CUP

INGREDIENTS

2 cups chopped or sliced white button mushrooms

¼ cup chopped onion

4 tablespoons olive oil, divided

1 tablespoon chopped parsley

½ teaspoon fresh thyme leaves or ¼ teaspoon dried thyme

¼ teaspoon salt, or to taste

Coarsely ground pepper to taste

1 tablespoon rinsed and drained, finely diced, oil packed sun-dried tomatoes

DIRECTIONS

1 In a skillet, combine the mushrooms, onion, and 1 tablespoon of the olive oil; cook until golden and until most of the liquid has evaporated; add the parsley, thyme, salt, and pepper.

2 In a food processor, puree the mushroom mixture. With the motor running, gradually add the remaining 3 tablespoons of olive oil through the feed tube. Transfer to a small bowl, and stir in the sun-dried tomatoes. Serve the spread on veggies or fruit slices, or on allowed crackers or melba rounds.

PER SERVING (1 TABLESPOON): *Calories 34 (From Fat 31); Fat 4g (Saturated 1g); Cholesterol 0mg; Sodium 38mg; Carbohydrate 1g (Dietary Fiber 0g); Protein 0g.*

GREEN LIGHT

Apple–Cheese Spread

PREP TIME: 10 MIN (PLUS 4 HOURS CHILLING TIME)	COOK TIME: NONE	YIELD: 1⅓ CUPS

INGREDIENTS

½ cup low-fat cottage cheese

4 ounces (½ of an 8-ounce package) Neufchatel cheese, softened

½ cup finely shredded reduced-fat cheddar cheese

1 tablespoon brandy, optional

½ cup shredded apple

1 tablespoon finely chopped almonds, toasted

DIRECTIONS

1 Place the cottage cheese and Neufchatel cheese in a blender; process until smooth. Spoon into a small bowl. Add the remaining ingredients (except the almonds) to the cottage cheese and stir well. Top with the chopped almonds.

2 Cover and chill thoroughly, at least 4 hours.

NOTE: Serve with apple or pear wedges, veggies slices, or melba toast rounds. (Just remember that melba toast rounds count as a carbohydrate — 9 rounds equals 1 carb choice.)

VARY IT: Try different varieties of apples, like Fuji, Braeburn, and Granny Smith, for delicious variations.

PER SERVING (1 TABLESPOON): *Calories 25 (From Fat 15); Fat 2g (Saturated 1g); Cholesterol 5mg; Sodium 32mg; Carbohydrate 1g (Dietary Fiber 0g); Protein 2g.*

Mango Salsa

PREP TIME: 5 MIN | **COOK TIME: 0 MIN** | **YIELD: 6 SERVINGS**

INGREDIENTS

1 mango, peeled and diced

½ cup peeled, diced cucumber

1 tablespoon finely chopped jalapeno

⅓ diced red onion

1 tablespoon lime juice

⅓ cup roughly chopped cilantro leaves

Salt and pepper

DIRECTIONS

1 Combine the mango, cucumber, red onion, lime juice, and cilantro leaves, and mix well.

2 Salt and pepper to taste.

PER SERVING: *Calories 38 (From Fat 0); Fat 0g (Saturated 0g); Cholesterol 0mg; Sodium 1mg; Carbohydrate 9g (Dietary Fiber 1g); Protein 1g.*

GREEN LIGHT

🍅 Avocado Salsa

INGREDIENTS

1 ripe avocado, peeled, seeded and diced into quarters

2 tablespoons finely diced red onion

½ cup quartered grape tomatoes

1 jalapeno, seeded and finely diced

2 tablespoons lime juice

2 tablespoons chopped cilantro

½ teaspoons ground cumin

Kosher salt, to taste

Pepper, to taste

DIRECTIONS

1 Combine all ingredients in a bowl and mix together gently.

2 Refrigerate.

PER SERVING: *Calories 36 (From Fat 30); Fat 3g (Saturated 1g); Cholesterol 0mg; Sodium 13mg; Carbohydrate 2g (Dietary Fiber 1g); Protein 0g.*

Chapter 14

Making Some Main Dish Mainstays

The heart and soul of any meal is the all-important entree. With its accompanying vegetables and side dishes, this main dish is the focal point of a healthy low-carb meal. These entree recipes are easy to prepare and focus on a lean protein accompanied by fruits and vegetables. Planning ahead and having ingredients ready overcomes the temptation to call pizza delivery or grab fast food.

Low-carb entree dishes are easy to make on the Whole Foods Weight Loss Eating Plan. Just let Green Light foods be the focus of your meals. When planning your meals, make sure each meal has a lean meat, fish, or poultry, at least one serving of the free veggies, and at least one serving of the free fruits if desired.

REMEMBER

You aren't held to a specific amount. For instance, you can choose to eat grilled chicken, a leafy green salad, green beans, and a bowl of cantaloupe, and you're still in the Green Light section. Another meal selection may be baked cod, a mixed fruit cup, steamed broccoli and carrots, and fresh spinach and orange salad.

Beyond Fish Sticks: Your Green-Light Guide to Seafood

Fish is a delicious part of just about every healthy eating plan known to humanity. Quick and easy to prepare, preparing seafood can be as simple as sautéing your favorite fish with a tiny bit of olive oil and a few simple spices and finishing it with a touch of lemon. Or, if you'd rather have a recipe to follow, try one of the recipes in this section, all of which are easy to prepare.

TIP

Start simple and expand your tastes. White–flesh fish (like cod, sole, halibut, and catfish) tend to be milder and are good fish if you're not used to eating seafood. Work up toward fresh tuna and salmon ("fishier" fish).

REMEMBER

Shellfish are an excellent source of protein and add almost no fat to your diet. The American Heart Association recommends eating two fish (particularly fatty fish) meals (8 to 12 ounces total) per week. Fatty fish like salmon, mackerel, herring, lake trout, sardines, and albacore tuna are high in heart healthy omega–3 fatty acids.

KEEP FISH SAFETY IN MIND

Mercury is a naturally occurring heavy metal that can build up in the bodies of fish in the form of methylmercury, which is highly toxic. Older, larger, predatory fish and other marine mammals contain high levels of mercury, polychlorinated biphenyls (PCBs), dioxins, and other environmental contaminants. This includes shark, swordfish, king mackerel, and tilefish from the Gulf of Mexico. Fish that are lower in mercury are canned light tuna, salmon, pollock, and catfish.

The U.S. Food and Drug Administration (FDA) advises children (age 2 and younger) and pregnant women to

- Avoid eating those fish with the potential for the highest level of mercury.

- Eat a variety of fish and shellfish that are lower in mercury.

- Check local advisories about the safety of fish caught by family and friends in local lakes, rivers, and coastal areas.

For middle-aged and older men and postmenopausal women, the benefits of eating fish far outweigh the potential risks when the amount of fish eaten is within the recommendation of at least 8 and up to 12 ounces per week. Eating a variety of fish helps minimize any potentially adverse effects due to environmental pollutants.

Baked Catfish Delight

PREP TIME: 30 MIN (PLUS 1 HR STANDING TIME)	COOK TIME: 50 MIN	YIELD: 4 SERVINGS

INGREDIENTS

4 catfish fillets (1 pound)

¼ cup lemon juice

¼ teaspoon Italian seasoning

Vegetable cooking spray

½ cup green onions, chopped

1 medium sweet red pepper, seeded and chopped

1 clove garlic, minced

1 small tomato, diced

¼ teaspoon salt

⅛ teaspoon pepper

1 cup shredded part-skim mozzarella cheese

DIRECTIONS

1 Rinse the fillets with cold water, and pat dry. Place in a shallow dish. Pour the lemon juice over the fillets; sprinkle with Italian seasoning. Cover and refrigerate 1 hour.

2 Preheat the oven to 350 degrees. Coat a large skillet with cooking spray and place over medium heat until hot. Add the onions, sweet red pepper, and garlic; sauté until the vegetables are tender, approximately 6 minutes. Add the tomato and sauté until thoroughly heated. Remove the mixture from the heat.

3 Remove the fillets from the lemon juice; place in a 12-x-8-x-2-inch baking dish. Sprinkle with salt and pepper. Bake, uncovered, for 15 minutes. Spoon the reserved vegetable mixture evenly over the fillets; sprinkle with cheese. Bake for an additional 10 minutes or until the fish flakes easily when tested with a fork.

TIP: Catfish is a great starter fish. Keep it low-carb with this easy recipe. Serve it with a side of light Low-Carb Crunch Coleslaw (refer to Chapter 15) or salad for a real treat.

PER SERVING: *Calories 236 (From Fat 124); Fat 14g (Saturated 5g); Cholesterol 67mg; Sodium 323mg; Carbohydrate 6g (Dietary Fiber 1g); Protein 25g.*

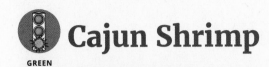

Cajun Shrimp

GREEN
LIGHT

PREP TIME: 5 MIN (PLUS 15 MIN STANDING TIME)	COOK TIME: 4 MIN	YIELD: 4 SERVINGS

INGREDIENTS

3 green onions, minced

2 tablespoons lemon juice

¾ teaspoon garlic powder

2 teaspoons paprika

¼ teaspoon salt

¼ teaspoon black pepper

¼ teaspoon cayenne pepper

1 tablespoon olive oil

1½ pounds medium shrimp, shelled with tails intact, deveined (see Figure 14-1)

Lemon wedges (optional)

DIRECTIONS

1 Combine the onions, lemon juice, garlic powder, paprika, salt, black pepper, and cayenne pepper in a 2-quart glass dish; stir in the oil. Add the shrimp; turn to coat. Cover and refrigerate at least 15 minutes.

2 Thread the shrimp onto metal or wooden skewers (if using wooden skewers, soak them in hot water for 30 minutes before use to prevent burning). Grill the shrimp over medium-hot coals about 2 minutes per side until opaque. Serve immediately with lemon wedges.

VARY IT! Use a bottled zesty cocktail sauce mixed with the olive oil as a marinade. Stir-fry shrimp in a skillet sprayed with nonstick cooking spray until the shrimp are opaque, just a couple of minutes.

NOTE: You can see a photo of Cajun Shrimp in the color insert.

PER SERVING: *Calories 168 (From Fat 45); Fat 5g (Saturated 1g); Cholesterol 252mg; Sodium 437mg; Carbohydrate 3g (Dietary Fiber 1g); Protein 28g.*

Cleaning and Deveining Shrimp

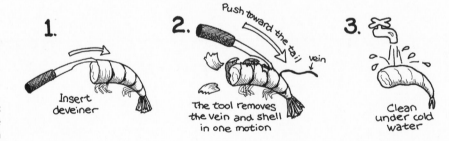

FIGURE 14-1: Follow these steps to devein shrimp.

Illustration by Liz Kurtzman

GREEN LIGHT

Onion–Lemon Fish

PREP TIME: 10 MIN	COOK TIME: 20 MIN	YIELD: 6 SERVINGS

INGREDIENTS

2 medium onions, thinly sliced

1 large lemon, thinly sliced

½ cup white wine

Small bay leaf

½ teaspoon whole peppercorns

1 cup water

1½ pounds fish fillets

DIRECTIONS

1 Combine all the ingredients except the fish fillets in a large skillet and gently simmer for 10 minutes. Add the fish.

2 Cover and continue to cook 10 minutes longer.

NOTE: I like to serve this fish with a quick dill sauce I whip up myself. Combine ⅓ cup plain low-fat yogurt with ½ teaspoon dried dill, plus fresh dill, if available. Let stand in the refrigerator for an hour or so to meld the flavors. Delicious!

PER SERVING: *Calories 102 (From Fat 11); Fat 1g (Saturated 0g); Cholesterol 53mg; Sodium 84mg; Carbohydrate 3g (Dietary Fiber 1g); Protein 19g.*

Bertie Jo's Salmon Wellington

PREP TIME: 20 MIN	COOK TIME: 25 TO 30 MIN	YIELD: 6 SERVINGS (* 1 CARBOHYDRATE CHOICE PER SERVING)

INGREDIENTS

6 salmon fillets, 4 ounces each

6 ounces light cream cheese, room temperature

½ cup sliced almonds

½ package puff pastry *

DIRECTIONS

1 Preheat the oven to 400 degrees.

2 Slice the salmon fillets lengthwise to make a pocket for stuffing if they're thick enough. If the fillets are thin, just leave them flat.

3 Mix the cream cheese with the almonds. Gently work the stuffing into the pocket of the salmon fillet. For thin fillets, spread the cream cheese–almond mixture on half of the fillet and fold the other half over it.

4 Divide the puff pastry sheet into 6 portions. Roll out to ⅛-inch thickness. Working quickly, wrap each fillet completely in the pastry dough. Seal the edges with water. Bake until the dough is browned, approximately 25 to 30 minutes.

PER SERVING: *Calories 475 (From Fat 265); Fat 30g (Saturated 7g); Cholesterol 86mg; Sodium 292mg; Carbohydrate 20g (Dietary Fiber 2g); Protein 32g.*

Oven-Fried Fish

GREEN LIGHT

PREP TIME: 10 MIN	COOK TIME: 25 MIN	YIELD: 6 SERVINGS (* CARB CHOICE PER SERVING NEGLIGIBLE)

INGREDIENTS

½ cup crushed corn flakes cereal*

½ teaspoon celery salt

⅛ teaspoon onion powder

⅛ teaspoon paprika

Dash of pepper

1 pound catfish or other fish fillets

¼ cup low-fat milk

Vegetable cooking spray

DIRECTIONS

1 Combine corn flakes, celery salt, onion powder, paprika, and pepper in a shallow dish. Dip fillets in milk; dredge in cereal mixture.

2 Place fillets in a baking dish coated with cooking spray. Bake at 350 degrees for 20 to 25 minutes or until fish is lightly browned and flakes easily when tested with a fork.

PER SERVING: *Calories 132 (From Fat 59); Fat 7g (Saturated 2g); Cholesterol 39mg; Sodium 82mg; Carbohydrate 4g (Dietary Fiber 0g); Protein 13g.*

Cooking Chicken, Beef, and Pork Entrees

Chicken is popular and easy to prepare. You can combine it with tasty vegetables and sauces to make a healthy meal. The chicken producers have made your culinary life easier by offering chicken in an almost endless variety of ways including individually quick-frozen pieces, boneless, skinless, marinated, pre-roasted, fresh, organic, free range . . . the list goes on. Use whatever chicken products best fit your lifestyle and budget. The more processed a chicken is, the more expensive. Find your comfort level with a balance between the two.

WARNING

Watch out for marinated meats, including chicken, in your local grocery store. They may be convenient, but they're often *loaded* with extra sugar and salts that are completely unnecessary and very unfriendly to low-carb dieters.

REMEMBER

Don't be afraid of lean beef. You can serve it two to three times per week accompanied by a variety of vegetables and fruits. Look for the leanest ground beef. Don't be afraid to ask your butcher or meat-department manager to trim roasts and steaks before wrapping and weighing them for you. The leaner the better, and who wants to pay for excess fat? (See Chapter 5 for more details on beef grading.)

With all your protein food sources, you want to eat a variety. You don't want a steady diet of the same kind of meat so mix up your meals. The following recipes give you plenty of choices.

Grilled Chicken Breasts with Grapefruit Glaze

PREP TIME: 10 MIN	COOK TIME: 20 MIN	YIELD: 4 SERVINGS

INGREDIENTS

2 cloves garlic, minced

1 teaspoon grapefruit zest (from about half grapefruit)

½ cup grapefruit juice (from one grapefruit)

1 tablespoon cooking oil

2 tablespoon honey

½ teaspoon salt

¼ teaspoon fresh-ground black pepper

4 bone-in, skinless chicken breasts (about 2 ¼ pounds in all)

DIRECTIONS

1 Light the grill. In a small bowl, combine the garlic, grapefruit zest, grapefruit juice, oil, honey, salt, and pepper.

2 Grill chicken breasts over moderately high heat, brushing frequently with the glaze, for 8 minutes. Turn and cook, brushing with more glaze, until the chicken is just done, 10 to 12 minutes longer. Remove.

3 In a small stainless-steel saucepan, bring the remaining glaze to a boil. Boil for about 1 minute, remove from the heat, and pour over the grilled chicken.

TIP: To enhance flavor, marinate the chicken in half the glaze for an hour or so. Use the other half of the glaze to brush while grilling.

VARY IT: Use a combination of citrus juices, such as orange, lemon, or lime, instead of all or part of the grapefruit juice.

PER SERVING: *Calories 271 (From Fat 54); Fat 6g (Saturated 1g); Cholesterol 134mg; Sodium 401mg; Carbohydrate 12g (Dietary Fiber 0g); Protein 41g.*

Baked Chicken with Winter Vegetables

GREEN LIGHT

PREP TIME: 30 MIN	COOK TIME: 1 HR	YIELD: 8 SERVINGS

INGREDIENTS

⅓ pound fresh or frozen Brussels sprouts, cleaned and stemmed

2 medium tomatoes, cut into wedges

⅓ pound carrots, peeled and cut into ¼-inch diagonal slices

1 acorn squash (about 8 ounces), peeled, seeded, and cubed

¼ cup chopped onion

1 teaspoon dried basil leaves

½ teaspoon dry mustard

¼ teaspoon salt

¼ teaspoon pepper

3½-pound broiler fryer chicken, cut up and skinned

DIRECTIONS

1 Preheat oven to 350 degrees. Combine sprouts, tomatoes, carrots, squash, onion, basil, mustard, salt, and pepper in a large bowl; toss well. Set aside.

2 Trim the excess fat from the chicken. Rinse the chicken with cold water; pat dry. Place the chicken in an oven browning bag prepared according to the package instructions. Place the reserved vegetable mixture in the bag around the chicken. Seal the bag according to the package instructions, cutting slits in the top of the bag. Place the bag in a 13-x-9-x-2-inch baking dish; bake for 1 hour or until chicken and vegetables are tender.

TIP: Brussels sprouts have a bad reputation with some people. But if you clean them properly, they can be an easy, delicious part of your regular diet. Remove their discolored leaves, cut off the stem ends, and wash them thoroughly. Cut a shallow X in the base of each sprout. This X allows the sprout to pick up the flavor of the cooking sauce or broth and become extremely tender.

NOTE: Check out the color insert for a photo of Baked Chicken with Winter Vegetables.

PER SERVING: *Calories 183 (From Fat 54); Fat 6g (Saturated 2g); Cholesterol 68mg; Sodium 156mg; Carbohydrate 9g (Dietary Fiber 3g); Protein 24g.*

**GREEN
LIGHT**

Bertie Jo's Company Chicken

| PREP TIME: 10 MIN | COOK TIME: 3 HR | YIELD: 6 SERVINGS |

INGREDIENTS

3 strips lean bacon, cut in half

6 chicken breast halves, boneless, skinless, split in two

Two 25-ounce jars dried beef

1 can Healthy Recipe cream of mushroom soup

8 ounces sour cream

DIRECTIONS

1 Preheat the oven to 275 degrees. Lay the bacon across the chicken lengthwise. Wrap the chicken and bacon in the beef slices (one on each side); secure with toothpicks.

2 Combine the soup and sour cream. Pour over the chicken. Bake uncovered for approximately 3 hours, basting occasionally. Don't overbake.

PER SERVING: *Calories 275 (From Fat 120); Fat 13g (Saturated 7g); Cholesterol 98mg; Sodium 671mg; Carbohydrate 5g (Dietary Fiber 0g); Protein 32g.*

Wine-Braised Chicken with Mushrooms

PREP TIME: 30 MIN	COOK TIME: 50 MIN	YIELD: 4 SERVINGS

INGREDIENTS

2½-3 pounds, bone-in skinless chicken thighs

Kosher salt

Freshly ground black pepper

3 tablespoons Dijon mustard, plus more as needed

½ cup seasoned Italian-style bread crumbs

2 tablespoons olive oil, plus more if needed

2 cloves garlic, thinly sliced

¾ cup white wine, amount varies depending on size of pan

8 ounces cremini or white button mushrooms, sliced

DIRECTIONS

1 Position the rack in the middle of the oven and heat to 350 degrees. Season chicken with salt and pepper. Generously coat both sides of the thighs with mustard and then dip in breadcrumbs, one at a time, turning meat over to ensure that it's evenly covered. Let chicken rest for at least 10 minutes to allow the coating to set.

2 In Dutch oven over medium heat, heat olive oil until shimmering. Add the breaded chicken. Cook until breading is dark golden brown, 3 to 5 minutes. Resist the urge to move the chicken too soon to ensure the beading stays put.

3 Flip pieces carefully with a fork. Cook another 3 to 5 minutes, adding more oil if necessary to keep pan from drying out and chicken from sticking. Don't worry if a little breading comes off — you can press it back on or leave to help thicken the braising liquid. Transfer chicken to baking sheet or platter.

4 If pan is looking dry, add another glug of oil. Stir in sliced garlic and cook until fragrant, 30 seconds to 1 minute. Add splash of wine and scrape any browned bits on the bottom of the pan. Add the sliced mushrooms, season with a generous pinch of salt, and stir. Cook for 1 to 2 minutes, just to jump-start the cooking process.

5 Nestle chicken pieces on top of mushrooms and pour in rest of wine around the chicken.

6 Cover pan with a lid and transfer to oven. Cook for 30 minutes and then remove lid. Cook an additional 15 to 20 minutes, until an instant-read thermometer reads 165 Fahrenheit. Serve warm with the mushrooms and plenty of juices for dipping.

NOTE: When pouring in the rest of the wine around the chicken, the amount you need varies based on the pan size, but make sure it's enough to cover the mushrooms and just reach the bottom of the chicken. Note: Dark meat is forgiving and will be fine up to as high as 195 Fahrenheit.

NOTE: FLIP to the color insert for a photo of Wine-Braised Chicken with Mushrooms.

PER SERVING: *Calories 235 (From Fat 99); Fat 11g (Saturated 2g); Cholesterol 72mg; Sodium 298mg; Carbohydrate 7g (Dietary Fiber 1g); Protein 20g.*

GREEN LIGHT

Betty's Busy-Day Roast

INGREDIENTS

6-pound beef roast

2 teaspoons salt

2 teaspoons pepper

1 tablespoon garlic salt

¼ cup Worcestershire sauce

DIRECTIONS

1 Preheat the oven to 225 degrees. Trim the excess fat from the roast. Cover with salt, pepper, and garlic salt.

2 Place the roast in a roasting pan, pour the Worcestershire sauce over it, and cover tightly. Bake for 8 hours. Skim the fat from the pan juices; reserve 1 cup of the juice to serve over the meat.

TIP: Make more roast than you'll need. The leftovers make great lettuce-wrap fillings and salad ingredients. Just slice it and place it on top of your favorite greens or cut it in chunks and serve it in butter lettuce cups.

PER SERVING (4 OUNCES): *Calories 265 (From Fat 111); Fat 12.5g (Saturated 5.5g); Cholesterol 82mg; Sodium 613.5mg; Carbohydrate 1g (Dietary Fiber 0g); Protein 33g.*

GREEN LIGHT

Eggplant Casserole

PREP TIME: 20 MIN	COOK TIME: 1 HR	YIELD: 8 TO 10 SERVINGS

INGREDIENTS

1½ pounds extra-lean ground beef

½ teaspoon rosemary

½ teaspoon oregano

½ teaspoon basil

1 teaspoon salt

½ teaspoon pepper

Cooking spray

1 eggplant

1 onion, thinly sliced

10 fresh mushrooms, sliced

16 ounces cottage cheese

3 eggs

½ pound reduced-fat Monterey Jack cheese, grated

DIRECTIONS

1 Preheat the oven to 400 degrees. Brown the meat until crumbly; drain off any fat. Add the rosemary, oregano, basil, salt, and pepper. Set aside.

2 Spray a 13-x-9-x-2-inch casserole dish with cooking spray. Slice the eggplant ¼-inch thick. Quarter the slices and arrange them on the bottom of the casserole dish. Top with the meat mixture. Place the onion slices on top of the meat. Add a layer of mushrooms.

3 Beat the cottage cheese and eggs together. Spoon over the casserole. Sprinkle with grated cheese. Bake, uncovered, for 1 hour.

TIP: Substitute tempeh for the ground beef to turn this recipe into vegetarian. Add Green Beans with Onions and Peach Salad Cups from Chapter 15 to this dish to make a tasty, filling meatless meal.

PER SERVING: *Calories 241 (From Fat 118); Fat 13g (Saturated 7g); Cholesterol 105mg; Sodium 666mg; Carbohydrate 7g (Dietary Fiber 2g); Protein 25g.*

No-Fail Meatloaf

PREP TIME: 15 MIN	COOK TIME: 60 TO 90 MIN	YIELD: 8 SERVINGS (*½ CARBOHYDRATE CHOICE PER SERVING)

INGREDIENTS

1½ pounds extra-lean ground beef

Three 8-ounce cans tomato sauce

1 egg, beaten

1 cup dried bread crumbs*

1 tablespoon dried onion

1½ teaspoons salt

¼ teaspoon pepper

4½ teaspoons Truvia brown sugar blend

2 tablespoons prepared mustard

2 tablespoons Worcestershire sauce

3 tablespoons vinegar

DIRECTIONS

1 Preheat oven to 350 degrees. Lightly mix the ground beef, 1 can of the tomato sauce, egg, bread crumbs, onion, salt, and pepper. Form a loaf from the mixture. Place in a shallow baking dish.

2 In a small bowl, combine the Truvia brown sugar blend, mustard, Worcestershire sauce, vinegar, and the remaining two cans of tomato sauce. Pour over the meatloaf and bake uncovered 60 to 90 minutes.

TIP: To make this meatloaf a Green Light food, cut out the bread crumbs or substitute 1 slice of whole wheat bread, toasted and torn into pieces to only add a negligible amount of carb.

VARY IT: To reduce the sodium, use a tomato sauce with no salt added.

PER SERVING: *Calories 232 (From Fat 65); Fat 7g (Saturated 3g); Cholesterol 50mg; Sodium 1,171mg; Carbohydrate 24 g (Dietary Fiber 1g); Protein 17g.*

GREEN LIGHT

Spicy Beef and Mushroom Brochettes

PREP TIME: 10 MIN	COOK TIME: 8 TO 10 MIN PLUS REFRIGERATION TIME	YIELD: 3 CUPS

INGREDIENTS

1 pound top sirloin beef, cut into 1-inch cubes

30 Monterey White or Brown mushrooms

1 red pepper, cut into 1-inch pieces

1 green pepper, cut into 1-inch pieces

½ cup canola oil

2 tablespoons Chef Paul Prudhomme's Blackened Steak Magic

6 wooden or metal skewers

DIRECTIONS

1 Place all ingredients in plastic resealable bag. Mix well. Place in refrigerator and marinate minimum 1 hour. Stir occasionally.

2 Soak wooden skewers in warm water for 10 to 20 minutes before grilling to prevent skewers from burning or use metal skewers.

3 Thread beef cubes, mushrooms, and peppers alternately onto prepared wooden or metal skewers. Cover and refrigerate until ready to cook. Discard any remaining marinade.

4 Grill over medium heat, turning several times until mushrooms are browned and beef is done, approximately 8 to 10 minutes. Serve hot.

NOTE: Refer to the color insert for a photo of Spicy Beef and Mushroom Brochettes.

PER SERVING (4 OUNCES): *Calories 326 (From Fat 176); at 20g (Saturated 3g); Cholesterol 76mg; Sodium 106mg; Carbohydrate 9g (Dietary Fiber 2g); Protein 30g.*

Stuffed Cube Steaks

PREP TIME: 15 MIN	COOK TIME: 45 MIN PLUS	YIELD: 6 SERVINGS (*½ CARBOHYDRATE CHOICE PER SERVING)

INGREDIENTS

6 beef cube steaks (1¾ pounds)

Salt

Pepper

½ cup low-calorie French-style salad dressing

1 cup shredded carrot

¾ cup finely chopped onion

¾ cup finely chopped green pepper

¾ cup chopped celery

¼ cup water

¼ teaspoon salt

½ cup canned beef broth

4 teaspoons cornstarch*

¼ teaspoon Kitchen Bouquet

DIRECTIONS

1 Pound or tenderize steaks to ¼-inch thickness. Sprinkle generously with salt and pepper; brush with salad dressing. Place in shallow dish; marinate for 30 to 60 minutes at room temperature.

2 In medium saucepan, combine carrot, onion, green pepper, celery, water, and salt. Simmer, covered, until vegetables are crisp-tender, about 7 to 8 minutes. Drain.

3 Place about ⅓ cup vegetable mixture on each steak. Roll up jelly-roll fashion; secure with wooden picks. Place meat rolls in 10-inch skillet; pour beef broth over. Simmer, covered, until tender, about 35 to 40 minutes.

4 Transfer meat to serving platter; remove picks. Skim fat from broth; reserve ¾ cup broth. Blend cornstarch with 2 tablespoons cold water; stir into reserved broth. Cook and stir till thick and bubbly; stir in kitchen bouquet. Pour over steak rolls.

TIP: Kitchen Bouquet is usually available in grocery stores or gourmet stores or online.

PER SERVING: *Calories 637 (From Fat 238); Fat 26g (Saturated 10g); Cholesterol 233mg; Sodium 678mg; Carbohydrate 12g (Dietary Fiber 1g); Protein 85g.*

Bun-Less Bacon Cheeseburgers

PREP TIME: 10 MIN	COOK TIME: 10 MIN PLUS	YIELD: 6 SERVINGS

INGREDIENTS

1 pound extra-lean ground beef

1 egg, beaten

½ cup reduced-fat sharp cheddar cheese, grated

3 tablespoons onion, finely chopped

1½ tablespoons ketchup

1½ tablespoons Worcestershire sauce

1½ teaspoon salt

¼ teaspoon pepper

6 slices turkey bacon or other lean bacon

DIRECTIONS

1 Mix well all ingredients except bacon. Form into 6 thick patties. Wrap bacon around each patty and secure with toothpicks.

2 Broil either under a broiler or on a grill until the bacon appears well done, approximately 10 minutes, turning once during cooking.

PER SERVING: *Calories 179 (From Fat 97); Fat 11g (Saturated 4g); Cholesterol 75mg; Sodium 502mg; Carbohydrate 3g (Dietary Fiber 0g); Protein 17g.*

GREEN LIGHT

Pork Chops with Apples

| PREP TIME: 10 MIN | COOK TIME: 45 MIN | YIELD: 4 SERVINGS |

INGREDIENTS

Four (4-ounce) lean boneless center-cut pork chops

Vegetable cooking spray

1 medium onion, chopped

1¼ cups water

1 teaspoon chicken-flavored bouillon granules

¼ teaspoon pepper

3 medium cooking apples, peeled and sliced

½ teaspoon ground cinnamon

DIRECTIONS

1 Sear pork chops on both sides of chop in large skillet coated with vegetable cooking spray for about 2 to 3 minutes per side, then remove. Add onions for a quick brown.

2 Combine water, bouillon granules, and pepper, stirring until granules dissolve; add to skillet. Add apples and cinnamon.

3 Simmer 15 minutes and then add the pork back into the sauce for just a few minutes to warm up.

PER SERVING: *Calories 196 (From Fat 44); Fat 5g (Saturated 2g); Cholesterol 65mg; Sodium 191mg; Carbohydrate 15g (Dietary Fiber 2g); Protein 23g.*

CONSIDER PORK IN YOUR LOW-CARB DIET

Though you may have heard it called "the other white meat," pork is considered red meat. Pork is a good source of certain nutrients as well as high-quality protein. Consumed in moderation, it can make a good addition to a healthy diet. Minimally processed, lean, fully cooked pork eaten in moderation can provide certain benefits when added to your diet. The healthiest pork options are lean cuts such as tenderloin, loin chops, and sirloin roast. Try the Pork Chops with Apples recipe for a tasty introduction to a pork entree.

Going Meatless: Vegetarian Options

Many folks are considering a plant-based diet to improve their health. So does that mean they're becoming a vegetarian or vegan? Not necessarily.

As Chapter 2 discusses, the western diet is dreadfully low in plant foods such as veggies, fruits, beans, and nuts. Those foods represented only 11 percent of a person's dietary intake; and, half of that 11 percent was contributed by french fries and ketchup! Whole grains were represented by a meager 4 percent. The rest of the western dietary intake was animal products and processed foods, which is hardly a recipe for good health, and the national health report card shows it.

Thus, increasing plant foods in your daily diet is a good idea. If you find the whole vegetarian/vegan thing a little intimidating, just start with a meatless meal or a meatless day. Here I give you some vegetarian entrees that you can match up with some vegetarian side dishes from Chapter 15 for a healthy and filling meatless meal.

REMEMBER

Take time to evaluate the quality of your plant foods. The Whole Foods Weight Loss Eating Plan in this book helps you do that. For example, white rice and white bread are plant-based foods, so that's good, right? Not so fast. They're both processed and are depleted of many healthy nutrients. In addition, because of their processing, they have a high glycemic index, which means they can make blood sugar levels spike and increase hunger, leading to overeating. Appendix A discusses the science of the glycemic index in greater detail.

If you're a vegetarian or vegan, lower your intake of processed carbs and reduce your portion sizes of the starchy carbohydrates. The important thing is to remember that you want the carbohydrates you eat to be good ones.

GETTING MORE PROTEIN AS A VEGETARIAN

If you're a vegetarian, you may consider these other protein sources:

- **Eggs or egg whites:** Eggs are a nutritious source of protein and relatively inexpensive. Each egg provides 6 to 8 grams of protein and has all the essential amino acids. Egg whites have fewer calories, but you'll also miss out on vitamin D, omega-3 fatty acids, and B vitamins housed in the yolk.

- **Dairy products:** Milk, cheese, and yogurt are excellent sources of protein and calcium. You'll find the most protein in cottage cheese or plain Greek yogurt with both containing 13 grams of protein or more per serving.

GREEN LIGHT

Zucchini-Tomato Bake

PREP TIME: 10 MIN	COOK TIME: 40 MIN	YIELD: 8 SERVINGS

INGREDIENTS

4 tablespoons plant butter

1 onion, chopped

2 large zucchini, sliced in ¼-inch slices

3 tomatoes, chopped

¼ pound mushrooms

½ teaspoon basil

3 tablespoons chopped parsley

Garlic salt and pepper to taste

¼ cup Parmesan cheese

¼ pound reduced-fat sharp cheddar cheese, grated

DIRECTIONS

1 Preheat the oven to 350 degrees. In a nonstick skillet, melt the plant butter over medium high heat. Sauté the onion and mushroom in the plant butter. Add the zucchini and sauté until tender. Mix in the tomatoes, basil, parsley, garlic salt, pepper, and Parmesan cheese.

2 Place the vegetable mixture in a 1½–quart casserole dish sprayed with nonstick vegetable spray. Top with the cheddar cheese. Bake for 20 to 30 minutes.

TIP: Serve with Savory Carrots and Melon Salad from Chapter 15 for a filling and tasty meatless meal.

PER SERVING: *Calories 126 (From Fat 81); Fat 9g (Saturated 3g); Cholesterol 12mg; Sodium 248mg; Carbohydrate 7g (Dietary Fiber 2g); Protein 7g.*

BE AS VEGETARIAN AS YOU WANT

If you're thinking of experimenting with going vegetarian, you may want to consider one of the following forms of vegetarian diets to see which one works for you:

- **Lacto vegetarian** includes consuming milk and other dairy products in addition to plant foods.

- **Lacto-ovo vegetarian** includes consuming eggs as well as milk and other dairy products in addition to plant foods.

- **Pescovegetarian** eats no red meat and no dairy but does consume fish as well as plant foods. If you're contemplating this avenue, be sure to include nonfried sea-food in your diet every day. Legumes and soy products should probably make an appearance in your diet to ensure you get enough calcium.

- **Pollovegetarian** eats no red meat and no dairy but does eat poultry and plant foods. Count your poultry as your lean protein, and add soy products or a calcium supplement to ensure that you're getting adequate calcium each day.

**GREEN
LIGHT**

🍅 Harold's Stir-Fry

| PREP TIME: 10 MIN | COOK TIME: 10 MIN | YIELD: 6 SERVINGS |

INGREDIENTS

2 large zucchini, sliced

½ large green pepper, sliced

½ large onion, sliced

2 garlic cloves, chopped

1½ tablespoon olive oil

1 teaspoon powdered
vegetable stock bouillon cubes

Salt and pepper

1 Roma tomato, seeded and
chopped

DIRECTIONS

1 Heat a nonstick skillet over medium heat until hot. Sauté the
zucchini, green pepper, onion, and garlic in the olive oil. Cover
the skillet, and reduce the heat to medium. Cook, stirring frequently, until the squash is barely tender, approximately 3 to
5 minutes. Don't overcook.

2 Add the vegetable stock bouillon cubes, salt, and pepper. Stir
in the tomatoes. Cook about 1 minute more.

VARY IT! You may add 1 tablespoon of grated fresh ginger and
1 tablespoon of soy sauce for a little extra kick.

TIP: Serve with a Baked Stuffed Potato and Sweet and Spicy Oranges
from Chapter 15 for a meatless meal bursting with flavor.

PER SERVING: *Calories 57 (From Fat 33); Fat 4g (Saturated 1g); Cholesterol
0mg; Sodium 164mg; Carbohydrate 6g (Dietary Fiber 2g); Protein 2g.*

Two-Squash Toss

| PREP TIME: 10 MIN | COOK TIME: 12 MIN | YIELD: 6 SERVINGS |

INGREDIENTS

3 small yellow squash, cut into ½-inch slices

2 medium zucchini, cut into ½-inch slices

One 2 ounce jar sliced pimiento drained

½ teaspoon dried Italian seasoning

¼ teaspoon salt

½ teaspoon garlic powder

3 tablespoons water

2 teaspoons plant butter

DIRECTIONS

1 Combine yellow squash, zucchini, pimiento, Italian seasoning, salt, and garlic powder in a 2½-quart casserole.

2 Add water and dot with plant butter.

3 Cover with heavy-duty plastic wrap and vent, microwave on high for 8 to 10 minutes or until vegetables are tender, stirring at 3 minute intervals. Check for your preferred doneness at the 3 minute intervals. Let stand covered 2 minutes.

TIP: Make a meal with Corn Medley and Carol's Broiled Cinnamon Peaches from Chapter 15 for another meatless meal.

PER SERVING: *Calories 52 (From Fat 15); Fat 2g (Saturated g); Cholesterol 3mg; Sodium 124mg; Carbohydrate 9g (Dietary Fiber 2g); Protein 3g.*

Vegetable Couscous

PREP TIME: 20 MIN	COOK TIME: 20 MIN	YIELD: 8 SERVINGS (*½ CARBOHYDRATE CHOICE PER SERVING)

INGREDIENTS

Vegetable cooking spray

½ tablespoon olive oil

2 medium-size yellow squash, diced

1 medium-size zucchini, diced

8 small fresh mushrooms, sliced

1 small sweet red pepper, seeded and diced

¼ cup, plus 1 tablespoon reduced-calorie

Italian salad dressing, divided

¼ cup water

½ teaspoon salt

½ cup couscous, uncooked*

DIRECTIONS

1 Coat a large skillet with cooking spray, add the olive oil, and place over medium heat until hot. Add the yellow squash, zucchini, mushrooms, and sweet red pepper; sauté until crisp-tender. Combine the squash mixture and 3 tablespoons of the salad dressing in a large bowl; toss well. Set aside, and keep warm.

2 Combine the water, the remaining 2 tablespoons salad dressing, and the salt in a small saucepan; bring to a boil. Remove from the heat, and stir in the couscous. Continue to stir until all the liquid is absorbed (about 3 minutes). Add to the reserved vegetable mixture, and stir well.

TIP: Serve with the Pinto Bean Salad and Skillet Corn from Chapter 15 and finish with Apple Treats from Chapter 13 for a filling meatless meal.

NOTE: You can see a photo of this recipe in the color insert.

PER SERVING: *Calories 80 (From Fat 21); Fat 2g (Saturated 0g); Cholesterol 0mg; Sodium 220mg; Carbohydrate 13g (Dietary Fiber 2g); Protein 3g.*

Chapter **15**

Adding Side Dishes to Your Meal

If entrees are the main event, side dishes are a welcome distraction. Try these low-carb comfort foods to add interest to your meal and remind you of home. You can also spend a carbohydrate choice or two to add to your meal — just don't exceed your limit of five carbohydrate choices for the whole day.

Besides increasing the nutrition power in your meal, fruits and vegetables help give your meals contrast in flavor, texture, color, and shape. They also fill up your tummy without filling up your calorie and carb load for the day. Look for the freshest fruits and veggies to add the most flavor to your meals, but the canned, frozen, or dried varieties work well, too. Vary the vegetables you eat to add the most interest — sticking to any eating plan is tough if it's boring. Check out Chapter 5 for more information on how fruits and veggies can be your partners in low-carb eating.

The role of the side dish is to round out and complete the meal or complement a bold entree. Or, you can spice up a plain dinner with flavorful sides. Use two to three side dishes in this chapter to make a complete and filling meal.

Pairing Veggie Side Dishes to Your Low-Carb Meals

Vegetables are nutrition superstars. They're low in calories and fat, cholesterol-free, and high in vitamins, minerals, phytochemical cancer fighters, and heart-protective antioxidants. Veggies are nature's defense mechanism, protecting you against disease when you eat them. And, as I discuss in Chapter 2, veggies are sorely neglected in the western diet. Adding these vegetable side dishes to your main course gives your meal and your health a powerful nutritional boost.

TIP

Cook your vegetables crisp and not mushy. Overcooking vegetables makes them soggy and causes them to lose important nutrients.

REMEMBER

Vegetables are the true superstars of nutrition. Paired with a lean protein, they complete any meal, stave off rumbling tummies, and provide great fiber for good health.

This section includes vegetable side dishes from the Green Light food lists meaning they're *free* on the Whole Foods Weight Loss Eating Plan, meaning you can eat as much as you want. However, a few side dishes include starchy carb veggies such as pinto beans, baked potato, corn, and even sweet potatoes. Eating a starchy carb is a good place to spend one or two of those five carb choices you're allowed each day.

🍅 Pinto Bean Salad

PREP TIME: 10 MIN	COOK TIME: NONE	YIELD: 8 SERVINGS (*½ CARBOHYDRATE CHOICE PER SERVING)

INGREDIENTS

Two 15-ounce cans pinto beans*

1 cup shredded Romaine lettuce

½ cup chopped celery

⅓ cup chopped purple onion

¼ cup chopped sweet red pepper

3 tablespoons red wine vinegar

2 tablespoons vegetable oil

2 teaspoons minced fresh cilantro

¼ teaspoon garlic salt

Lettuce leaves

½ cup shredded reduced-fat cheddar cheese

DIRECTIONS

1 Place the pinto beans in a colander, and rinse under cold water for 1 minute. Set the colander aside, allowing the beans to drain 1 minute.

2 Combine the beans, lettuce, celery, onion, and red pepper in a large bowl; set aside. Combine the vinegar, oil, cilantro, and garlic salt in a jar; cover tightly, then shake vigorously. Pour the vinegar mixture over the reserved bean mixture; toss gently to coat well. Cover and chill thoroughly.

3 To serve, spoon the bean mixture into a lettuce-lined salad bowl and sprinkle with cheese.

TIP: This quick salad is a welcome addition to any luncheon. Make sure your cilantro is fresh; consider throwing in more than the recipe calls for if you're a cilantro fan.

PER SERVING: *Calories 119 (From Fat 48); Fat 5g (Saturated 1g); Cholesterol 5mg; Sodium 196mg; Carbohydrate 13g (Dietary Fiber 3g); Protein 5g.*

Skillet Onion Slices

| PREP TIME: 15 MIN | COOK TIME: 15 MIN | YIELD: 6 SERVINGS |

INGREDIENTS

¼ cup low-calorie Italian salad dressing

⅓ cup water

½ teaspoon salt

3 medium onions, cut in ½-inch slices

2 tablespoons snipped parsley

2 tablespoons shredded Parmesan cheese

Paprika

DIRECTIONS

1 In your largest skillet, heat the salad dressing, water, and salt. Place the onion slices in a single layer in the skillet. (Don't worry if the onions overlap a bit.) Cover and cook over low heat for 10 minutes.

2 Turn the onion slices; sprinkle with parsley, cheese, and paprika. Cook, covered, 5 minutes; cook, uncovered, 5 minutes more.

NOTE: This recipe is fantastic with Vidalia onions or other sweet onions when they're in season, but you can enjoy this recipe anytime.

PER SERVING: Calories 30 (From Fat 14); Fat 2g (Saturated 1g); Cholesterol 2mg; Sodium 305mg; Carbohydrate 3g (Dietary Fiber 1g); Protein 1g.

Green Beans with Onions

GREEN LIGHT

PREP TIME: 10 MIN	COOK TIME: 8 TO 10 MIN	YIELD: 4 SERVINGS

INGREDIENTS

9-ounce package frozen cut green beans

½ teaspoon dried marjoram leaves, crushed

8-ounce can peeled, small pear onions, drained

1 tablespoon plant butter

DIRECTIONS

1 Cook the beans according to the package instructions, except add marjoram to the cooking liquid. Add the onions to the beans during the last few minutes of cooking time.

2 Continue cooking until the onions are heated through. Drain thoroughly; stir in the plant butter. Transfer the vegetables to a serving dish.

TIP: This is a super-quick side dish that makes mouths smile. Try these easy green beans with Betty's Busy Day Roast in Chapter 14.

NOTE: Plant (nut/seed) butter refers to a product that contains at least 90 percent nut/seed ingredients. Many plant butters feature oils from almonds, olives, and avocados. You can find a variety of plant butters in the dairy case of your local supermarket.

PER SERVING: *Calories 43 (From Fat 12); Fat 1g (Saturated 0g); Cholesterol 0mg; Sodium 21mg; Carbohydrate 7g (Dietary Fiber 2g); Protein 1g.*

GREEN LIGHT

 # Spaghetti Squash

PREP TIME: 10 MIN	COOK TIME: 30 TO 40 MIN	YIELD: 6 SERVINGS

INGREDIENTS

1 large spaghetti squash

Nonstick vegetable spray

3 tablespoons plant butter

Salt and pepper, to taste

½ cup Parmesan cheese

DIRECTIONS

1 Preheat the oven to 350 degrees. Cut the squash in half, lengthwise. Place on a baking dish sprayed with nonstick vegetable spray, with the cut side of the squash down on the baking dish, and bake until tender to the touch, approximately 45 to 60 minutes. Remove from the oven.

2 Using a fork, scrape the flesh from the cut side of the cooked squash to make "spaghetti." Continue scraping the squash to the rind. Season the spaghetti with plant butter, salt, pepper, and Parmesan cheese.

NOTE: Spaghetti Squash gets its name from the unique way it's served. You take the cooked flesh of the squash and shred it with a fork, making it look like long threads of spaghetti.

PER SERVING: *Calories 151 (From Fat 75); Fat 8g (Saturated 2g); Cholesterol 5mg; Sodium 334mg; Carbohydrate 17g (Dietary Fiber 4g); Protein 5g.*

GREEN LIGHT

Summer Squash Medley

INGREDIENTS

Vegetable cooking spray

1 tablespoon plant butter

1 large clove garlic, minced

1 small sweet red pepper, seeded and cut into strips

2 small yellow squash, cut into ¼-inch diagonal slices

2 small zucchini, sliced

2 green onions, thinly sliced

1 cup cherry tomatoes, halved

¼ teaspoon dried whole oregano

¼ teaspoon salt

⅛ teaspoon pepper

DIRECTIONS

1 Coat a large skillet with the cooking spray; add the plant butter and place over medium heat until the plant butter melts.

2 Add the garlic; cook 1 minute, stirring constantly. Add the sweet red pepper, yellow squash, and zucchini; cover and cook 6 minutes. Stir in the onions, tomatoes, oregano, salt, and pepper; cover and cook 2 to 3 minutes or until vegetables are crisp-tender.

NOTE: Despite its name, summer squash is available year-round in most parts of the United States. This flavorful side dish is great with a broiled chicken breast or grilled sirloin. Add a mixed green salad for a filling nutritious meal.

TIP: Refer to the color insert for a photo of Summer Squash Medley.

PER SERVING: *Calories 62 (From Fat 29); Fat 3g (Saturated 1g); Cholesterol 0mg; Sodium 186mg; Carbohydrate 8g (Dietary Fiber 3g); Protein 2g.*

Microwave Zucchini

GREEN LIGHT

PREP TIME: 2 MIN	COOK TIME: 6 MIN	YIELD: 4 SERVINGS

INGREDIENTS

2 zucchini

2 teaspoons plant butter

Garlic salt, to taste

Freshly ground pepper, to taste

2 tablespoons Parmesan cheese, grated or shredded

DIRECTIONS

1 Wash the zucchini thoroughly. Slice each zucchini lengthwise into 2 pieces. Lay them cut side down on a microwave-safe dish.

2 Microwave on high for 2 to 4 minutes, or until barely yielding to the touch. Turn the zucchini over. Pierce with a fork, and add plant butter. Sprinkle generously with garlic salt and pepper, and then Parmesan cheese. Microwave about 1 minute longer.

TIP: If you ever have unexpected guests, you can quickly expand this side dish by adding more zucchini. In Step 2, microwave the batch for 1 to 2 minutes per zucchini and adjust the seasoning as desired. So, for three zucchini, microwave 3 to 6 minutes, and so on.

PER SERVING: *Calories 42 (From Fat 25); Fat 3g (Saturated 1g); Cholesterol 2mg; Sodium 132mg; Carbohydrate 3g (Dietary Fiber 1g); Protein 2g.*

GREEN LIGHT

Savory Carrots

| PREP TIME: 10 MIN | COOK TIME: 8 TO 10 MIN | YIELD: 6 SERVINGS |

INGREDIENTS

¾ cup water

1 pound carrots, peeled and sliced

4 green onions with tops, sliced

2 tablespoons Brummel and Brown

½ teaspoon salt

DIRECTIONS

1 Bring water to a boil in a medium saucepan. Add the carrots and onions. Cover; cook over medium heat 15 to 20 minutes.

2 Remove from the heat; drain. Add the Brummel and Brown and salt. Toss lightly to coat.

TIP: You can use baby carrots in this recipe and avoid the peeling and slicing with the full-sized carrots.

NOTE: Brummel and Brown is a buttery spread made by blending plant-based oils, purified water, and real yogurt. It has half the fat and calories of real butter and no trans fat, no partially hydrogenated oils, and no cholesterol. You can find it in the dairy section of your local supermarket.

PER SERVING: *Calories 48 (From Fat 16); Fat 2g (Saturated 0g); Cholesterol 0mg; Sodium 220mg; Carbohydrate 8g (Dietary Fiber 2g); Protein 1g.*

Candied Sweet Potatoes

PREP TIME: 9 MIN	COOK TIME: 14 MIN	YIELD: 4 SERVINGS (*1 CARBOHYDRATE CHOICE PER SERVING)

INGREDIENTS

2 large sweet potatoes (1 ¾ pounds)*

4 ½ teaspoons Truvia Brown Sugar Blend

1 tablespoon plant butter

1 tablespoon unsweetened orange juice

DIRECTIONS

1 Wash sweet potatoes and pat dry; prick each sweet potato several times with a fork. Arrange sweet potatoes 1 inch apart on a layer of paper towels in microwave oven. Microwave uncovered on high for 8 to 10 minutes or until sweet potatoes are tender, turning and rearranging potatoes after 4 minutes. Let potatoes stand 5 minutes.

2 Peel sweet potatoes and cut into ½-inch slices.

3 Combine brown sugar blend and plant butter in a 2-quart casserole. Microwave uncovered on high for 1 to 1½ minutes or until brown sugar blend and plant butter melt, stirring after I minute. Stir in orange juice.

4 Add sweet potato slices and toss gently. Cover with wax paper and microwave on high 1 to 2 minutes or until potatoes are thoroughly heated.

5 Toss gently before serving. Serve immediately.

NOTE: Candied sweet potatoes on a low-carb diet, you ask? Yes! The Truvia Brown Sugar Blend and the small amount of unsweetened orange juice keep the added carbs low. Sweet potatoes are an excellent source of vitamin C, beta-carotene, and fiber. More importantly, they rank low in glycemic load. Eaten in moderation, they can be low-carb-friendly, because they pack such a nutritional punch. This recipe is a good place to spend one of your five carb choices.

TIP: If you have trouble with the sweet potatoes holding their shape after microwaving, you can first peel and slice the sweet potatoes before microwaving. Then place them in a skillet to simmer with a bit of water for 5 minutes. This will allow the sweet potatoes to hold their shape and still endure a little microwave zapping down the line.

PER SERVING: *Calories 79 (From Fat 18); Fat 3g (Saturated 2g); Cholesterol 8mg; Sodium 41mg; Carbohydrate 12g (Dietary Fiber 2g); Protein 1g.*

GREEN LIGHT

Asparagus with Lemon Sauce

| PREP TIME: 5 MIN | COOK TIME: 12 MIN | YIELD: 6 SERVINGS |

INGREDIENTS

One 10 ounce package frozen asparagus spears

1 tablespoon, plus 2 teaspoons Truvia Spoonable

1 egg

1 tablespoon plant butter

¼ cup lemon juice

2 teaspoons grated lemon rind

DIRECTIONS

1 Cook asparagus according to package directions; drain well. Transfer cooked asparagus to a serving dish, and keep warm.

2 Using a whisk, combine Truvia and egg to blend. Melt plant butter over low heat in a small skillet; add egg mixture. Whisk over medium heat until mixture thickens.

3 Whisk in lemon juice, and cook over medium heat until thickened and bubbly. Pour over asparagus and sprinkle with lemon rind. Serve immediately.

PER SERVING: *Calories 42 (From Fat 23); Fat 3g (Saturated 1g); Cholesterol 27mg; Sodium 32mg; Carbohydrate 2g (Dietary Fiber 1g); Protein 2g.*

Stir-Fried Asparagus

GREEN LIGHT

INGREDIENTS

1 pound fresh asparagus

2 tablespoons canola, corn, or peanut oil

½ teaspoon salt, or to taste

2 garlic cloves, thinly sliced

½ cup water

1 red bell pepper seeded, cored, and sliced into 2-inch-long julienne strips

1¼ teaspoons cornstarch, dissolved in 1 tablespoon water

DIRECTIONS

1 Cut or snap the tough ends from the asparagus. Remove the leaf scales from the bottom of the spears. Wash thoroughly under running water and drain. Roll-cut into 1½-inch lengths.

2 Pour the oil into a wok or stir-fry pan and place over high heat. Add the salt and garlic and stir around the pan until the oil is hot; the garlic will begin to sizzle. Add the asparagus and stir for about 1 minute. Pour in the water and cook, covered, over medium-high heat for about 2 minutes or until the asparagus are tender-crisp.

3 Stir in the red pepper and stir for 30 seconds to 1 minute, or until the pepper loses its raw look. Stir up the cornstarch slurry and pour it into the pan, stirring until the liquid thickens. Remove from the heat, taste, and add salt as desired. Serve hot.

NOTE: This simple stir-fry relies on the sweet freshness of springtime asparagus for flavor rather than on heavy spices. This dish pairs well with Onion-Lemon Fish or Grilled Chicken Breasts with Grapefruit Glaze in Chapter 14.

PER SERVING: *Calories 63 (From Fat 41); Fat 5g (Saturated 1g); Cholesterol 0mg; Sodium 203mg; Carbohydrate 5g (Dietary Fiber 2g); Protein 2g.*

Corn Medley

PREP TIME: 10 MIN	COOK TIME: 5 TO 7 MIN	YIELD: 6 SERVINGS (*1 SERVING EQUALS ONE CARBOHYDRATE CHOICE)

INGREDIENTS

10-ounce package frozen whole kernel corn*

½ cup chopped celery

1 teaspoon powdered chicken bouillon

⅓ cup water

2-ounce can sliced mushrooms, drained

1 or 2 medium Roma tomatoes, diced

Salt and pepper to taste

Splash of balsamic vinegar (optional)

DIRECTIONS

1 In a medium saucepan, combine the corn, celery, bouillon, and ⅓ cup water. Bring to a boil. Cover and simmer until vegetables are tender, about 5 to 7 minutes.

2 Stir in the mushrooms and diced tomatoes; heat through. Season to taste with salt and pepper. Add a splash or two of balsamic vinegar, if desired.

TIP: Frozen corn works much better than its canned cousin. The frozen variety seems crisper, fresher, and even a bit sweeter.

VARY It: To make it vegetarian and vegan, replace the chicken bouillon with a vegetable stock cube.

PER SERVING: *Calories 48 (From Fat 4); Fat 0g (Saturated 0g); Cholesterol 0mg; Sodium 190mg; Carbohydrate 11g (Dietary Fiber 2g); Protein 2g.*

🍅 Skillet Corn

PREP TIME: 15 MIN	COOK TIME: 12 TO 15 MIN	YIELD: 6 SERVINGS (*1 SERVING EQUALS ONE CARBOHYDRATE CHOICE)

INGREDIENTS

10 ears fresh corn*

½ cup 2 percent milk

1 teaspoon salt

⅛ teaspoon pepper

1 tablespoon plant butter

DIRECTIONS

1 Shuck corn and remove silk from ears. Cut kernels from cobs. Scrape cobs gently with back of knife to get juice.

2 Add milk, salt, and pepper to corn, and stir.

3 Melt plant butter in a heavy skillet. Pour corn mixture into skillet. Simmer until tender, stirring frequently.

PER SERVING: *Calories 192 (From Fat 48); Fat 5g (Saturated 2g); Cholesterol 7mg; Sodium 440mg; Carbohydrate 38g (Dietary Fiber 5g); Protein 7g.*

Baked Stuffed Potatoes

PREP TIME: 1 HR, 10 MIN	COOK TIME: 20 MIN	YIELD: 6 SERVINGS (*1 SERVING EQUALS ONE CARBOHYDRATE CHOICE)

INGREDIENTS

3 medium baking potatoes*

⅓ cup skim milk

½ teaspoon salt

Dash pepper

Dash paprika

Reduced-fat sharp cheddar cheese, grated

DIRECTIONS

1 Scrub potatoes; puncture skin with fork. Bake at 425 degrees for 1 hour. Cut potatoes in half lengthwise. Scoop out inside; mash.

2 Add milk, salt, and pepper to potato mash. Beat till fluffy, adding additional skim milk if needed. Pile lightly into shells; sprinkle with grated cheese. Return to oven until hot, about 10 minutes. Sprinkle with paprika.

PER SERVING: *Calories 111 (From Fat 15); Fat 2g (Saturated 1g); Cholesterol 5mg; Sodium 268mg; Carbohydrate 20g (Dietary Fiber 2g); Protein 5g.*

Low-Carb Crunchy Coleslaw

| PREP TIME: 15 MIN | COOK TIME: 0 MIN PLUS REFRIGERATION | YIELD: 8 SERVINGS |

INGREDIENTS

4 cups shredded cabbage

½ cup shredded carrots

⅓ cup lite mayo

2 tablespoons prepared mustard

2 tablespoons vinegar

½ teaspoon salt

DIRECTIONS

1 Combine all ingredients in a medium bowl. Toss gently to coat.

2 Cover and chill.

PER SERVING: *Calories 38 (From Fat 23); Fat 3g (Saturated 0g); Cholesterol 3mg; Sodium 280mg; Carbohydrate 4g (Dietary Fiber 1g); Protein 1g.*

Getting Some Natural Sweetness — Including Fruit Side Dishes

Fruit, with its naturally sweet flavor, is a great way to spark up a meal. Use lemon slices, small bunches of grapes, or small watermelon wedges to give a simple meal immediate pizzazz. Keep fresh fruit washed and handy, so it's readily available to the whole family for quick snacking. These great recipes give you useful ideas for incorporating fruits into your diet all day long.

Fruit always makes a nice side dish to any meal. It adds refreshing flavor to a meal and is a nice complement to savory dishes. These recipes contain a variety of options: fresh fruit, fruit in salads, and cooked fruit.

REMEMBER

Fruit salads are as satisfying as vegetable salads and can be used for any brunch, lunch, or dinner menu. Fruit can also be featured as the main ingredient in desserts, offering several nutritional benefits. Thanks to the natural sweetness of most fruit, you don't need to add any sugar. Fruit desserts also provide more vitamins, more fiber, and fewer calories than other types of desserts. The Peach Salad Cups in the following section have occasionally made an appearance on the dessert menu.

A WINTER FRUIT BOWL: JUST COMBINE AVAILABLE FRESH FRUIT WITH CANNED FRUIT

Because many fruits are unavailable during the winter, you can combine available fresh fruit with canned fruits and still enjoy your favorites all winter long. For example, mix available fruits like fresh kiwi and mango with year-round canned fruits like pineapples and mandarin oranges to make a large colorful and flavorful fruit bowl perfect for any fall or holiday meal. Try this combination of ingredients:

- 1 can, 11 ounces mandarin oranges, drain well

- 1 can, 20 ounces pineapple chunks, canned in own juice, drain well

- ½ pound fresh strawberries, sliced thin

- 3 kiwi fruits, skins removed and sliced into rounds and then halves

- 1 mango, sliced into bite sized chunks

Drain well and set all ingredients in a bowl so they can mingle. If desired, pour ½ cup or less Honey-Lime Dressing (see Chapter 12) over the fruit. Mix everything well together. Refrigerate for 2 hours or overnight for flavors to mingle. Mix well before serving.

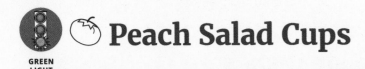

Peach Salad Cups

| PREP TIME: 20 MIN | COOK TIME: NONE | YIELD: 4 SERVINGS |

INGREDIENTS

2 medium to large peaches (about 6 to 8 ounces each), peeled, halved, and pitted

1 tablespoon lime juice, divided

½ cup fresh raspberries (or strawberries, quartered)

2 tablespoons unsweetened peach nectar

¼ teaspoon almond extract

1 packet of stevia (optional)

Curly leaf lettuce leaves (optional)

DIRECTIONS

1 Carefully scoop out the pulp from the peach halves, leaving a ¼-inch-thick shell. Chop the pulp, and set it aside. Brush the peach shells with 2 teaspoons lime juice to prevent browning. Set aside.

2 Combine the reserved pulp, the berries, the peach nectar, the remaining 1 teaspoon of lime juice, and the almond extract in a small bowl. Toss gently to coat. If it tastes a little too tart, add a packet of stevia. Spoon 3 tablespoons of the peach–berry mixture into each peach shell. Serve on curly-leaf lettuce leaves, if desired.

TIP: This recipe works best with ripe, in-season peaches. You can make it ahead — just cover and refrigerate until ready to serve.

TIP: Use a grapefruit knife to scoop out the peach pulp.

PER SERVING: *Calories 49 (From Fat 1); Fat 0g (Saturated 0g); Cholesterol 0mg; Sodium 0mg; Carbohydrate 13g (Dietary Fiber 3g); Protein 1g.*

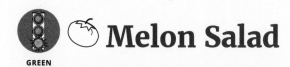

Melon Salad

PREP TIME: 15 MIN	COOK TIME: 0 MIN	YIELD: 8 TO 10 SERVINGS

INGREDIENTS

½ cantaloupe, cut into bite-size chunks

½ honeydew, cut into bite-size chunks

¼ seedless watermelon, cut into bite-size chunks

⅓ cup honey

2 tablespoons fresh lime juice

2 tablespoons fresh lemon juice

Mint sprigs (optional)

DIRECTIONS

1 Mix melon chunks gently together in large bowl.

2 Dissolve the lime and lemon juices into the honey. Add to fruit until desired sweetness.

TIP: When fruit is in season and full of flavor, keep this dish on hand for mealtime, snack time, or any time.

PER SERVING: *Calories 101 (From Fat 2); Fat 0g (Saturated 0g); Cholesterol 0mg; Sodium 6mg; Carbohydrate 26g (Dietary Fiber 1g); Protein 1g.*

Sweet and Spicy Oranges

PREP TIME: 20 MIN	COOK TIME: 0 MIN	YIELD: 8 SERVINGS (*½ CARBOHYDRATE CHOICE PER SERVING)

INGREDIENTS

8 large navel oranges

Few drops orange extract

1 tablespoon water

¼ cup powdered sugar*

¼ teaspoon cinnamon

DIRECTIONS

1 Finely grate the rind of 2 oranges; set the rind aside. Remove and discard the peel and pith of all oranges. Slice the oranges crosswise into ¼-inch-thick slices and arrange on a serving platter.

2 Mix the orange extract with water and sprinkle over the orange slices. Sift the powdered sugar over the top, and sprinkle with the reserved rind. Cover and refrigerate at least 2 hours. Sprinkle with cinnamon just before serving.

TIP: The rind, which is the top layer of orange peel that's scraped off, gives this dish its zesty tang. When you scrape the rind off the outside with a grater, avoid pushing through to the *pith* (the thick white fibrous layer before you get to the meat of the orange). The rind provides a great flavor while the pith is very bitter.

PER SERVING: *Calories 80 (From Fat 1); Fat 0g (Saturated 0g); Cholesterol 0mg; Sodium 58mg; Carbohydrate 20g (Dietary Fiber 4g); Protein 2g.*

GREEN LIGHT

🍅 Carol's Broiled Cinnamon Peaches

| PREP TIME: 10 MIN | COOK TIME: 5 TO 10 MIN | YIELD: 8 SERVINGS |

INGREDIENTS

Two 15-ounce cans peach halves canned in extra-light syrup

2 tablespoons plant butter

2 teaspoons Truvia brown sugar blend

DIRECTIONS

1 Drain the peaches. Place the peaches cut side up in a broiler pan. Dot the center of each peach with the plant butter. Sprinkle lightly with the brown sugar substitute. Sprinkle with cinnamon.

2 Broil approximately 5 to 10 minutes until browned.

VARY it: If you have an extra dairy serving left over, add ½ cup light vanilla ice cream with no sugar added.

PER SERVING: *Calories 43 (From Fat 14); Fat 2g (Saturated 0g); Cholesterol 0mg; Sodium 34mg; Carbohydrate 8g (Dietary Fiber 1g); Protein 0g.*

HOW TO MAKE VEGETARIAN OPTIONS VEGAN

If you're practicing a vegan lifestyle, ensure that you're getting enough soy products to maintain adequate calcium intake. Count soymilk as dairy and count all legumes as lean proteins. Consider taking a vitamin B_{12} supplement because vitamin B_{12} is only available from animal foods. Getting complete protein containing all the essential amino acids is also a concern with the vegan diet. Eating a variety of plant-protein sources ensures getting all the essential amino acids. The Registered Dietitian Nutritionists (RDNs) at the Cleveland Clinic listed these well-known vegan/vegetarian protein sources:

- **Beans:** A half cup of any bean variety packs 6 to 9 grams protein plus 6 to 8 grams of fiber.

- **Lentils:** Adding a half cup of cooked lentils (brown, green, or red) to soups, curries, tacos, or salads adds about 12 grams of protein to your meal.

- **Edamame:** Lightly boiled or steamed soybeans — often served in their shell — make a great snack or appetizer.

- **Tofu:** Made from soybeans, tofu is so versatile that you can use it in place of meat in a recipe or even as a base for creamy desserts. It provides 8 grams of protein per 3.5-ounce serving.

- **Tempeh:** Made from soybeans that are fermented and pressed into a block, tempeh is high in protein, prebiotics, and other nutrients. Because it's more compact than tofu, it's higher in protein — three ounces will provide 15 to 16 grams. Tempeh's firm but chewy texture makes it a good addition to sandwiches and salads. Or, crumble it to substitute for ground meat in recipes.

- **Grains:** Not only do grains count as a carbohydrate, they also pack a protein punch. A half-cup serving of oats adds 5 grams of protein to your morning meal. A quarter cup (uncooked) of barley or quinoa also adds 5 to 6 grams. Teff, millet, amaranth, and other ancient grains are also great options to mix up your meals.

- **Green peas:** Peas sometimes get a bad rap, but they're a great source of protein. One cup of cooked peas has 8 grams.

- **Nuts:** Technically a legume, the peanut packs the most protein out of all the commonly consumed nuts (9 grams per quarter-cup serving). Almonds and pistachios are close behind with 7 and 6 grams, respectively.

- **Seeds:** Seeds are a great source of protein and unsaturated fats. Sunflower seeds contain 8 grams of protein per ounce and pumpkin seeds contain 7 grams per ounce. Sprinkling hemp seeds on your morning oatmeal or toast adds 10 grams protein per ounce.

- **Plant-based beverages:** Some milk substitutes, such as soy milk and pea milk, have nearly as much protein as cow's milk. Look for unsweetened or lightly sweetened varieties.

- **Nutritional yeast:** The secret ingredient in many vegan "cheese" sauces, nutritional yeast is a great source of protein and B vitamins. One tablespoon sprinkled on top of your meal adds 2 grams of protein.

- **Vegetables:** Though not the most abundant sources of protein, if your diet is heavy in vegetables, you'll get a decent amount of protein. For example, a cup of cooked Brussels sprouts contributes 4 grams of protein. Leafy greens like spinach, watercress, and bok choy have a high protein content per calorie.

MEAT SUBSTITUTES: Faux meat products can make the transition to a plant-based diet easier for meat lovers, but they aren't all healthy. Choose options with minimal ingredients, ample protein, and reasonable amounts of saturated fat and sodium. Many of these food products are made from soybeans and some are listed on the ingredient panel as texturized vegetable protein (TVP). *TVP* is nothing more than heavily processed soybeans and isn't a good choice. Be sure to scrutinize the ingredient panel of meat substitutes. Some of these products have preservatives, sugar, inflammatory oils, or other ingredients you don't want.

Chapter **16**

No Sacrifices Made: Tasty Desserts and Refreshing Beverages

Does being on a low carb diet mean never eating a sweet treat again? Well, not on the Whole Foods Weight Loss Eating Plan. That's where those one to five carb choices that I discuss in Chapter 6 come into play. Everyone likes a little sweet at the end of a satisfying meal or a nice hot beverage on a rainy or snowy day. Most of the recipes in this chapter are Green Light, meaning you don't count them at all, and you can even eat them freely as a snack, but a few of them do count in your Yellow Light category so you will need to make room for them. (*Note:* Any recipe not with a Green Light icon is a Yellow Light food.)

Ending Your Meal on a Sweet Note: Low-Carb Desserts

Desserts can be heavenly and are a highly anticipated ending to a meal. However, topping off an impressive meal with a disastrously rich dessert can leave you feeling stuffed and sluggish. Fresh fruit can be a far better conclusion for all your guests. Fruit in either cup, salad, or sherbet form can serve as a "lightener" during, as well as after, a meal. If you want a little richer post-meal treat, dessert may be a good place to spend one or two of those five carbohydrate choices you're allowed each day. But it's nice to know that with these great fruit dessert recipes, you don't have to!

REMEMBER

No foods (not even desserts) are absolutely off-limits on this dieting plan. If you watch your portion sizes and try the helpful tips that limit unnecessary sugars, you can still enjoy sweet treats and tasty snacks.

You can eat sweets and sugar, if you count the carbohydrate they contain. The issue is that sugars and sweets don't have vitamins and minerals, but they do have a lot of calories, even in small servings. My best recommendation is to avoid hidden sugars in food, especially refined, pre-packaged, and processed foods. Make the sugar you eat count. Did you really enjoy that fat-free cookie? Probably not, but it likely contained 12 grams of carbs, which is equivalent to eating an entire tablespoon of sugar. You'd probably be more satisfied with ¾ cup of fresh strawberries, which contain the same number of carbs, have way more fiber and nutrients, and are pretty darn filling. And don't forget, strawberries are free to you — whereas the fat-free cookie will cost you one carb choice for the day.

Fruits are the original nutritious fast foods and make great grab-and-go desserts. They're healthy, packaged in individual servings, and can serve as a wonderful tasty dessert. Buy your fruits in season at the peak of ripeness. Nothing is sweeter than fresh watermelon, cantaloupe, peaches, cherries, and berries.

GREEN LIGHT

Poached Pears with Raspberry-Almond Purée

PREP TIME: 20 MIN	COOK TIME: 40 TO 50 MIN (PLUS COOLING TIME)	YIELD: 4 SERVINGS

INGREDIENTS

1½ cups water

Sugar-substitute equivalent to ¾ cup sugar

½ teaspoon cinnamon

Juice from 1 lemon, approximately 3 tablespoons

4 whole pears, peeled, stems left on

10 ounces frozen raspberries, thawed

¼ teaspoon almond extract

4 teaspoons chopped almonds

DIRECTIONS

1 Bring water, sugar substitute, cinnamon, and lemon juice to a boil in a covered, deep saucepan. Add the pears to the boiling liquid. If the pears aren't covered, add water until they are. Return to a simmer, cover, and cook 20 to 30 minutes or until firm-tender. Cool in cooking liquid, until cool enough to handle.

2 Gently core the pears from the bottom, removing the seeds. Puree the raspberries and almond extract in a blender.

3 Serve raspberry purée over or under the pears. Sprinkle with chopped almonds.

PER SERVING: *Calories 165 (From Fat 19); Fat 2g (Saturated 0g); Cholesterol 0mg; Sodium 1mg; Carbohydrate 38g (Dietary Fiber 5g); Protein 2g.*

🍅 Peach Yogurt Freeze

PREP TIME: 40 MIN	COOK TIME: 5 MIN (PLUS FREEZING TIME)	YIELD: 8 SERVINGS

INGREDIENTS

1 envelope unflavored gelatin (¼ ounce)

½ cup cold water

2 eggs

1 tablespoon, plus 2 teaspoons Truvia Spoonable

½ cup unsweetened orange juice

Two 16-ounce cartons low-fat vanilla yogurt

3 cups peeled, chopped fresh peaches

DIRECTIONS

1 Soften the gelatin in cold water in a small saucepan; let stand 1 minute. Cook over medium heat, stirring constantly, until gelatin dissolves. Set aside.

2 Beat the eggs and Truvia Spoonable until thick and lemon colored. Stir in the reserved gelatin mixture, the orange juice, and the yogurt. Place the peaches in an electric blender or food processor; process until smooth. Add the pureed peaches to the yogurt mixture; stir well.

3 Pour the peach mixture into the freezer can of a hand-turned or electric ice-cream freezer. Freeze according to the manufacturer's instructions. Scoop the peach mixture into individual dessert bowls, and serve immediately.

VARY IT: Experiment with whatever fruits are your favorite. It's great with strawberries or raspberries if you don't mind a few seeds.

TIP: To speed up the preparation, look for frozen fruit with no added sugar. It can save you valuable peeling and coring time.

NOTE: Each serving equals one serving of milk and free fruit.

PER SERVING (1 CUP): *Calories 108 (From Fat 19); Fat 2g (Saturated 1g); Cholesterol 56mg; Sodium 55mg; Carbohydrate 18g (Dietary Fiber 1g); Protein 6g.*

FROZEN DESSERT FREAKS, APPLY HERE

If you're a dessert freak, an ice-cream freezer is a great addition to your low-carb lifestyle. If you make your own yogurt, ice cream, or sorbet, you can control the amount of sugar you add to any recipe and ensure that you're using delicious fresh fruit every time. Or you may choose to use one of the great new natural sugar-substitutes I describe in Chapter 6. Most freezers come with a recipe book that includes sugar-free and low-sugar recipes.

GREEN LIGHT

🍅 Maple Apple Rings

PREP TIME: 25 MIN	COOK TIME: 15 MIN	YIELD: 4 SERVINGS

INGREDIENTS

4 medium baking apples, cored and thinly sliced into rings

3 tablespoons reduced-calorie maple syrup

1 tablespoon plant butter, melted

½ teaspoon ground cinnamon

⅛ teaspoon ground nutmeg

¼ cup sliced almonds

DIRECTIONS

1 Preheat oven to 350 degrees.

2 Arrange the apple rings evenly in a 1½-quart baking dish sprayed with nonstick cooking spray. Combine the syrup, plant butter, cinnamon, and nutmeg, stirring well. Spoon the syrup mixture evenly over the apples. Sprinkle the almonds over the syrup mixture. Cover the dish. Bake 15 minutes or until apples are tender.

VARY IT: Vary the baking time based on your preference. The apples are crisp-tender after about 15 minutes, but if you like really tender apples, go for 30 minutes.

PER SERVING: *Calories 161 (From Fat 57); Fat 6g (Saturated 1g); Cholesterol 0mg; Sodium 60mg; Carbohydrate 27g (Dietary Fiber 5g); Protein 2g.*

A NOTE ON LOW-CALORIE SWEETENERS

Low-calorie sweeteners add a taste to foods and beverages similar to sugar. Most don't contain calories and those that do are used in very small amounts because of their concentrated sweetening power. Thus, they add essentially no calories to foods and beverages. These sweeteners practically eliminate or substantially reduce the calories in some foods and beverages such as carbonated soft drinks, light yogurt, sugar-free puddings, and your favorite homemade desserts.

Low-calorie sweeteners result in a wide range of food choices that can help you manage your intake of calories and carbs. Using these sweeteners may help you in the early stages to reduce your carbohydrate intake. Currently researchers have discovered a wide range of natural sweeteners to replace the artificial sweeteners from times past. Always check the conversion table on the package to know how much low-calorie sweetener equals how much sugar.

🍅 Pineapple Sundaes

PREP TIME: 15 MIN | **COOK TIME: 20 MIN** | **YIELD: 6 SERVINGS**

INGREDIENTS

8-ounce can pineapple tidbits in own juice

1 tablespoon Truvia brown sugar blend

1 tablespoon water

2 teaspoons cornstarch

3 tablespoons raisins

2 teaspoons plant butter

¼ teaspoon ground cinnamon

⅛ teaspoon ground nutmeg

½ teaspoon vanilla extract

3 cups light vanilla ice cream

1 tablespoon unsweetened flaked coconut, toasted

DIRECTIONS

1 Drain the pineapple, reserving the juice. Set the pineapple aside. Combine the reserved juice, brown sugar blend, water, and cornstarch in a small non–aluminum saucepan; stir well. Cook over medium heat until thickened, stirring constantly. Stir in the pineapple, raisins, plant butter, cinnamon, and nutmeg. Cook over low heat, stirring frequently, until thoroughly heated. Stir in the vanilla.

2 To serve, place ½ cup light ice cream in individual dessert dishes. Spoon 3 tablespoons warm pineapple mixture over each serving of ice cream. Sprinkle ½ teaspoon coconut over each serving. Serve immediately.

NOTE: Pineapple is so naturally sweet, you don't need the heavy or even light syrup found in some canned fruit.

NOTE: The amount of cornstarch is negligible, so this recipe is a Green Light.

TIP: Look for it canned in its own juice. If you have some extra fat choices for the day, consider adding some toasted nuts on top.

NOTE: Each sundae equals one serving of milk and free fruit.

PER SERVING: *Calories 191 (From Fat 56); Fat 6g (Saturated 3g); Cholesterol 35mg; Sodium 62mg; Carbohydrate 32g (Dietary Fiber 1g); Protein 3g.*

GREEN LIGHT

Sparkling Fresh Fruit Cup

PREP TIME: 25 MIN	COOK TIME: NONE	YIELD: 8 SERVINGS

INGREDIENTS

4 medium-size fresh pears, cored and diced

2 tablespoons lemon juice

2 cups halved fresh strawberries

¾ pound fresh plums, pitted and thinly sliced

2 cups peeled, diced fresh peaches

2 cups sparkling apple cider, chilled

Fresh mint sprigs (optional)

DIRECTIONS

1 Place diced pears in a large bowl, and sprinkle with lemon juice; toss gently. Add strawberries, plums, and peaches; toss gently to combine.

2 To serve, place 1 cup fruit mixture in individual dessert cups. Pour ¼ cup sparkling apple cider over each serving. Garnish with fresh mint sprigs, if desired. Serve immediately.

VARY IT: If any fruit in the recipe isn't in season, feel free to substitute your favorites. You can even substitute canned fruit if absolutely necessary, but I recommend draining the fruit before combining it with the sparkling cider.

TIP: Substitute a stevia-sweetened ginger ale or lemon-lime soda for the sparkling apple cider.

PER SERVING: *Calories 138 (From Fat 8); Fat 1g (Saturated 0g); Cholesterol 0mg; Sodium 1mg; Carbohydrate 35g (Dietary Fiber 4g); Protein 1g.*

Cranberry-Grape Sorbet

PREP TIME: 15 MIN (PLUS FREEZING TIME)	COOK TIME: NONE	YIELD: 12 SERVINGS

INGREDIENTS

2½ cups cran-grape juice cocktail

½ cup sparkling apple juice

1 egg white

1 packet sugar substitute

DIRECTIONS

1 Pour the cran-grape juice cocktail into two freezer-safe trays; freeze until almost firm. Spoon the mixture into a large mixing bowl, and beat at high speed of an electric mixer until slushy. Gently stir in the sparkling apple juice. Again using an electric mixer, beat the egg white (at room temperature) at high speed for 1 minute. Add the sugar substitute, beating until soft peaks form. Carefully fold the beaten egg white into the juice mixture.

2 Pour into the freezer can of a hand-turned or electric ice-cream freezer. Freeze according to the manufacturer's instructions. Scoop the sorbet into individual dessert bowls, and serve immediately.

VARY IT: You can substitute diet grapefruit soda (like Fresca) or lemon-lime soda for the apple juice, if you prefer.

PER SERVING (½ CUP): *Calories 36 (From Fat 1); Fat 0g (Saturated 0g); Cholesterol 0mg; Sodium 6mg; Carbohydrate 9g (Dietary Fiber 0g); Protein 0g.*

**GREEN
LIGHT**

Frosty Fruit Cup

PREP TIME: 10 MIN (PLUS FREEZING TIME)	COOK TIME: NONE	YIELD: 8 SERVINGS

INGREDIENTS

15-ounce can pineapple chunks, in own juice

16 ounces diet lemon-lime carbonated beverage

2 tablespoons lime juice

Few drops green food coloring

1 cup seedless green grapes

2 cups cantaloupe balls

Mint sprigs, if desired

DIRECTIONS

1   Drain the pineapple, reserving the juice. Combine the reserved juice, carbonated beverage, lime juice, and food coloring; stir. Pour into a 3-cup refrigerator-safe tray; freeze just to a mush, about 2 to 2½ hours. A few stirs every 30 minutes or so will help keep it slushy.

2   Combine the pineapple chunks, grapes, and cantaloupe. Break the frozen mixture apart with a fork, if necessary. Spoon into 8 sherbet glasses; top with fruits. Garnish with mint sprigs, if desired.

PER SERVING: *Calories 61 (From Fat 2); Fat 0g (Saturated 0g); Cholesterol 0mg; Sodium 16mg; Carbohydrate 15g (Dietary Fiber 1g); Protein 1g.*

Baked Crimson Pears

| PREP TIME: 15 MIN | COOK TIME: 30 MIN | YIELD: 8 SERVINGS |

INGREDIENTS

4 fresh medium pears

1 cup low-calorie cranberry juice cocktail

3 inches stick cinnamon

10 drops red food color (optional)

DIRECTIONS

1 Peel, halve, and core pears; place in 1-quart casserole.

2 Mix cranberry juice cocktail, stick cinnamon, and red food coloring, if using; bring to boiling. Pour over pears.

3 Bake, covered, at 350 degrees for 10 minutes. Turn pears; bake, covered, 10 minutes. Turn pears; bake, uncovered, till tender, 5 to 10 minutes more. Remove cinnamon stick. Serve in juice.

PER SERVING: *Calories 107 (From Fat 2); Fat 0g (Saturated 0g); Cholesterol 0mg; Sodium 4mg; Carbohydrate 28g (Dietary Fiber 5g); Protein 1g.*

Chocolate-Almond Crisps

PREP TIME: 15 MIN	COOK TIME: 40 MIN	YIELD: 12 SERVINGS (*1 CARBOHYDRATE CHOICE PER SERVING)

INGREDIENTS

2 egg whites at room temperature

¾ cup, plus 2 tablespoons sifted powdered sugar*

3 tablespoons, plus 1½ teaspoons unsweetened cocoa

¼ cup semisweet chocolate mini-morsels*

¼ cup finely chopped blanched almonds

½ teaspoon almond extract

Vegetable cooking spray

DIRECTIONS

1 Preheat oven to 300 degrees.

2 Beat egg whites at high speed of electric mixer for 1 minute. Combine the sugar and cocoa; gradually add the sugar mixture to the egg whites, 1 tablespoon at a time, beating until stiff peaks form and the sugar dissolves, 2 to 4 minutes. Fold in mini-morsels, almonds, and almond extract.

3 Drop by teaspoonfuls, 1 inch apart, onto cookie sheets that have been lined with parchment paper. Bake for 40 minutes or until set. Cool slightly on cookie sheets; gently remove to wire racks, and cool completely. Store in an airtight container.

NOTE: These tasty morsels are great for chocoholics everywhere. And you can't get a better source of vitamin E than almonds.

PER SERVING (3 CRISPS): *Calories 80 (From Fat 23); Fat 2.5g (Saturated 1g); Cholesterol 0mg; Sodium 7mg; Carbohydrate 3g (Dietary Fiber 0g); Protein 2g.*

🍅 Peanutty Cupcakes

PREP TIME: 25 MIN

COOK TIME: 20 MIN

YIELD: 12 CUPCAKES
(*1 CARBOHYDRATE
CHOICE PER SERVING)

INGREDIENTS

2 ounces Neufchatel cheese, softened

3 tablespoons no-sugar-added creamy peanut butter

1 tablespoon honey

½ cup quick cooking oats, uncooked*

¾ cup boiling water

⅓ cup vegetable oil

Brown sugar substitute equivalent to ½ cup packed brown sugar

1 egg

½ teaspoon vanilla extract

¾ cup all-purpose flour

½ teaspoon baking soda

1 teaspoon ground cinnamon

½ teaspoon ground cloves

¼ teaspoon ground nutmeg

⅛ teaspoon salt

DIRECTIONS

1 Preheat oven to 375 degrees. Combine the Neufchatel cheese, peanut butter, and honey in a small bowl, stirring well; set aside. Combine the oats and boiling water in a small bowl, stirring well. Set aside, and let cool.

2 Gradually combine the oil and brown sugar substitute, beating well at medium speed. Add the egg and vanilla, beating well. In a separate bowl, combine the flour, baking soda, cinnamon, cloves, nutmeg, and salt. Alternately add the flour mixture and oatmeal mixture to the creamed mixture, beginning and ending with the flour mixture. Mix well after each addition, scraping the sides of the bowl often.

3 Spoon ⅔ cup of batter into each of 12 paper–lined muffin cups. Put ½ tablespoon of the peanut butter mixture on top of the batter. Bake for 20 minutes. Remove the cupcakes from pans, and let cool on wire racks.

TIP: Reusable, nonstick baking sheets work great for lining cookie sheets. A product from France made by Silpat replaces pan-greasing or cooking spray. The Silpat sheet makes for easy cleanup. You can find them in most kitchen stores.

PER SERVING: *Calories 160 (From Fat 90); Fat 10g (Saturated 2g); Cholesterol 21mg; Sodium 116mg; Carbohydrate 19g (Dietary Fiber 1g); Protein 3g.*

Key Lime Pudding Cakes

PREP TIME: 15 MIN	COOK TIME: 5 MIN (PLUS 4 MIN STANDING TIME)	YIELD: 6 SERVING (*½ CARBOHYDRATE CHOICE PER SERVING)

INGREDIENTS

1 tablespoon, plus 2 teaspoons Truvia Spoonable

⅓ cup all-purpose flour*

¼ teaspoon salt

2 eggs, separated, at room temperature

¾ cup skim milk

2 tablespoons key lime juice

1 tablespoon lime zest

Vegetable cooking spray

Lime slices, fresh berries, fresh mint sprigs for garnish (optional)

DIRECTIONS

1 Combine the Truvia Spoonable, flour, and salt in a medium bowl; set aside. Beat the egg yolks at the high speed of an electric mixer until thick and lemon colored; add the milk and lime juice, beating well. Mix in the dry ingredients; beat well. Set aside.

2 Beat the egg whites at the high speed of an electric mixer until soft peaks form. Gently fold the egg whites and lime zest into the milk–egg yolk mixture. Pour the batter evenly into six 6-ounce custard cups that have been coated with cooking spray.

3 Place 3 custard cups in the microwave. Microwave, uncovered, at medium-high (70-percent power) for 2 to 2½ minutes, rotating a half-turn after 1 minute. Let stand 2 minutes. Repeat with the remaining custard cups. If desired, garnish with berries, lime slices, and fresh mint sprigs. Serve warm.

NOTE: Refer to the color insert for a photo of Key Lime Pudding Cakes.

PER SERVING: *Calories 68 (From Fat 16); Fat 2g (Saturated 1g); Cholesterol 71mg; Sodium 134mg; Carbohydrate 9g (Dietary Fiber 0g); Protein 4g.*

Thumbprint Cookies

INGREDIENTS

Nonstick cooking spray

8-ounce package Sweet 'n Low sugar-free low-fat yellow cake mix*

3 tablespoons orange juice

2 teaspoons grated orange peel

½ teaspoon almond extract

4 teaspoons peach all-fruit spread

2 tablespoons almonds, chopped

DIRECTIONS

1 Preheat oven to 350 degrees. Spray baking sheets with non-stick cooking spray.

2 Beat the cake mix, orange juice, orange peel, and almond extract in a medium bowl with an electric mixer at medium speed for 2 minutes, until the mixture looks crumbly. Increase the speed to medium and beat 2 minutes or until smooth dough forms. Dough will be very sticky. Coat your hands with nonstick cooking spray. Roll the dough into 1-inch balls.

3 Place the balls 2½ inches apart on prepared baking sheets. Press the center of each ball with your thumb. Fill each thumbprint with ¼ teaspoon fruit spread. Sprinkle with nuts. Bake 8 to 9 minutes or until cookies are light golden brown and lose their shininess. Don't overbake. Remove to wire racks; cool completely.

VARY IT: Try any flavor of all-fruit spread that appeals to you. Raspberry and apricot make delicious variations.

TIP: The cake mix is available online if you have trouble finding it at your supermarket.

PER SERVING: *Calories 87 (From Fat 44); Fat 5g (Saturated 1g); Cholesterol 0mg; Sodium 15mg; Carbohydrate 12g (Dietary Fiber 1g); Protein 1g.*

GREEN LIGHT

Cranberry Ice Delight

PREP TIME: 5 MIN (PLUS FREEZING TIME)	COOK TIME: 8 MIN	YIELD: 6 SERVINGS

INGREDIENTS

2 tablespoons, plus 1 teaspoon Truvia Spoonable

½ envelope unflavored gelatin, approximately 1½ teaspoons

Dash salt

2 cups reduced-calorie cranberry juice cocktail, divided

1 tablespoon lemon juice

DIRECTIONS

1 In a saucepan, combine the Truvia Spoonable, gelatin, and salt. Stir in 1 cup of the cranberry juice cocktail. Heat and stir over medium heat until the Truvia Spoonable and gelatin dissolve. Remove from the heat. Stir in the additional 1 cup of cranberry juice cocktail and 1 tablespoon lemon juice.

2 Freeze in a 3-cup refrigerator tray until firm. Break into chunks; in a chilled bowl, beat with an electric mixer until smooth. Return the cranberry mixture to the tray; freeze until firm. To serve, break into chunks with a fork and spoon into individual dessert dishes.

TIP: Don't forget to chill the beater along with the mixing bowl; otherwise, you'll have a super-slushy mess on your hands.

PER SERVING: *Calories 26 (From Fat 0); Fat 0g (Saturated 0g); Cholesterol 0mg; Sodium 27mg; Carbohydrate 6g (Dietary Fiber 0g); Protein 1g.*

Drinking Your Way in a Low-Carb Diet

The job of beverages in a meal is to complement not overpower the food. Who doesn't enjoy a soothing tea during a meal or a relaxing coffee at the end of the meal?

WARNING

Beverages are a major source of excess sugars in the western diet. Replacing those beverages with a noncalorie or low-calorie drink is important to maintaining your low-carb diet. Coffee, tea, water, and diet beverages with healthy sweeteners like stevia leaf extract, erythritol, or monk fruit that I discuss in Chapter 6 can fill the gap.

The beverage recipes in this section are great additions to any breakfast, lunch, or dinner. Enjoy these nourishing beverages any time.

INFUSE YOUR WATER WITH YOUR FAVORITE TASTES

From a health standpoint, water is the best beverage, but many people just don't like the taste of plain water. If that's you, try fruit-, vegetable-, and herb-infused waters as good alternatives. Even though many flavored bottled waters are available to buy, you can make your own. Some good combinations include any of the following (or create your own):

- Strawberry, lemon, and mint
- Orange and lime slices
- Strawberry and pineapple
- Cucumber and lemon slices

Wash all your produce before infusing even if you're going to peel it. Cut up or slice thinly your fruit and veggies, place them in the bottom of a fruit jar or pitcher, and add fresh water. Refrigerate at least a couple of hours (overnight is better).

Some nifty fruit infuser water bottles are available if you're looking for a gift for a friend or yourself. If you prefer to drink a soda every day, switching from a regular soda to a zero-calorie alternative makes sense. But be wary of how many carbonated beverages you drink a day. Some evidence shows that carbonated beverages, regular or diet, can make you hungrier. An occasional regular soda or other carbonated beverage isn't going to harm you; however, if you choose a regular soda, be sure to count the carbs as one or more of your carb choices. **Remember:** A 12-ounce can of regular soda has 40 grams of carb (sugar) and counts as 3 carb choices!

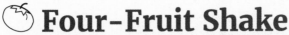# Four-Fruit Shake

PREP TIME: 5 MIN	COOK TIME: NONE	YIELD: SIX SERVINGS (*¼ CARBOHYDRATE CHOICE PER SERVING)

INGREDIENTS

1 cup unsweetened orange juice

1 cup skim milk

1½ cups fresh or frozen strawberries, washed and hulled

8-ounce can unsweetened crushed pineapple, undrained

1 medium-size ripe banana*

¼ teaspoon coconut extract

1 cup ice cubes

Fresh strawberry slices, optional

DIRECTIONS

1 Combine the orange juice, milk, strawberries, pineapple, banana, and coconut extract in an electric blender; process until smooth.

2 Add the ice cubes, and process until smooth. Pour into glasses and garnish with strawberry slices, if desired. Serve immediately.

VARY IT! For an ultra-smooth shake, substitute crushed ice for ice cubes. Your blender will do less work and thank you for it.

VARY IT! Keep your proportions of fruit and liquid the same, but feel free to substitute any fruits you have on hand. Just remember to count the banana (if you're using one) in your carbohydrate count for the day. One of my favorite variations substitutes freshly peeled kiwi for half the strawberries. Mango and papaya are also great choices. Blueberries make an excellent addition as well, and kids love the funky color to spice up their breakfast routine.

PER SERVING (1 CUP): *Calories 85 (From Fat 4); Fat 0g (Saturated 0g); Cholesterol 0mg; Sodium 23mg; Carbohydrate 19g (Dietary Fiber 2g); Protein 2g.*

Peppermint Cocoa

PREP TIME: 3 MIN	COOK TIME: 5 TO 7 MIN	YIELD: FOUR SERVINGS (¼* CARBOHYDRATE CHOICE PER SERVING)

INGREDIENTS

3 tablespoons unsweetened cocoa

3 teaspoons Truvia Spoonable

⅛ teaspoons salt

⅓ cup water

2 cups skim milk

¼ teaspoon peppermint extract

DIRECTIONS

1 In a large saucepan, combine the cocoa, Truvia Spoonable, salt, and water; mix well.

2 Cook over medium heat, stirring constantly, until the mixture comes to a rolling boil. Gradually stir in the milk and peppermint. Heat just to boiling. Serve hot.

TIP: For a special holiday treat, look for sugar-free candy canes and use them to decorate and stir your cocoa at the same time.

PER SERVING (½ CUP): *Calories 54 (From Fat 5); Fat 1g (Saturated 0g); Cholesterol 3mg; Sodium 137mg; Carbohydrate 9g (Dietary Fiber 1g); Protein 5g.*

GREEN LIGHT

Hot Tomato Refresher

PREP TIME: 5 MIN	COOK TIME: 8 TO 10 MIN	YIELD: 12 SERVINGS

INGREDIENTS

Two 24-ounce cans vegetable juice cocktail

2 tablespoons lemon juice

2 teaspoons Worcestershire sauce

½ teaspoon ground allspice

Lemon slices (optional)

DIRECTIONS

1 In a large saucepan, combine all the ingredients, except the lemon slices. Heat through, but don't boil.

2 Just before serving, float thin lemon slices atop the hot beverage, if desired.

VARY IT! You can add 1½ cups of vodka to create a warm wintry Bloody Mary. Just make sure you count one carb choice for each serving.

PER SERVING (4 OUNCES): *Calories 25 (From Fat 0); Fat 0g (Saturated 0g); Cholesterol 0mg; Sodium 299mg; Carbohydrate 5g (Dietary Fiber 1g); Protein 1g.*

Pineapple–Peach Smoothie

PREP TIME: 15 MIN	COOK TIME: NONE	YIELD: 3 SERVINGS

INGREDIENTS

½ cup canned pineapple chunks in juice, undrained

½ cup unsweetened pineapple juice

2 canned peach halves in water, drained and diced

1 cup low-fat plain yogurt

1 cup low-fat milk

2 ½ teaspoons Truvia Spoonable

DIRECTIONS

1 Combine pineapple chunks, pineapple juice, and peaches in an electric blender or food processor; cover and process until pureed.

2 Add yogurt, milk, and Truvia Spoonable; continue to process until smooth and thickened.

3 Pour into individual glasses, and serve immediately. Refrigerate any leftovers.

NOTE: The color insert has a photo of a Pineapple-Peach Smoothie.

PER SERVING: *Calories 155 (From Fat 17); Fat 2g (Saturated 1g); Cholesterol 9mg; Sodium 96mg; Carbohydrate 26g (Dietary Fiber 1g); Protein 8g.*

4

Sticking to the Plan

Chapter **17**

Eating Out without Apologies

E ating away from home is so common that it's almost an assumption. A friend of mine says that when she tells her family it's time to eat, they all get in the car! Eating away from home has increased dramatically, and many people feel that you can't possibly eat out and follow a healthy diet at the same time.

In the past, eating out was rare for the typical family and considered a special occasion. When families did go out to eat, it was usually to an independently run restaurant with a variety of foods on the menu. However, today Americans eat out more than ever before. The traditional family meal with all family members present, eating together, and leaving the table at the same time is unfortunately the exception rather than the rule. Work schedules, school schedules, sports games, band practice, and other activities have family members leaving and arriving home in different time zones. People eat in the car, at the counter, in front of the TV, and wherever else is convenient; people run errands on their lunch hour and eat snacks at their desks.

Knowing how to find healthy, low-carb options no matter where you eat is crucial. In this chapter, I tell you everything you need to know to do exactly that.

Making Smart Choices in Restaurants

If you eat out frequently, it just stands to reason that every meal can't possibly be a "treat." Instead of being "special," those away-from-home meals need to reflect how you would eat at home when you can. Why? Because when you eat at home, you have a more balanced diet. But you still need to watch portion sizes — portions at home have gotten bigger, just as they have in restaurants. When you eat out, *especially* if you eat out often, you have to be more discerning in your food selections and more resistant to those restaurant marketing messages trying to get you to eat more than you need. When you eat out, enjoy being waited on and be happy you don't have to clean up, but stay in control of what you eat.

TIP

Train yourself to give the menu a more critical review and look beyond traditional entrees for food choices on the menu. Often an appetizer and soup or salad are very satisfying choices. Look for fresh fruit cups for dessert instead of loading up on rich, heavy cakes and pies.

The following sections can make the decision of choosing what you'll eat in restaurants easier by providing tips on what to look for on the menu and why being aware of portion control is so important.

Studying the menu in advance

Planning ahead makes all the difference when you first begin a new dieting regimen, and choosing a low-carb life style is no exception. Create a plan *before* you order, at least until low-carb eating becomes second nature.

When you aren't hungry, study the online (or carry-out) menus of restaurants you like to frequent. Keep the following pointers in mind:

>> **Train yourself to fully examine the menu, not just pick the first thing that grabs your eye.** Pizza joints have salads bars, Mexican restaurants usually have soup and salads, and you can skip the fried rice in a Chinese restaurant.

>> **Look at the different types of dishes.** Think beyond the traditional entree. Mark items on the menu that you would enjoy eating but are also more nutritious.

   Also, look at the appetizer list. Mark the ones that aren't heavy with starch or fat. Look at the soup and salad list and then the entree items.

>> **Inspect how the dishes are prepared.** Look for broiled, grilled, or baked items. Keep your balance. Look for more lean protein, fruits, and vegetables (ask for veggies without butter).

Many chain restaurants now have calorie counts and other nutritional informa-tion listed directly online or on the physical menu. Even though the carb count may not be available, you can still utilize this information. The calorie levels are based on 2,000 calories per day for women and up to 2,500 calories per day for men. So, if you're eyeing that taco salad thinking it's a healthy choice, but you see it contains 1,000 calories, maybe you should rethink that choice. That's half of your daily allotment. Make your choice around 600-700 calories per meal and look at the carb choices in that meal. Choose the meal with the fewer starchy carb choices. Consider the fajita salad as an alternate — just don't eat the bowl.

Go for a test meal. Select a restaurant and decide to make healthy choices. Use the carry-out or online menu to pre-select your order. Bring a supportive dining partner and make your order for the healthier choice. Do the same thing at a fast-food restaurant. Go through a drive-thru and make the healthiest choice possible. The more times you do that, the easier it'll be to do it the next time.

If you aren't sure which options to choose on the menu, check out the following sections for tips on great low-carb ordering in a restaurant.

Appetizers

Select a smarter appetizer. Start your meals with a bowl of broth-based (not cream-based) soup, salad, fresh fruit, or raw vegetables. Other good choices are tomato juice, clear broth, bouillon, consommé, marinated vegetables, a fresh fruit cup, or steamed fresh seafood.

Salads

Almost any salad in a restaurant is better than no salad at all. Look for tossed vegetables, like the traditional lettuce/sliced-tomato/cucumber combo. Or protein-based dishes that include cottage cheese. If you can't be sure that the restaurant serves light or low-calorie dressings, opt for lemon juice or vinegar. And always get it on the side. Forego any croutons or bread that may come with the salad unless you've factored them into your carb choices.

Entrees

Order roasted, baked, broiled, or grilled meat, poultry, fish, or seafood. Look for lean meats with the fat trimmed. For more on the best lean proteins, check out Chapter 5. Order your gravy or sauce on the side. Instead of a dinner entree, con-sider combining a salad with a low-fat appetizer.

Vegetables

French fries aren't vegetables! They used to be (in their raw form, as potatoes), but after they're peeled and fried, they lose their vegetable status. Look for raw, stewed, steamed, boiled, or stir-fried vegetables. Just about any veggie is a good veggie, until you deep-fry it, so avoid the onion rings, fried mushrooms, fried okra, and so on.

Desserts

Cut back on the sweet stuff. Instead try fresh fruit or fresh fruit juice, fat-free or low-fat yogurt, or gelatin desserts. If you must have a sweet ending to your meal, split the dessert with one or more of your friends. Order one dessert for the table and give everyone a taste.

Beverages

Go for black coffee, plain tea, sugar-free soda, or water with lemon. Avoid sugary soft drinks.

Assessing portion sizes

Restaurants are known for big portions and enticements to eat more. Value-added meals with extra-large soft drinks and fries are hard to turn down. You're better off reducing your portion size from the beginning by not ordering the large size. Recent studies indicate that people eat as much as they're served. If a regular-size burger will satisfy your hunger, but you order the jumbo burger, you'll eat all of the larger burger. Find out how to recognize that comfortable feeling at the end of a meal and avoid that stuffed feeling. Note how much better your afternoon goes when you don't overeat.

Try to keep the portion sizes appropriate. If you know the portions are too large, set some aside to take home at the beginning of the meal, not at the end. Take out the food you're reserving for later and then eat the rest.

If you've forgotten what a portion should look like, check out the guidelines for portion sizes in Chapter 4. Start measuring foods at home until you have a good understanding of a reasonable portion.

Splitting entrees

Splitting an entree with a dining partner is a good way to have a satisfying meal, reduce calories, and save money. But first ask the waiter if the restaurant allows it. Some restaurants allow you to split the entree but will bring doubles of the side items like bread or potatoes. That won't help you. Other restaurants offer half portions of the regular items.

Reducing liquid calories

Watch out for beverages. Studies show that people don't adjust their food intake for liquid calories. In other words, people don't eat less just because they're consuming extra calories in sugar-sweetened soft drinks or other drinks. Calories from drinks are purely additive to the diet. Choose plain tea, coffee, or water instead.

If you enjoy alcohol with your meal, remember alcoholic beverages count as carb choices. Review Chapter 4 for more information on alcohol. A glass of wine or a low-carb beer will cost a carb choice, but it may just be what you're needing. Mixed drinks will also count as a carb choice; just be sure the mixer is low-carb.

Knowing how to order

Don't be afraid to ask questions. You'd certainly ask questions before plunking down cash for a home or a new car. Is your body any less important or valuable?

TIP

Here are a few tips on the right questions to ask:

>> **If you don't know what's in a dish or don't know the serving size, ask.** Don't worry about taking the time to ask. Others may have questions too.

>> **Ask for the chips or bread to be brought with the meal rather than ahead of the meal, or not at all, so you won't fill up on these items before you even see your food.** Order a low-carb appetizer, soup, or juice if you're hungry.

>> **Ask for a fruit cup as an appetizer or the breakfast melon for dessert.** Read the menu creatively.

>> **Confirm that you can order foods that aren't breaded or fried because they add carbs and fat.** If the food comes breaded, peel off the coating.

>> **Ask for substitutions.** Instead of french fries, request a double order of a vegetable. If you can't get a substitute, just ask that the high-fat carb food be left off your plate.

>> **Offer to place your order first when eating with friends.** Many people change their minds to higher calorie choices after listening to others order.

>> **Ask for low-calorie items, such as salad dressing, even if they're not on the menu.** Vinegar and a dash of oil or squeeze of lemon are a better choice than high-fat dressings.

>> **Ask for fish or meat broiled with no extra butter.** Add a fruit or melon salsa on the side if you want a little more pizzazz.

> **>> Ask for sauces, gravies, and salad dressings on the side.** Try dipping your fork tines in the salad dressing, then spear a piece of lettuce. Or add a teaspoon of dressing at a time to your salad. You'll use less this way.

Making Sensible Fast-Food Selections

The average American eats in a fast-food restaurant four times a week. One popular fast-food chain has you eating out 20 times a month as its goal. In order for them to reach that goal, they employ high-powered advertising and enticements. What's a person to do? Raising your awareness of the situation is the first defense. Then arm yourself with good strategies to improve your food selection. Don't let someone else control your food choices.

If you're having fast food for one meal, let your other meals that day contain healthier foods like fruits and vegetables. Count your carbohydrate choices appropriately. The following sections offer fast-food suggestions.

Pizza restaurants

Pizza can be a good fast-food choice. When ordering pizza, go for thin-crust pizza with vegetable toppings. Try to order by the slice. Limit yourself to one or two slices or a personal-pan pizza. If you plan for leftovers, put them away and out of sight before you dig in.

Here's one easy meal plan:

>> Two slices from a 14-inch thin-crust Canadian bacon, pineapple, and veggie pizza

>> Tossed salad with low-fat Italian dressing

>> Diet soft drink, unsweetened tea, or water with lemon

This makes for a delicious and filling meal, and it will only cost you two carbohydrate choices. (For more on carb choices, check out Chapter 6.)

Burger joints

Probably the most-common fast-food experience is the ever-present burger restaurant. The hamburger is the quintessential American food. Here's how you can continue to indulge, the low-carb way:

>> Junior-size cheeseburger with lettuce, tomatoes, pickles, and onions

>> Lettuce-wrapped burger or bunless burger with sautéed onions and mushrooms

>> Kid-size or small french fries

>> Side salad with low-fat dressing

>> Fresh orange juice, unsweet tea, water with lemon, or diet soft drink

Buffet-style restaurants

Be cautious of all-you-can-eat buffets or smorgasbords. The temptation to try some of everything may overwhelm your good intentions to make good food choices. Try to choose restaurants that can provide you with foods to meet your needs.

TIP

But if you do end up at a buffet table, try this trick: Picture your plate and mentally divide it into quarters. Select fruit, vegetables, and lean proteins for three-fourths of the plate. The last quarter is reserved for any starchy carbs or sweet items. See Figure 17-1 for an example of what your buffet plate should look like. Always eat more healthy foods than the less healthy ones.

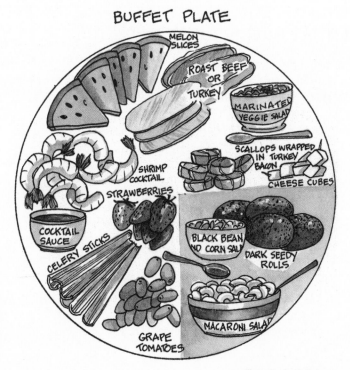

FIGURE 17-1:
Fill three-fourths of your plate with fruits, vegetables, and lean proteins, and you can put any starchy carbs or sweets in the remaining quarter.

Illustration by Liz Kurtzman

Evaluating Carry-Out Options

Many take-out counters in specialty food stores and supermarkets offer lightly stir-fried or roasted vegetables. This healthy indulgence costs about the same price as a high-calorie dessert. Look for fresh fruit whole or cut up. Alternately, keep fruit handy with you at all times — at home, on your desk, in your car. That way, even if the restaurant doesn't offer it, you don't have to go without.

Eating on the road or in the air

Plan a picnic at a rest stop rather than stopping for fast food. You'll be able to stretch your legs and take in some fresh air. Carry bottled water, diet colas, or fruit juice in your cooler rather than sugary soft drinks. Pack fresh fruit for snacking. Notice how more alert you are when driving after a healthy low-carb meal than a heavy starchy carb meal.

Most sandwich shops, airports, mall food courts, and outdoor refreshment stands offer fresh fruit. Pack snacks when you travel, though, just in case you can't find a healthy snack. They really come in handy if you miss a flight, get stuck without an in-flight meal, or just plain don't like the food they serve. For more on great snacks and low-carb dieting, check out Chapter 10.

Smart eating on the go

Eating smart while you're traveling can really help minimize the adverse affects of the stress that usually goes along with it. And just because you're on the go doesn't mean you can forget all your rules of healthy eating.

TIP

Here are some tips to keep you on the right road:

>> **Practice portion control.** Try to eat the same portion as you would at home. If the serving size is larger, share some with your dining partner, or put the extra food in a container to go.

>> **Eat slowly.** Your brain needs a few minutes to catch up with your stomach. Make sure you give it time to tell you you're full.

>> **Reduce stress.** Find ways to reduce stress that don't involve food. (Go for a walk or do some stretches.)

>> **Keep a food log and evaluate your choices against the Whole Foods Weight Loss Eating Plan.** Mark the food groups you're neglecting. Pay special attention to between-meal eating.

» **Be wary of impulse eating.** Today's lifestyle allows for eating any time anywhere. Keeping your food log may help you to better structure your eating pattern around your lifestyle.

» **Avoid skipping meals.** Don't skip meals — if you do, you're more likely to fill the void with snacks that provide calories, but few nutrients.

» **Reward yourself — but not with food.** Buy yourself a little souvenir like a magnet to remind you of your success.

» **Eat preventively.** If you know that an eating situation will test your willpower, then eat a little snack before you leave the house — cottage cheese and fruit, a small cheese wedge and grapes, peanut butter and apple wedges, or a glass of skim milk or 100-percent fruit juice.

» **If your food choices were less than ideal, then compensate by choosing healthier foods at your other meals.** Remember, healthy eating isn't made up of one food or one meal. It's your overall food intake that counts.

» **Exercise.** Walk off your extra food intake.

Seeing How Ethnic Foods Stack Up

One major reason people choose to eat out (after convenience, of course) is to get a different variety of foods than they prepare for themselves at home. This doesn't have to be a license for eating to oblivion, however. Most ethnic restaurants have plenty of healthy choices. Every culture has as its foundation an array of whole minimally processed foods. When those cultures become more westernized, deep-frying, breading, sweet sauces, desserts, and other unhealthy choices show up in the cuisine. The following sections examine a few common ethnic restaurants and identify the low-carb options.

Chinese

Authentic Chinese food features plenty of vegetables and lean meat, but watch out for deep-fried meats in sugary sauces like the one on the ever popular General Tsao's chicken or sweet-and-sour pork. Limit your intake of the starchy, Asian-style sticky white rice. Opt for oriental noodles, like lo mein instead. Try to avoid the deep-fried foods, like egg rolls; the sweet sauces can have a lot of sugar. Just remember to order whole foods without sauces or breading.

Greek/Mediterranean

The Mediterranean Diet has garnered the respect of the medical community because of its ability to lower the risk of heart disease and type 2 diabetes. In fact, Greek and Mediterranean restaurants of all cultures are becoming more popular.

Mediterranean diets have a moderate amount of fat, but most of the fat comes from healthy fats, such as olive oil and other oils, and the polyunsaturated fats found in fish, canola oil, walnuts, and other foods. Actual Mediterranean cuisine encompasses the Mediterranean basin, which covers several vastly different geographical areas including Spain, Italy, Greece, Egypt, Turkey, Syria, and Israel among many others.

Several cornerstones of Mediterranean cuisine include olive oil, vegetables, fruit, fresh seafood, wine, lamb, beef, lemon juice, fresh cheese, artisan breads, and dried spices. When eating Mediterranean food, choose low carb by avoiding bread, pasta, potatoes, processed cereals, and rice. Switch instead to quinoa, whole grains, beans, and lentils because they're tasty and filling. Also, remember the plate rule that starches and sweets should take up no more than a quarter of your plate.

Check out the newest edition of *Mediterranean Diet Cookbook For Dummies* by Meri Raffetto (John Wiley & Sons, Inc.) for more information about this diet if you're serious about trying it.

Indian

Because of the climate, India grows a lot of rice, which is a staple of the diet. Dishes also utilize a variety of local vegetables and fruit. Other popular ingredients are mustard seeds and paste, chilies (both green and red), as well as *paanch phoran,* which is mix of five spices — white cumin seeds, onion seeds, mustard seeds, fennel seeds, and fenugreek seeds. Yogurt, coconut, maize, and gram flour are also common ingredients. Milk and dairy products play a huge role in the preparation of sweets in India. Mustard oil is extremely popular and used for both deep frying and cooking.

Sweets are popular in India, and the region is renowned for its sugary treats. Be wary when eating a low-carb Indian diet because many food choices can derail your plan. Ask questions when eating in Indian restaurants.

Good choices include the following:

>> *Bihari kebab,* thinly sliced beef fillets placed on wooden skewers and cooked on a grill

>> Coconut curry chicken thighs

>> Foods with lots of veggies, fruit, lean meats, and spicy low-carb soups

Italian

Pasta dishes and bread can quickly exceed your carb limit. Thin-crust pizza with vegetable toppings is a good choice. Look for antipasto for a great selection of meats, cheeses, and marinated vegetables. It's usually on the appetizer menu. Try seafood, like savory *cioppino* (a spicy fish stew), and meat dishes, like osso bucco, braised beef shanks, or chicken cacciatore. All are great with a big salad. Skip anything parmigiana-style unless you confirm that the cutlets aren't breaded. Shirataki noodles are long, white noodles also known as *konjac* or miracle noodles. They're a popular low-carb alternative to pasta because they're very filling yet have few calories.

Mexican

Most Mexican restaurants in the United States serve high-starch, high-fat foods like refried beans, rice, enchiladas, and flour and corn tortillas. You usually start your meal with a basket of chips and salsa. The chip basket may get refilled two or three times before your food is served. These foods are denser in calories than they are in nutrients — certainly a set-up for disaster. Try sticking with grilled seafood and chicken dishes, black beans, and entrees such as fajitas. Ask the waiter to bring the chips *with* the meal instead of before. It only takes a big hand-ful of chips to equal a carbohydrate choice.

Order bean burritos, soft tacos, fajitas, and other nonfried items when eating Mexican food. Limit refried beans or ask for boiled beans. Pile on extra lettuce, tomatoes, and salsa. Watch out for deep-fried taco salad shells — a taco salad can have more than 1,000 calories if you eat the bowl!

To get you started, try this meal:

>> Chicken fajitas (ask for soft corn tortillas instead of flour and eat only two)

>> Grilled peppers and onions and salsa

>> Boiled beans (skip the rice)

>> Tea, plain

The tortillas will cost you two carb choices, and a ½ cup of beans count for one carb choice and a whopping 8 grams of fiber. For more on the benefits of fiber, take a look at Chapter 6.

Thai/Vietnamese

The Thai and Vietnamese cuisines have some similarities and differences. They both share rice and noodle dishes, and they both use a lot of herbs and spices. However, they have some differences, which Table 17-1 lists.

TABLE 17-1 **Differences between Thai and Vietnamese Cuisines**

Thai Cuisines	Vietnamese Cuisines
Has strong flavors due to the use of stronger usage of spices.	Tends to have more mild flavors.
Generally has copious amounts of spicy chili peppers.	Uses hot peppers on occasion usually as toppings.
Has more of an Indian and Malay influence and has more of a curry-based dish with rice.	Has more of a French influence and common dishes are rice noodle dishes.

Most restaurants accommodate low-carb requests by substituting vegetables for rice or providing additional protein in place of starch. Sugar and starch are the primary carb culprits in curry, but you have almost as many options as you do vegetable choices when you replace them. Nonstarchy vegetables have serious thickening power when you cook them in curry sauce and puree them. Just about any legume or pulse, such as beans and lentils, and most cruciferous and fibrous vegetables, such as broccoli and carrots, can thicken about three times as much liquid when pureed. Chicken lettuce wraps and some soups can be carb-friendly foods. You don't know unless you ask.

Chapter **18**

Psyching Yourself Up

A healthy diet isn't complicated — it's a matter of choice. You've probably thought about eating healthier, exercising more, and getting more fit before, but for some reason, you never seem to get there. Maybe you haven't thought the process through thoroughly enough, or maybe you've tried to do a complete overhaul of your life when making small steps would be better. Whatever the reason, today you have the opportunity to make a permanent, life-long change. Read on!

Preparing Your Mind

Analyze your motivation by writing down every benefit you can think of for changing your diet. Is it to lose weight? Is it to have more energy and feel better? Is it to improve a problem with your health? Think of every possible reason. These are *your* reasons and not someone else's. No benefit is too small or insignificant if it's important to you.

TIP

Pick out two or three reasons that are the most important to you. Write them down on slips of paper and put them in places where you can see them every day — on the mirror, on the refrigerator, in your purse or billfold, or in a drawer at work. Or open a new note in your Notes app on your phone and refer to it on a regular basis. Review them every morning when you get up, every evening before going to bed, and several times in between. Stay focused, and you'll achieve your goal.

Ask yourself:

>> Why am I doing this?

>> For whom am I doing this?

>> What are my expectations from doing this?

Analyzing Your Eating: Mindful or Mindless?

Paying attention to your experience of eating can help you improve your diet, manage food cravings, and lose weight. You may say, "I eat when I'm hungry and that's it." But are you really hungry?

REMEMBER

Recognize the two types of hunger:

>> **Physical hunger** is true hunger, which is characterized by an empty feeling in your stomach and discomfort that can only be relieved by eating.

>> **Psychological hunger** is associated with cravings, emotional eating, and boredom eating.

People's busy daily lives often make mealtimes rushed affairs. You may find yourself eating in the car during your commute, at the desk in front of a computer screen, or on the couch watching TV. Many people eat mindlessly, shoveling food down regardless of whether they're still hungry or not. This mindless eating satisfies emotional needs — to relieve stress or to cope with unpleasant emotions such as sadness, anxiety, loneliness, or boredom.

REMEMBER

Mindful eating is the opposite of this kind of unhealthy mindless eating. Mindful eating is about focusing all your senses and being present as you shop for, cook, serve, and eat your food. Mindful eating helps you become more attuned to your body and how eating certain foods make you feel. Being mindful can help you to avoid overeating, make it easier to change your dietary habits for the better, and enjoy the improved well-being that comes with a healthier diet.

Visualizing Your Success

Take five minutes every day to visualize how you want to live your life. Develop a mental image of yourself being healthy and making the right choice. Think about the following images:

>> Imagine yourself feeling well — alive, healthy, energetic — looking forward to each day.

>> See yourself going about your daily activities accomplishing your work and feeling good about it.

>> Imagine yourself selecting fruits, vegetables, lean proteins, and low-fat dairy foods because you *want* to not because you *have* to.

>> Think about how good the food tastes and imagine healthy nutrients feeding your cells and nourishing your body.

Recognizing Your Level of Commitment

To fully establish your commitment to making changes, you need to understand your readiness for taking serious action. Refer to Parts 1 and 2 for more ways to make important lifestyle changes.

In making your commitment to change, it's helpful to understand how ready you are to make the change. Researchers James O. Prochaska and Carlo C. DiClemente developed a Stages of Change model to help assess your readiness or someone else's readiness for making changes. They've identified six stages to change: pre-contemplation, contemplation, preparation, action, maintenance, and termination.

WARNING

Some people remain in the same stage for months or even years at a time. Understanding the Stages of Change model helps you be more patient with yourself when making a change. For example, if you try to force yourself to jump from contemplation to maintenance, you'll just end up frustrated. On the other hand, if you take a moment to assess where you are in the change process, you can adapt your approach.

REMEMBER

People don't move easily from one stage of change to the other. They often bounce back and forth between two stages before they move forward to the next stage. They may go through the entire process three or four times before they make it through without a setback.

Read the descriptions of the stages in the following sections and determine your level of commitment to change.

Ignorance isn't always bliss: The pre-contemplation stage

People in this stage aren't receptive to solutions because they can't see the problem. As the saying goes, "Denial ain't just a river in Egypt." They may go on a diet because of pressure from their partners, parents, or friends. They're typically very resistant to change and are anxious to rationalize the situation. When a discussion does begin, they change the subject or blame someone or something else. You may hear them say things like:

"I'm eating this stuff because my husband wants me to."

"It's in my genes. My whole family is fat."

"I have a low thyroid, and everything I eat goes to fat."

"I can't eat better because my wife won't cook it for me."

"I can't eat better because we have to keep all these snacks in the house for the kids."

"My knees are bad and I can't exercise. Everyone knows you can't lose weight if you don't exercise."

"I can't afford to eat healthy food."

They feel the situation is hopeless. Sometimes they can't even articulate the problem. They just feel there is nothing they can do to overcome the barriers in their life.

If you're in this stage, begin by asking yourself these questions:

>> Have I ever tried to change this behavior?

>> How do I recognize that I have a problem?

>> What would have to happen for me to consider my behavior a problem?

So how does this work, anyway? The contemplation stage

People in this stage start to recognize and acknowledge that they have a problem. They begin to think about solving it. They struggle to understand the problem, to see its causes, and wonder about possible solutions. They know they want to get healthy and they know how to do it, but they aren't sure if they're ready to start. They have indefinite plans to take action within the next few months. It isn't uncommon for people in this stage to say things like:

"I really want to lose weight, and someday I'm going to do it."

"When I get through with this project, then I'm really going to start exercising and eating better."

"After I graduate from college and get out from under this stress, I'm going to take better care of myself."

When people in this stage start to transition to the preparation stage of change, their thinking is marked by two changes: They begin to think more about the future than the past; then they start to feel anticipation, anxiety, and excitement, and activity starts to occur to prepare for the change.

You may view change as a process of giving something up rather than a means of gaining emotional, mental, or physical benefits. If you're contemplating a behavior change, ask yourself these important questions:

>> Why do I want to change?

>> Is there anything preventing me from changing?

>> What are some things that can help me make this change?

How do I do it? The preparation stage

People in the preparation stage are planning to take action and are making the final adjustments before they begin to change their behavior. They've purchased the walking shoes, joined the gym, stocked up on healthier food, or adjusted their schedule. However, they may not have fully resolved their ambivalence about making the change. They may still need a little convincing.

During the preparation stage, you may begin making small changes to prepare for a larger life change. For example, if losing weight is your goal, you may switch to lower-carb foods or read self-help books.

TIP

Doing the following can also help you get ready:

>> Gather as much information as you can about ways to change your behavior. Refer to Chapter 6 for specific tips.

>> Write down your goals. Check out Chapter 4 for ways you can set and record your goals.

>> Prepare a plan of action. Chapter 22 provides more information.

>> Find resources such as support groups, counselors, or friends who can offer advice and encouragement. See the section, "Rallying Support," later in this chapter for more details.

Practice makes perfect: The action stage

This stage is when people actually modify their behavior and their surroundings. They take the action for which they have been preparing. They start walking. They avoid the pastry cart. They make a healthier food choice. They switch to sugar-free beverages.

This stage requires the greatest commitment of time and energy. Their changes in lifestyle become visible to others. If you're taking action toward achieving a goal, congratulate yourself and reward yourself for any positive steps you take. Reinforcement and support are extremely important in helping maintain positive steps toward change. Take the time to periodically review your motivations, resources, and progress in order to refresh your commitment and belief in your abilities.

Creating a habit: The maintenance stage

Change never ends with the action stage. The new behavior has to become a habit. Without a strong commitment to maintenance, there will be relapse, usually to pre-contemplation or contemplation. But relapse is okay if you learn from it.

REMEMBER

The key to success is to not let these setbacks undermine your self-confidence. If you lapse back to an old behavior, take a hard look at why it happened. What triggered the relapse? What can you do to avoid these triggers in the future? Even though relapses can make you feeling disappointed, frustrated, or like a failure, the best solution is to start again with the preparation, action, or maintenance stages of behavior change.

TIP

Maintaining the new behavior and avoiding temptation involves developing coping strategies. Try replacing old habits with more positive actions. During this stage, people become more assured that they'll be able to continue their change.

Maintenance on the Whole Foods Weight Loss Eating Plan isn't triggered by reaching a weight or fitness goal. On this plan, maintenance simply means that you're following through on all the good habits you've started. You aren't finished; your job isn't over at this point. You must maintain these habits to secure the benefits.

Making it permanent: The termination stage

The termination stage is where you no longer need to attend to the task of maintaining the change. It should be a celebratory stage, but not many people reach this stage. This stage is characterized by a complete commitment to the new habit and a certainty that you'll never go back to your old ways. However, for the majority of people staying in the maintenance period indefinitely is normal. That's because it takes a long time for a new habit to become so automatic and natural that it sticks forever with little effort.

Taking It Up a Notch: Moving from One Level of Commitment to the Next

As you progress through each stage, you gain important skills, learning, and insights. Whatever stage you find yourself in today, you have made significant effort and progress toward your goals.

By reading this book, you're at the very least in the contemplation stage. Do the following assignments to help move you into the preparation stage.

Write out answers to the following:

» Choosing healthier foods will give me the following benefits:

» I'll make the following changes to achieve a healthier diet:

Follow through on making those changes, and you're now in the action stage. You're developing a self-image that is fit, and you're becoming proactive in maintaining your fitness. You see yourself in control of your health and able to rise above influences that make you less healthy.

Recording your food choices is a great way to identify good habits and a great way to identify problem areas. Keep a record of everything you eat for a week, including portion sizes and the food category of free, caution, or stop. Think about where you were, who was with you, and how you felt. You only hurt yourself if you're not honest.

After you've recorded your food choices for the week, answer these questions:

>> What days did you make the best food choices and why?

>> What days did you *not* make good food choices and why?

>> Was a certain time of day harder for you to make a good food choice?

>> What changes can you make to ensure success in the future?

Identify your danger zones. Does sitting in the kitchen cause you to raid the pantry? Does lingering at the dinner table make you long for dessert?

Rallying Support

Don't go it alone. Find someone to be in your corner, someone who is nonjudgmental and positive-minded, someone who believes in you. Carefully, and I mean *carefully*, identify one or more friends or family members who will support your efforts. Some people think the best way to get support is to announce to the world that they're on a diet. They think that publicly making this announcement will ensure their compliance.

Be careful if you tell people you're going on a diet. This declaration can easily backfire on you and turn into resentment as well-meaning friends turn into food cops, policing every bite of food you put into your mouth. They may not understand your eating plan because everyone seems to have a preconceived idea of what you should or should not eat. (For some reason, they feel no obligation to justify their *own* food choices, of course.)

My personal recommendation is to keep your plans private except for one or two sincere supporters. You know what you can eat and not eat and how much. Just make good choices and think about something else.

After identifying your support people, list two or more ways they can help you. Talk to them about it ahead of time and determine how they can help. Come up with a secret sign language that lets them tell you if you're about to go overboard.

When you've prepared your mind, assessed your level of commitment, gained knowledge and insight into your behavior, and created your support system, you're ready to go. *Remember:* This is a lifetime project, so don't get upset if you have an occasional slip. One bad day is no reason to quit. Forgive yourself, learn from the experience, and continue to move forward.

REMEMBER

Your goals are making the right food choices and getting regular exercise. Don't set yourself up for failure by trying to achieve a predetermined number. Concentrate on developing a healthy lifestyle and then reap the benefits.

TIP

If you want to keep a record of the results of your good habits, use the following chart:

Measurement	Today	After 6 Weeks	After 12 Weeks
Body Mass Index (BMI; see Chapter 4 for more information)			
Weight			
Pants size			
Waist measurement			
Bust/chest measurement			
Hip measurement			
Upper-arm measurement			
Thigh measurement			
Calf measurement			

TIP

To monitor your medical benefits, make an agreement with your healthcare provider. After they do the baseline lab work that includes blood sugar, total cholesterol, HDL cholesterol, LDL cholesterol, triglycerides, blood pressure, and weight, tell them that you want to try lifestyle changes. Set an appointment to return in three months (or sooner if you need support) for repeat lab work to evaluate your results.

Chapter **19**

Setting Yourself Up to Succeed

I s your home your own worst enemy? Chances are, the source of some of your greatest temptations is right in your own kitchen. The typical kitchen tends to have too many high-calorie, high-carbohydrate, and high-fat foods and too few fruits and vegetables, whole grains, lean meat, and low-fat dairy products.

You need to build an environment that supports your new healthy lifestyle. Although you may be tempted to give the whole place an overhaul, your spouse and kids or other housemates may be saying, "We aren't on a diet. Don't get rid of *our* food." You don't have to toss out everyone's favorite food. Think about giving your kitchen a makeover rather than an overhaul. Tolerate some high-calorie foods in the house, but focus on eating healthier snacks. Make those healthy choices available to everyone. You may be surprised at how often other family members choose a healthy food when they have a choice.

This chapter gives you some tips and pointers to help you be successful in your quest to better health. You'll find out how to avoid those foods that pull you off track, how to organize your kitchen for ready access to low-carb foods, and how to handle food safely in the process.

Identifying Your Trigger Foods

Most people have their own high-calorie foods that they just can't seem to resist. With trigger foods, a small bite just doesn't work. They're the sorts of foods that, when you start eating them, you just can't stop. If you know the food is in the house, you're constantly drawn to it as if it were a magnet. These foods are called *trigger foods* because they pull the trigger on overeating and increase your hunger all day long.

You may not be aware that a certain food is a trigger food for you until you really think about it. Getting in touch with how certain foods make you feel is important. When you keep a record of your food intake, record how you feel after eating a food. If a food tastes wonderful, you can't seem to get enough of it, and eating it intensifies your hunger for all foods the rest of the day, then that food is a trigger food.

TIP

Follow these suggestions for dealing with your own trigger foods:

>> **Exclude all trigger foods from your shopping and house.** If doing so is too brutal for the rest of the family, include a few of them along with healthier snack choices. Divide the trigger foods into portions and store the portions in the freezer. If you do indulge, it will already be portioned out for you.

>> **Avoid excess hunger.** When you're hungry, resisting anything especially trigger foods, is difficult. Plan healthy between-meal snacks and never skip a meal.

>> **Avoid letting stress contribute to overeating.** Maintain your regular meals, exercise, and sleep. Go for a walk rather than grabbing for the cookie jar. See Chapter 20 for tips on managing stress.

>> **Make trigger foods less accessible.** Hide them. Store them in the highest cabinet or in the back of the freezer.

>> **Develop some great-tasting treats from fruits, sugar-free gelatin, and sugar-free puddings.** Start with recipes in Part 3 and then develop your own.

TIP

If you have a sweet tooth, include a lot of fruit in your diet to satisfy it. Fresh fruit at the peak of ripeness is wonderfully delicious and sweet. If fresh isn't available, try frozen or canned fruits in juice or water. Mix several kinds together or try frozen bing cherries by themselves for an instant treat. Try topical fruits like mangos, and unsweetened versions of dried fruits, like raisins and dried pineapple. Combine your fruit snack with some spoonfuls of cottage cheese for greater satiety value.

Stocking the Fridge

The refrigerator is often the center of the kitchen, which in turn is the center of the home. Try to keep these staples on hand so you can whip up low-carb meals in minutes:

>> Low-fat or nonfat milk (or dairy alternatives), yogurt, and cheeses

>> Fresh eggs as well as egg-substitutes or egg whites

>> Tub or spray margarines that are olive oil–based, yogurt-based or plant oil–based with no trans-fatty acids

>> Low-fat deli meats and turkey bacon

>> Low-fat or oil-free salad dressing, avocado oil, olive oil, sesame seed oil, grapeseed oil

REMEMBER

Fruits and veggies are the original fast foods. They're packaged ready to go, and you don't need a knife and fork. However, when first introducing your family to fruits and vegetables as snacks, you may need to increase their accessibility. Make them convenient by cutting them up and having them ready to go and storing them in plastic bags or containers. Take a look at Appendix B for a ready-made grocery list full of fresh fruits and veggies.

TIP

Keep a variety of fresh fruits and veggies on hand and ready to go. Here are a few ideas to get you started:

>> **Buy apples, pears, or other in-season fruits.** Use the apple wedger with your kids' help to cut the apples in wedges.

>> **Buy a whole watermelon.** Keep a bowl of watermelon chunks for an easy snack, or make up several small watermelon wedges to use as a quick side dish to a sandwich or meal.

>> **Prep your veggies as soon as you get home from the grocery store.** If you buy a head of cauliflower or broccoli, cucumbers, peppers, and so on, clean and slice them immediately. Store them in the fridge so they'll be ready for snacking when you are.

Filling the Freezer

You can buy several items to keep in the freezer to make your low-carb life easier. But make sure you save room to make meals ahead and freeze them, so you'll have healthy low-carb meals ready to go all the time.

Here's the short list of freezer must haves

>> Low-carb frozen entrees

>> Individual frozen pizzas

>> Frozen unbreaded fish fillets

>> Lean cuts of meat and skinless poultry

>> Light or sugar-free frozen yogurt or ice cream

>> Sugar-free fudge bars or ice cream bars

>> 100-percent fruit juice concentrates

>> Frozen vegetables without sauces

TIP

Keep some blueberries, seeded cherries, or grapes in the freezer. These are great bite-sized treats and are much better for you than popsicles, frozen novelties, or even juice pops. Choose a diet lemon-lime soda, grapefruit-flavored soda, or club soda to pour over a bowl of frozen fruit for a quick, delicious fruit salad.

Organizing the Cupboards and Pantry

Your pantry should have a range of foods, from dried beans and grains to ready-to-go, almost out-of-the-can foods for quick meals. However, that doesn't mean stock up on mac and cheese or packaged dinners. You should choose canned and jarred foods that are processed as little as possible. Look for canned beans and tomatoes, but skip the spaghetti dinner in a box. You can get roasted red peppers or chilies in a jar, but avoid the urge to get canned soup.

WARNING

Getting help with already prepped ingredients is fine, but be wary if the only prep you do is heating it in a microwave. If that's the case, the food is likely loaded with preservatives, trans fats, and chemicals your body doesn't need and won't tolerate well over the long haul.

The following lists gives you items to keep in your cupboards and pantry because they're important carb-friendly meals: healthy oils, marinated foods, and canned and jarred foods.

Oils and vinegars

Look for healthy oils, like olive oil, canola oil, and peanut oil or light combination oils. These choices are better than corn oil or any kind of shortening. For details on which oils are healthy, check out Chapter 8.

TIP

Nonstick vegetable oil spray is a great addition to any pantry. You can find it in a variety of flavors, including olive oil, garlic, butter, and the like. You can buy oil misters to create your own versions. They're available at virtually any store that sells cookware. You can use any kind of oil you have at home. Just make sure you clean the mister occasionally instead of just refilling it, because the dregs can get rancid if you don't.

Many types of vinegar are available. Vinegars are by nature acidic. Adding an acidic food to a meal lowers the glycemic index of the meal. Keep a variety of vinegars on hand to enhance different flavors in salads. Look for different varieties (such as apple cider, balsamic, garlic, raspberry, champagne, cabernet, or zinfandel) to make your own dressings or add a quick no-carb sauce to a meal.

Marinated foods

Marinated vegetables are great as snacks and side dishes. The vinegar they contain helps lower the glycemic index of the foods you eat along with them. You can eat most of these items right out of the jar, and they make great additions to veggie trays, antipasti, and salads. All the following are green light foods on the Whole Foods Weight Loss Eating Plan:

>> Artichoke hearts

>> Capers

>> Horseradish, Dijon, spicy, or plain mustard

>> Marinated vegetables (okra, beans)

>> Olives

>> Pickles, pickle relish

>> Roasted peppers

>> Red and white table wine (for cooking)

>> Sun-dried tomatoes

Canned and jarred foods

Look for these items to help you whip together easy weeknight meals:

>> 100-percent fruit preserves

>> Canned chicken or beef bouillon

>> Canned or dried beans such as pinto, navy, kidney, limas, garbanzo, peas

>> Canned fruit packed in light syrup or juice

>> Canned new white potatoes

>> Canned tomatoes and tomato paste

>> Canned tuna, salmon, or sardines (in water)

>> Canned vegetables (asparagus, carrots, green beans, mushrooms)

>> Fat-free refried beans

>> Ketchup

>> Natural or low-sugar peanut butter

>> Salsa

Grains

These grains are handy additions to your pantry, but remember your portion sizes because these foods count as carbohydrate choices:

» High-fiber, no sugar, cereals

» Low-carb flours (almond, flax, oat, psyllium husk, pumpkin, or sunflower flours)

» Low-sugar granola or make the Homemade Granola in Chapter 11

» Oatmeal

» Whole-grain pasta, long-grain rice, wild rice

» Whole-grain flours and cornmeal

Check out Chapter 6 for the details on how to use your five carb choices each day.

Snacks

Use these snacks sparingly. They can help in a pinch when you need a sweet-tooth fix:

» Low-sugar cookies, like vanilla wafers, animal crackers, or gingersnaps

» Low-fat microwave popcorn

» Sugar-free gelatin and puddings

» Sugar-free hot cocoa mix

» Whole-grain crackers

Seasonings

Variety may be the spice of life, but what would food be without seasoning? Keep these seasonings on hand for quick additions to marinades, sauces, and one-pot meals:

» Bouillon cubes or sprinkles

» Garlic and onion, fresh, minced, and powder

» Reduced-sodium soy sauce or Worcestershire sauce

» Salt-free seasonings

» Sugar substitutes, natural (allulose, erythritol, monk fruit, stevia leaf extract, xylitol; see Chapter 6)

Paying Attention to Safety

Food-borne diseases cause an estimated 600 million illnesses globally according to the World Health Organization. Don't make the mistake of only associating those illnesses with travel, restaurants, and public eating places. Even though illnesses occurring in these public places get all the press, food-related illnesses can occur right in your own home.

REMEMBER

The cardinal rule of food safety is simple: Keep hot foods hot; keep cold foods cold; and keep hands, utensils, and the kitchen clean. The following tips can help:

>> Allow sufficient cooking time for food to reach safe internal temperatures during cooking, and hold the food at a high enough temperature to prevent bacterial growth until it is served. Use a food thermometer to check temperatures.

>> Go directly home upon leaving the grocery store and immediately unpack foods into the refrigerator or freezer upon your arrival.

>> Wash the countertops, your hands, and utensils in warm, soapy water before and after each step of food preparation or use the popular bleach wipes to clean the countertops.

TIP

Allowing refrigerated foods to warm up to room temperature and allowing cooked foods to cool down to room temperature creates a temperature range conducive to bacteria growth known as the *danger zone*. Between the temperatures of 40 and 140 degrees is the prime growing temperature for bacteria. No food should be kept at that temperature for longer than two hours. The *2-40-140 rule* will help you to remember the time and temperature danger zone for foods: No more than 2 hours between 40 degrees F and 140 degrees F.

Here are a few other safety tips that can help keep you and your family safe from food-borne illnesses:

>> **When in doubt, throw it out.** Throw out foods with danger-signaling odors. But be aware that most food poisoning bacteria are odorless, colorless, and tasteless. Don't even taste a food that is suspect.

>> **Use separate cutting boards for meat and poultry.** Don't use wooden cutting boards because bacteria can live in the grooves. Sterilize cutting boards in the dishwasher. Consider buying separate colors for meat and fresh foods like veggies and bread. Also, use separate knives for cutting meat, poultry, veggies, and cheese. Wash with hot water after each use.

>> **Wash and disinfect sponges and towels regularly.** Launder in a bleach solution.

>> **Avoid cross-contamination by washing all surfaces (including your hands) that have been in contact with raw meats, poultry, or eggs.** Sanitize before processing and in between processing new foods.

>> **Thaw meats or poultry in the refrigerator, not on the kitchen counter.** If you must thaw foods quickly, use cool running water or the microwave.

>> **Don't put cooked food on a plate that was used for raw meat or poultry.** If you bring your raw steaks, chicken, or burgers to the grill on a platter, get a fresh platter for the final product.

>> **Mix foods with utensils, not your hands.** And keep hands and utensils away from your mouth, nose, and hair.

Your refrigerator temperature should be kept at 34 to 40 degrees F. If there is a lot of opening and shutting of the refrigerator door in your household, keep the temperature near the lower end (34 degrees). Put food in the refrigerator quickly to prevent the growth of bacteria; don't let leftovers sit out for more than two hours (hot dishes for more than an hour). Store foods in plastic bags or covered containers. Keep meat separate from vegetables to prevent cross-contamination.

TIP

Keep your freezer at sub-freezing — 0 degrees Fahrenheit. Wrap food in plastic wrap and foil, or store in airtight plastic bags or sealed tubs with the date marked. Place new items in the back, and rotate existing food to the front to help use them in a timely manner. If possible, use leftovers before uncooked meat.

Nonperishable doesn't mean a food lasts forever; it will perish at some point. Most dry goods now have expiration dates on them. Always follow those dates when they're available. When they're not available, here are a few guidelines:

>> **Canned foods:** Stored properly, most unopened canned foods keep for at least one year. If the top of a can is bulging, throw it out.

>> **Bottled foods:** Sealed, they last a few months. After they're opened, be sure to refrigerate them. Depending on the food, they can last one week to two months when opened.

>> **Boxes and bags of food:** Sealed, they last for three months to one year; open, they last one week to three months. Store open products in airtight containers to extend their longevity and to prevent odor crossover and insect invasion.

TIP

Whole-grain flours and cornmeal may keep best in the freezer. Put the whole package in a large airtight plastic bag before freezing. When baking, take out the portion you need and let it reach room temperature before using.

Chapter **20**

Falling Off the Wagon and Getting On Again

G uess what? Falling off the wagon is normal, and nearly everyone who is striving to live and eat healthier has done it at least once if not several times. Viewing failure as a weakness or allowing it to lower your self-esteem or self-worth doesn't make sense. And it's certainly not a reason to give up. People who are the most successful at changing a behavior go through the process three or four times before they can make it through without one slip. Slip-ups give you the opportunity to figure out where you went wrong and prevent it from happening again.

This chapter explains how to grant yourself some mercy and how you can sit back, take a breath, and figure out how this setback occurred. You can then make a plan of action and start again. The next time you'll be armed for success.

Forgiving Yourself

Okay, so you blew it. You totally lost control, threw caution to the wind, and pigged out. What are you going to do now? You're feeling low, and your opinion of yourself is negative, but hold it right there. You're headed on a guilt trip, so slam on the brakes, bang a U-turn, and head the other way. You've just been granted new insight into your behavior. Use it to avoid this problem in the future.

REMEMBER

Forgiving yourself doesn't mean accepting the behavior or making excuses for it. You need to learn from your mistake, gain more self-control, and grow in your capacity to overcome it. Not forgiving yourself makes these goals harder to reach and gives the event power over you. Release yourself from the powerful grip of your own mistakes by doing the following:

>> **Be willing to take immediate corrective action.** If you brought tempting foods into your home, throw them out. Pick up all the trash and garbage in your house, including your tempting foods, and immediately carry it to the trash. If you pigged out at a restaurant, then go for a walk or work out until you're hot and sweaty.

>> **Think about how you would respond to someone who did the same thing.** Would you berate that person to the same extent that you berate yourself? Of course you wouldn't. Is your mistake worse than someone else's? Think especially of how you would respond to someone you love if you learned they were treating themselves in the way you treat yourself.

>> **Confess your mistake to a trusted partner, friend, or counselor.** Talk about it. Discuss why it happened and how bad you felt about it. Develop a plan to avoid the mistake in the future.

>> **Practice loving yourself.** You're worthy of good treatment in your body, mind, emotions, and spirit. Get past this and move on.

Analyzing the Fall

So, you pulled into the drive-thru and ordered a milkshake. You feel terrible about it. Think about the conditions that led to that behavior:

>> Were you hungry?

>> Were you angry?

>> Were you feeling sorry for yourself?

>> Were you feeling you deserved it because of something good you did?

>> Were you influenced by the restaurant sign that reminded you of a TV commercial advertising milkshakes?

>> Was someone with you that influenced your decision?

Take time to carefully analyze what motivates you to get off track. Do you use food as comfort for depression or anger? Do you use food as a reward? Do you realize how susceptible you are to the power of suggestion? Were you unrealistic in your goal? If none of these apply and you were truly hungry, evaluate your pattern of eating. Maybe you need to eat more, earlier in the day, to prevent afternoon hunger. When you discover the motivation behind a poor food choice, you can plan an alternative defense.

The following sections give you the tools to overcome those negative behaviors that harm your success. Soon you'll have a plan of defense, a less stressful life, a positive attitude, and more self-control. You'll reap the benefits of your organization and planning. But, most of all, you'll move yourself up on your priority list and start taking better care of *you*.

Planning alternative defenses

When you determine what motivates you to overeat or not exercise, develop an alternate strategy. The key to any successful strategy is planning. If you don't plan how you'll deal with difficult situations, they'll happen to you. Acting is much better than reacting, so, figure out your trigger situations and make a plan to head them off. If you can't go into the employee lounge without putting money in the vending machine, don't go in the employee lounge. Bring your lunch and eat at your desk or outside. Or take a healthy snack from home when you go into the employee lounge.

TIP

You may have to try out several strategies before you find the one that works the best for you. Don't be in a hurry. If you've been struggling with making or breaking a habit, here are some ways to coax it one step at a time:

>> **Set small incremental goals.** If walking a mile is just too much for you to handle, then walk for five minutes. When five minutes of walking starts to feel easy, then increase it by five more minutes, and so on.

>> **Set realistic expectations.** Don't go full-steam into an exercise program and become so sore you don't exercise again for a week.

>> **Be your own best cheerleader.** You'd do it for someone else — why not do it for yourself? Set up a reward system. Drop a dollar in a jar each time you exercise, or try a new activity. Each time you work in all your veggies each day, drop in a quarter. Use the money to buy yourself a little nonfood reward like a book or magazine. If you want to wait and save for a bigger treat, reward yourself with a massage.

>> **Schedule time for yourself.** Set times for workouts and walks and actually follow through with it. Plan to take some time for a relaxing lunch to refresh your mind and renew your commitments. Or just plan time to read a chapter in a book with no distractions. Whatever you like to do that's relaxing and helpful to your goal of good health (both physical and mental), make time for it.

Conquering stress

A major factor in falling off the wagon is stress. When everything is perfect (and how often does that happen?), you eat right, exercise, and have a good attitude. But a minor crisis occurs and all your best-laid plans go out the window. You give in to the power of the crisis and may not even realize it because it short-circuits your thinking processes. In fact, you aren't thinking at all; you're *reacting.*

REMEMBER

People under stress put themselves at the bottom of their priority list. They sleep poorly (either too much or not enough), eat poorly, reduce or eliminate exercise, and drop out of social activities. If this sounds familiar, you're doing exactly the opposite of what you need to do. So, accept responsibility, admit the crisis is important, and start to deal with it. Take one day at a time and be flexible. Crises, small and large, in your life are permanent. Accept the crisis, do what you can about it, and move on. Don't try to resolve all your problems at once. Break them down into manageable parts. And, most of all, continue to take care of yourself.

When you recognize that stress, not hunger, is causing you to crave food, you may be able to avoid eating as a stress reaction. Or at least you may be able to find a healthy food to satisfy the craving.

People overwhelmed by stress often reach for sugary treats to get a sugar high and escape the emotion for the moment. This never works for long because, after the initial rush, you're left feeling a little sick and sometimes depressed and guilty. If stress in your life is contributing to poor eating, work on these five areas: attitude, organization, self-control, planning, and self-care.

Attitude

Thomas Edison said, "Genius is 99 percent perspiration and 1 percent inspiration." So, chalk up genius to the right attitude. The same is true with success in any endeavor, including low-carb dieting. Look into incorporating these practices into your goals:

>> **Adjust your attitude.** Instead of looking at stressful situations as problems, focus on the solutions. Problems can become opportunities to problem-solve and practice critical thinking. And more often than not, you discover more from mistakes and obstacles than you do from an easy well-planned life.

>> **Whenever possible, take charge.** Just the change in perspective of making things happen versus having things happen to you is less stressful. It may seem tough at first, but this single small thing can help you realize huge improvements in your life.

Organization

Being prepared is most of the battle. Get organized today, and you'll be a step closer to winning the battle. These tips can help your organization skills:

>> **Start with organizing the regular daily chores of life.** If searching for shoes every morning makes the kids late for school, then find them the night before. Enjoy the peaceful drive to school.

>> **Schedule your stress.** When you have this luxury, take advantage of it. If you have a big project due at work, it's probably not the best week to also get ready to go on vacation. If your in-laws are visiting, don't also try to organize the PTA bake sale, paint the house, and relandscape the yard. Whatever the events in your life, ask yourself, "Do I need to do this?" and, "Do I really need to do this now?" Find what works for you.

Self-control

Self-control means knowing when to say yes and when to say no:

>> **Just do it.** Procrastination breeds stress. If you're dreading something, then get after it and get it over with. If you're going to continue to think about doing it, just do it now, and get on with your day.

>> **Just say, "No."** You know they can and will find somebody else. The reason you're being asked is because the person before you said, "No." Only do what you truly want to do.

Planning

Inevitable obstacles are part of life, but the more you can anticipate, the better off you are. Keep the following suggestions in mind to prepare:

>> **Set realistic goals.** Don't take on too much. Whether it's the amount of weight you're going to lose or how many errands you're going to cram into a weekend, be realistic. There is no pressure like the pressure that you put on yourself. Understand what you can actually do in a day, and do it well.

>> **Practice it.** You can't predict every stressful event that comes up, but you can prepare for some of them. Being prepared reduces stress. If you know that you have to confront a co-worker, you can develop a plan ahead of time. Role-play with a friend to help you make it realistic. If you have to have a difficult conversation with your significant other, practice in the mirror. Find a strategy that works for you.

Self-care

You're the best person to take care of you, so start today:

» **Treat your body and mind right.** Eat a healthy diet, get enough sleep, and exercise regularly. Reward yourself with a relaxing bubble bath or massage. You'll reduce the stress in your life, gain energy and confidence, and be less susceptible to the side effects of stress.

» **Take breaks as often as you need to.** You may not be able to work in scheduled breaks throughout the day, but definitely take a few breaks, and then come back to your work refreshed. Often, you're able to complete a job much quicker if you have something fun to look forward to when you're done, like a walk around the building with a friend. Also, often a problem you're dealing with looks much different through a fresh pair of eyes, even if they're your own.

» **Give yourself a pep talk.** Keep telling yourself you can handle this, and you will get through it. Avoid putting yourself down with negative words about your abilities.

TAKING CARE OF YOUR EMOTIONAL HEALTH

When you say to someone, "you're the picture of health," the image you see is of someone who is physically healthy, but emotions are part of that image, too. You just don't see them, but they're also important . Your emotional health is the same as your *wellbeing*.

Living a problem-free life is impossible, but the way you bounce back from setbacks despite problems is important. Your emotional health is your resilience in getting up when life knocks you down. Keeping the mind and the body in sync is just as important as training and caring for your physical body. To care for your mind, do some activities that are designed to calm you and free your mind for positive thoughts. Meditate on the blessings in your life, pray and be thankful, keep a gratitude journal (putting pen to paper is putting action to meditation). Keep your mind and body in focus with tai chi, yoga, stretching, or a good massage. Stay focused on the good in your life.

Renewing Your Commitment

If you've tried everything but just can't seem to create the new habit, take an honest look at your motivation. Are you making the change because you really want to or because you think you should or have been told you should? Chapter 18 helps you access your motivation and analyze your relapse. It may take a couple of false starts before you finally begin making progress.

REMEMBER

If at first you don't succeed, try again. Very few people succeed at making permanent changes in their lives the first time out. Don't use failure as an excuse to quit. Everyone remembers baseball player Babe Ruth as the Home Run King. Few remember that he was also the Strike-Out King.

Learn from your mistakes, and move on. At each setback, or slipup, figure out what went wrong, and then develop a strategy for heading it off the next time.

Breaking the Cycle of Failure

If you're having trouble getting from where you are to where you want to be, you may be trapped in a cycle of failure. You may be hanging on to past events and attitudes that are constantly sabotaging your efforts. For new eating habits and exercise patterns to begin, old eating habits and exercise patterns must end. Your problem may not be how to get new, innovative, healthy thoughts and behaviors into your mind, but how to get old ones out.

REMEMBER

Success doesn't just happen. It's a constant progression of discovering what works, practicing it until it's a habit, and getting rid of what doesn't work. You can't move forward if you continue the old ways of doing things.

Here are a few ideas for getting your attitude moving in the right direction:

>> **Think about what negative behaviors and attitudes are preventing you from being successful.** Are you subconsciously sabotaging your efforts because you're unwilling to give up some habits? What do you need to let go of in order to move forward?

>> **Rethink and renew your commitment to yourself.** Do you really want to be a healthier person or is it someone else's idea? Are you fearful of the new person you will become?

>> **Think about what else you can do to improve yourself while creating a new lifestyle.** Study a new skill, read a book, take a class — exercise your mind as well as your body.

>> **Continue striving to be healthy.** Share your experiences with someone else who is trying to become healthy. You aren't going to be the same person in the future that you are today. Start accepting and adjusting to the new you.

5

Recognizing Factors Other Than Food

Know when dietary supplements may be necessary and what supplements you may need.

Set lifetime fitness goals and know how to reach them.

Achieve balance in your health practices and your life.

Chapter **21**

Taking Supplements When Food May Not Be Enough

The dietary-supplement industry is one of the fastest growing industries in modern times. It encompasses the manufacture and sale of vitamin, mineral, herbal, and botanical supplements. As much as 70 percent of the U.S. population is taking supplements, mostly vitamins, convinced that the pills will make them healthier and will make up for their poor eating habits. Classic vitamin deficiencies such as scurvy from vitamin C deficiency or pellagra from vitamin B_3 deficiency are almost unheard of today. But with people eating less-than-ideal diets and skimping on fruits and vegetables, marginal deficiencies aren't uncommon in some groups. Marginal deficiencies in several vitamins are risk factors for heart disease, cancer, and osteoporosis.

Americans are concerned about their health and easily fall prey to advertising promising miracle health benefits by simply taking a pill. This presents a new problem to be concerned about: the dangers of excess vitamins or minerals mainly through taking too many supplements. *Remember:* There is no magic bullet; the closest thing is a healthy diet.

In this chapter, I help you determine whether you need supplements and, if so, which ones you need.

Looking First at Food

If you eat a poor diet every day, vitamins are the least of your problems. You can't replace a healthy diet with a pill. Scientists don't know what ingredient in a healthy diet is responsible for which condition. They do know that people who consume five servings or more of fruits and vegetables have less disease. Often, when the nutrients are taken out of the diet and given as a supplement instead, the person experiences no benefit and, in fact, sometimes it may even be harmful.

If there *is* a magic bullet, it's a healthy diet based on whole foods like fruits, vegetables, grains, lean meats, and dairy products. In addition to the vitamin or mineral content, whole foods contain other nutrients your body needs. Besides calcium, a glass of skim milk contains protein, vitamin D, riboflavin, phosphorus, and magnesium. Whole foods contain soluble and insoluble fiber that helps to prevent heart disease, diabetes, and constipation. Whole foods contain substances called *phytochemicals,* which help protect you against cancer, heart disease, osteoporosis, and diabetes. If you depend on supplements instead of eating a healthy diet, you miss out on the benefits of phytochemicals.

REMEMBER

Supplements are exactly what the name implies, *supplements to* not *substitutes for* a healthy diet. Eat a healthy diet every day and then consider supplements when your health situation warrants it. Check out Part 2 for details on what foods constitute a healthy diet.

TECHNICAL STUFF

The science of nutrition has a principle called *nutritional synergy,* which means the whole is greater than the sum of the parts. So the all-around healthy diet produces healthy results. Isolated parts of the diet don't necessarily produce isolated health benefits. Herbals and dietary supplements isolate a particular food component, but they may not provide better health benefits because they don't have nutritional synergy. For example, people with certain types of cancer were shown to have low levels of beta-carotene and vitamin C. However, researchers were disappointed when studies showed no benefit (and even potential harm) from beta-carotene and vitamin C supplements. Beta-carotene and vitamin C are indicators of fruit and vegetable intake. Numerous studies do show that people who have diets high in fruits and vegetables have less incidence of cancer. People benefit from the nutritional synergy of a balanced, healthy diet.

Investigating Supplements

The term *supplement* describes any extra vitamins, minerals, antioxidants, or herbs that people take hoping to get health benefits. The following sections examine these four types of supplements in greater detail.

Vitamins

You need vitamins for normal body functions, mental alertness, and resistance to infection. They enable your body to process proteins, carbohydrates, and fats. Certain vitamins also help you produce blood cells, hormones, genetic material, and chemicals in your nervous system. Unlike carbohydrates, proteins, and fats, vitamins and minerals don't provide fuel (calories). However, they help your body release and use calories from food.

There are 14 vitamins that fall into two categories:

>> **Fat-soluble:** The fat-soluble vitamins include vitamins A, D, E, and K. They're stored in your body's fat. Some fat-soluble vitamins, such as vitamins A and D, can accumulate in your body and reach toxic levels.

>> **Water-soluble:** The water-soluble vitamins include vitamin C, choline, biotin, and the seven B vitamins — thiamin (B_1), riboflavin (B_2), niacin (B_3), pantothenic acid (B_5), pyridoxine (B_6), folic acid/folate (B_9), and cobalamin (B_{12}). There is some short-term storage of these vitamins, but because they're water-soluble, a person excretes any excesses of these vitamins in urine.

WARNING

Many people believe that because the excess is excreted, you can't have toxic effects from water-soluble vitamins, but that isn't true. Excess amounts from supplements of some water-soluble vitamins have been shown to have negative effects. From the time the excess water-soluble vitamin is ingested until the time the excess is excreted, negative effects can occur, particularly if you have taken that excess dose for several days or months.

Minerals

Your body also needs minerals. Major minerals — those needed in larger amounts — include calcium, phosphorus, magnesium, sodium, potassium, and chloride. Calcium, phosphorus, and magnesium are important in the development and health of your bones and teeth. Sodium, potassium, and chloride, known as electrolytes, are important in regulating the water and chemical balance in your body. In addition, your body needs smaller or trace amounts of chromium, copper, fluoride, iodine, iron, manganese, molybdenum, selenium, and zinc. These are all necessary for normal growth and health.

Antioxidants

Antioxidant supplements are popular and commonly considered healthy. Fruits and vegetables, which are rich in antioxidants, are associated with many health benefits, including a reduced risk of disease. The antioxidants in fruits and vegetables are known as phytochemicals. These plant substances include lycopene, zeaxanthin, lutein, beta-carotene, alpha-carotene, and so on; they're considered non-vitamin antioxidants. These substances can regulate and stabilize free radicals.

Free radicals can damage the body's cells, leading to disease and aging. Free radicals are produced naturally in your body from normal body processes. They're also produced in the environment from UV exposure, air pollutants, tobacco smoke, and industrial chemicals like pesticides. The antioxidants reduce the damaging effects of free radicals.

Antioxidant supplements contain 70 to 1660 percent of the daily value of the antioxidants. Diets high in fruits and vegetables have been proven to provide numerous health benefits. However, scientists aren't certain that supplements containing more than a 1,000 times of a nutrient is more beneficial. Early studies on antioxidant supplements have indicated that these substances can eliminate some of the health benefits associated with exercise, can increase the risk of many types of cancer, and can increase the risk of birth defects in some cases.

TIP

Because more research is needed, eat plenty of fruits and vegetables, and check with your healthcare provider or registered dietitian nutritionist before taking antioxidant supplements.

Herbs

Herbal supplements are part of a larger category of plant-derived substances known as *botanicals.* Botanicals can include bath and body products, lotions, salves, essential oils, and even insect repellent. Herbs are dried parts of plants and are usually taken to address specific health symptoms. You may hear of people taking ginkgo biloba for memory enhancement or St. John's wort to relieve symptoms of depression. But unlike vitamins and minerals, herbal products don't have nutritional value. They're a form of self-medication, and many people claim benefits from herbal cures. Because they're usually marketed as "natural," people tend to think of them as being safe.

WARNING

Ignore the myth that herbs can't be damaging because they're natural. Most prescription drugs have their origins in natural substances, and they can definitely do damage if not administered properly. High doses of ma huang (ephedra), guar gum, willow bark, comfrey, chaparral, and kava kava have been associated with harmful effects. *Don't take these herbal products.*

Although the U.S. Food and Drug Administration (FDA) regulates herbal supplements, the FDA doesn't regulate them as strictly as prescription or over-the-counter (OTC) drugs. They fall under a category called *dietary supplements.* No federal standards exist for herbal supplements to ensure dose, safety, or potency. Healthcare providers don't have a consistent agreement (with scientific fact to back it up) about what constitutes a safe and effective dose of herbal supplements. Even though some manufacturers do a good job, herbal products aren't produced according to standardized guidelines and may differ in content from producer to producer. They're often marketed for a perceived drug-like effect for a medical problem but are not regulated as drugs.

Establishing Your Needs

You've probably heard of the *recommended dietary allowance (RDA)*. These values, first published in 1941, provide nutrition guidance to health professionals and to the general public. The original intent of the RDAs was to prevent deficiency diseases, like scurvy and rickets, in the population. However, thanks to improvements in food production and supply, vitamin deficiencies are no longer a problem in the United States. You may notice that foods like white bread and sugary breakfast cereals are *fortified* with vitamins and minerals. These vitamins and minerals are the main nutritional value you'll get from these products.

In the mid-1990s a transition began from focusing on meeting minimum requirements to establishing optimal requirements to reduce the risk of chronic diseases such as heart disease, osteoporosis, certain cancers, and other diseases that are diet-related. Recognizing that today people's problem is excess not only in calories, but also in vitamins and minerals (mainly supplied by supplements), safe upper levels of supplements need to be determined.

These more comprehensive dietary guidelines called the *Dietary Reference Intakes (DRIs)* were introduced in order to broaden the existing RDA guidelines. The DRIs are intended to reduce the risk of diet-related chronic conditions, establish optimal values for adults and children, and set upper levels of intake. The categories are determined based on strong scientific evidence and are updated as the scientific evidence indicates. Check out Appendix C for the latest information on DRIs.

Avoiding excesses

Too much of a good thing can be a bad thing, especially where supplements are concerned. Vitamin excess is definitely possible with supplementation, particularly for fat-soluble vitamins.

Because supplements aren't regulated like prescription drugs are, if you're going to move beyond the average multivitamin/mineral and calcium supplement, you must do the research to answer these questions before you begin taking the supplement. Ask yourself these questions:

>> What is the upper limit for the supplements I'm interested in taking?

>> What benefit am I hoping to achieve by taking this supplement?

>> Will the supplement interfere with any of my other medications?

Two of the most troubling vitamin excesses occur with vitamins A and D. Excess vitamin D has been linked to hypercalcemia, which has been linked to breast cancer. However, recently vitamin D_3 has been found to have a wider margin of safety than originally thought. Vitamin A toxicity results when excessive amounts of vitamin A supplements are consumed. Excessive vitamin A is toxic to the liver, increases your risk of osteoporosis, and may cause birth defects. Hence, just avoid more than the RDA of Vitamin A. See the following section for the upper limits of some vitamins and minerals.

Knowing how much is too much

Because of the increasing practice of fortifying foods with nutrients as well as the increased use of dietary supplements, many people are at risk of consuming too much of certain vitamins and minerals. Scientists have determined how much is too much, and you need to be aware of these numbers so that you don't overdo it (check out Table 21-1 for the skinny on the limits). Keep in mind that these limits are based on the *total* intake of a nutrient — including what you get from food, fortified food, and supplements.

TABLE 21-1 **Supplements: How Much Is Too Much**

Supplement	Nutrient Upper Limits	Negative Symptoms or Reactions That May Occur Beyond the Upper Limit
Vitamin A	More than 3,000 mcg RAE/day	Liver toxicity, birth defects, increased risk of osteoporosis
Niacin	More than 35 mg NE/day *(This applies only to niacin in supplements or fortified foods. There is no upper limit for niacin in natural sources.)*	Flushing (reddening of the face and/or neck accompanied by the feeling of heat)
Vitamin B_6	More than 100 mg/day	Loss of feeling in the arms and legs

Supplement	Nutrient Upper Limits	Negative Symptoms or Reactions That May Occur Beyond the Upper Limit
Folic acid	More than 1,000 mcg DFE/day *(This applies only to synthetic folic acid or fortified foods. There is no upper limit for folic acid from natural sources.)*	Worsening of vitamin B_{12} deficiency
Vitamin C	More than 2,000 mg/day	Diarrhea
Vitamin D	More than 100 mcg/day	Hardening of the soft tissues (blood vessels, heart, lung, kidneys, and tissues around joints)
Vitamin E	More than 1,000 mg/day *(This applies only to vitamin E in supplements or fortified foods. There is no upper limit for vitamin E from natural sources.)*	Excessive bleeding
Calcium	More than 2,500 mg/day for age 19-50; 2,000 mg/day for age 51 and up	Kidney stones, a decrease in absorption of other nutrients
Phosphorus	More than 4,000 mg/day for up to age 70; 3,000 mg/day for over age 70	Elevated blood levels of phosphate
Magnesium	More than 350 mg/day *(This applies only to magnesium in supplements or fortified foods. There is no upper limit for magnesium in food and water.)*	Diarrhea, confusion, depression, disorientation
Iron	More than 45 mg/day	Constipation, nausea, vomiting, diarrhea
Selenium	More than 400 mcg/day	Loss of hair and nails
Zinc	More than 40 mg/day	Nausea, vomiting, lower HDL ("good") cholesterol, less resistance to disease

The highest level of nutrient intake is considered unlikely to pose any risk of adverse health effects to almost all individuals in the general population. If your intake of a given nutrient increases above the limit, then the risk of adverse effects is thought to gradually increase as well. This doesn't mean that all individuals will have problems at this level. It simply means that this is the level where your risk of developing negative side effects increases.

If you're consistently consuming a nutrient at the upper limit, view it as a warning flag rather than a cause for alarm. Taking high levels of individual nutrients hasn't been shown to be beneficial for healthy people. Check with your healthcare provider, pharmacist, or registered dietitian nutritionist to see if continuing to take the nutrient at the higher level is in your best interest.

LABELING CHANGES

Recently the FDA amended the regulations for the nutrition labeling of conventional foods and dietary supplements to include updated daily values (DV) as reference daily intakes (RDIs) for folate, niacin, vitamin A, vitamin D, and vitamin E. Except for niacin, which had its unit of measure established in the 1989 RDA as "niacin equivalent (NE)," the other four nutrients have new units of measure associated with the updated RDAs.

- **Folate,** whose unit of measure was just micrograms (mcg), is now referred to as micrograms DFE (meaning mcg dietary folate equivalents).

- The **vitamins A, D, and E** all had used a unit of measure known as international units (IUs). Those units of measure have been changed to the following:

  - Vitamin A micrograms RAE (retinol activity equivalents)

  - Vitamin D micrograms (mcg)

  - Vitamin E milligrams α-Tocopherol (mg)

You'll recognize these new units of measure in your reading of the Nutrition Facts Label on foods and dietary supplements.

Note: The *upper limits (ULs)* don't apply to anyone under the care of a healthcare provider who is taking a nutrient for medical treatment.

Determining if you need more

Many Americans get most of the vitamins they need from the foods they eat, but deficiencies involving even one vitamin can lead to problems. Inadequate levels of some vitamins can lead to chronic disease, including cancer and heart disease. Also, certain medical problems can alter your need for nutrients. Here's a list of health conditions and the vitamins that may alter their progression:

>> **Osteoporosis:** Vitamin D, along with calcium, has been shown to reduce bone loss and fracture risk in the elderly. For more on the dangers and prevention of osteoporosis, take a look at Chapter 7.

>> **Heart disease:** Folic acid, vitamin B_6, and vitamin B_{12} may decrease risk of heart disease. Results from studies on vitamin E preventing heart disease are less conclusive. Beta-carotene (vitamin A) may raise the risk in smokers.

>> **Cancer:** Lycopene, technically a non-vitamin antioxidant, may be even better than vitamin E in helping to prevent prostate cancer. It's found in tomatoes

and tomato products. Folic acid has been shown to decrease risk of colon cancer in both men and women and breast cancer in women who drink alcohol. Beta-carotene may increase risk of lung cancer in smokers.

>> **Birth defects:** Folic acid appears to reduce the risk of spinal birth defects in infants whose mothers take these supplements. Excessive vitamin A during pregnancy may cause negative side effects.

>> **Macular degeneration:** A common cause of vision loss in senior adults is age-related macular degeneration. Recent studies indicate that supplements of vitamin C, vitamin E, beta-carotene, zinc, and copper may slow the progression of the disease. Also, the phytochemicals lutein and zeaxanthin may prevent it. Because supplements of these nutrients can exceed recommended levels, you should check with your eye-care professional before taking them. Too much lutein can block the effects of lycopene, a phytochemical important in lowering cancer risk. Generally, people who have a lifelong habit of eating spinach or collard greens five or more times per week are almost 90 percent less likely to develop macular degeneration. If you have a family history of macular degeneration, start incorporating these vegetables into your diet.

>> **Diabetes:** All essential nutrients are important in diabetes. A well-balanced diet is the very best source of these nutrients for people with diabetes. A multiple vitamin-mineral supplement may also be helpful. Check with your healthcare provider, registered dietitian nutritionist, or certified diabetes educator before taking any additional supplements.

>> **Homocysteine:** *Homocysteine* is a factor in your blood that has been recognized as a risk factor for cardiovascular disease. High levels of homocysteine are predictive of adverse cardiac events in people with established coronary artery disease. The B-complex vitamins B_6, B_{12}, and folic acid can lower homocysteine levels and reduce your risk of adverse events. Check with your physician, cardiologist, or registered dietitian nutritionist to see if these supplements would benefit you.

>> **Hypertension:** Persons taking medication to lower their blood pressure may need a potassium supplement. Your physician should determine whether you need one. Foods supplying the nutrients potassium, magnesium, calcium, protein, and fiber have been shown to lower blood pressure. Supplements of these nutrients do not lower blood pressure.

>> **Lactose intolerance:** *Lactose intolerance* is a condition in which a person lacks the enzyme *lactase* to digest the milk sugar, *lactose*. People who are lactose-intolerant find ways to avoid the intake of dairy foods. It's recommended that persons with lactose intolerance take a 600 mg calcium supplement one or two times per day to supplement their diet.

TIP

The elderly, vegans, and alcoholics are especially at risk for inadequate intake of some vitamins. Supplements are often recommended for these persons, but they should also try to increase their dietary sources if possible. Look for the listed natural sources to get the following vitamins:

>> **Folic acid:** Dark green leafy vegetables, whole grains and fortified grain products, beans, avocados, bananas, orange juice, and asparagus

>> **Vitamin B$_6$:** Fish, poultry, legumes, whole grains, nuts, peas, and bananas

>> **Vitamin B$_{12}$:** Fish, meat, poultry, eggs, and dairy products (If you're a vegan and don't eat animal products, you'll need to take a supplement of vitamin B$_{12}$.)

>> **Vitamin C:** Citrus fruits, such as oranges and grapefruits, strawberries, melons, tomatoes, green and red peppers, and broccoli

>> **Vitamin E:** Margarine, nuts, vegetable oils, wheat germ, and whole grains

Navigating the Sea of Supplements

More than a third of the American population takes multivitamins and antioxidants regularly. If after talking with your healthcare provider, you decide to take one, you may wonder which to choose? Follow these guidelines:

>> **Choose a broad-spectrum supplement that contains vitamins and minerals.** It should supply 100 percent of the daily value for about ten vitamins and four or five minerals. Look for vitamin A, beta-carotene, vitamin C, vitamin D, vitamin E, sometimes vitamin K, B-complex vitamins, like thiamin (B$_1$), riboflavin (B$_2$), niacin (B$_3$), pantothenic acid (B$_5$), pyridoxine (B$_6$), cobalamin (B$_{12}$), and folic acid. Look for the minerals iron, zinc, calcium, and magnesium.

>> **Choose a calcium supplement separately.** Getting the daily amount of calcium you need in a multivitamin is difficult. If you do, the pill will be so large you can't swallow it. Buy your calcium as a separate supplement.

>> **Consider gender-specific or age-specific vitamins.** Multivitamins are marketed for everybody, but with new information on requirements, you may want to choose a product specifically formulated for men or women, or for people in your own age group, including teens, children, and people older than 50. The amount of iron recommended for younger women isn't recommended for men or postmenopausal women. Women typically need more calcium than men. Older women need more calcium than younger men.

The list goes on, but the closer you can get to your gender and stage of life, the more likely you'll find a multivitamin that fits your needs.

» **Save your money.** Price isn't an indicator of quality. Go for the lowest price available. Generic or store brands available in large national chain stores are usually modeled after popular brands and are less expensive. Compare the ingredients. They're often the same or nearly the same.

» **Avoid gimmicks that increase the price by including herbals and antioxidants in many multivitamin formulations.** Herbal supplements aren't essential for human nutrition and may have drug-like qualities. Besides, studies show that less than half of herbal supplements sold in the United States contain the amount of potency on the label.

» **Watch out for marketing hype such as claims of "high potency."** There is no legal definition of such a term.

» **Pay attention to expiration dates.** Supplements can lose potency over time especially in a hot and humid climate. Don't buy supplements that don't have an expiration date. And obviously don't buy supplements with an expiration date if they're already expired. If you find expired supplements on the shelves, turn them in to the store manager.

» **Look for "USP" or "ConsumerLab.com" on the label.** The USP seal or ConsumerLab.com seal ensures that the supplement:

- Actually contains the ingredients that it states on the label

- Contains the stated amount of those ingredients

- Will dissolve or disintegrate effectively so it will release the nutrients and it can be absorbed

- Has been screened for the contaminants like pesticides and bacteria

- Has been manufactured in sanitary conditions

These seals don't mean the claims are proven or that the product has been FDA approved. It also doesn't mean that by taking this product you don't have to eat well. It just means that the product is what it says it is, not that it does what it says it does.

TIP

If you have difficulty swallowing vitamins or other pills, ask your healthcare provider if a chewable or liquid form may be better for you. Children's chewable vitamins include adult dosing and RDA information right on the label. Calcium supplements are now available in chewable delicious flavors, like chocolate, caramel, and mochaccino.

REMEMBER

Store supplements in a safe place and keep them out of the sight and reach of children. Lock them in a cabinet or other secured location. Be especially careful with supplements containing iron. Iron overdose is a leading cause of poisoning deaths among children.

WARNING

Check with your healthcare provider, pharmacist, or registered dietitian nutritionist before taking anything other than a standard multivitamin/mineral supplement of 100-percent daily value or less. This is very important if you have health problems or are taking prescription medications. For instance, high doses of niacin can result in liver problems. An excess of vitamins E and K can interfere with blood-thinning medications such as anticoagulants and complicate the proper control of blood thinning. If you're already taking supplements and haven't told your healthcare provider, discuss it at your next visit.

REMEMBER

Although there are special conditions for some people that indicate a vitamin/mineral supplement, a well-balanced diet is still the best source of all essential nutrients. If supplements are indicated, they are to supplement the well-balanced diet not substitute for a well-balanced diet. Fix your diet first; then decide if you need to supplement.

Chapter **22**

Setting a Fitness Goal

eing healthy and fit is its own reward. Wake up rested, ready to start your day with plenty of energy and feeling good about yourself, which is the foundation of a balanced healthy life. But so often, people tie all their efforts to eat well and exercise to a number on a scale or to a particular body shape. This chapter helps you to appreciate other factors of good health.

If you're like most people, you may not think very much about what you eat. You get hungry and you eat until you're full. Pretty simple, right? However, the foods you choose to eat are very important in determining how you feel. Your food choices make a big impact not only in how much you weigh, but on how much energy you have, your mood, your risk of illness, and even your mental alertness. Eating well isn't a test of your willpower over junk food. Eating well is a *choice* to eat foods that nourish your body, feed your cells, and allow your body to repair and heal itself. This doesn't mean never eating foods you enjoy. It means selecting foods that balance your nutritional needs.

REMEMBER

Your diet may be the greatest individual factor affecting your overall health and quality of life.

Establishing Realistic Expectations

Most people have an unrealistic view of what they should weigh. You may feel a certain amount of excitement when you decide to make a lifestyle change to lose weight. You begin to have visions of what you weighed in high school and set out to lose 50 pounds. You may lose 20 pounds and feel like a failure because you didn't lose the other 30. But you lost 20 pounds! Who said you had to lose 50? Congratulate yourself for losing 20 and vow to keep it off.

TIP

Be patient in your expectations. Concentrate on eating well and getting more exercise and don't worry about the weight loss. People respond to weight loss in different ways. The minute some people alter their diet, they drop several pounds. Other people may need several weeks before they show a weight loss.

REMEMBER

Most early weight loss, regardless of when it occurs, is water loss. The loss in body fat starts after a couple of weeks. The more overweight you are when you start a weight-loss plan, the greater your initial weight loss will be. It isn't unusual for an extremely obese individual to drop 10 to 20 pounds in three weeks. But they won't continue to lose at that rate. A healthy and more permanent weight loss is 1 to 2 pounds per week. The closer you are to your ideal weight, the slower your weight loss will be. If you have only 10 pounds to lose, your weight loss may average only a half-pound per week. However, benefits such as more energy, better sleep, and better mood happen right away.

Putting your weight-loss goal in perspective is important. The following sections show you how to be realistic in setting your goals.

Accepting your size

Healthy and fit people come in all shapes and sizes. But most people measure their health in numbers — the number on the scale, the number of calories, or the number of fats or carbs they've eaten.

REMEMBER

You're a human, not a number. You can eat well, get regular exercise, and still be larger than average. And you're far healthier than your thin counterpart who eats poorly and is sedentary. Unfortunately, society judges the thinner person as healthier than you.

Rise above the propaganda and be proud of who you are. In accepting your size, don't accept poor eating habits and inactivity. Everyone deserves a healthy diet and the chance to be physically fit. If you're overweight, you're eating too much carbohydrate. If you adjust your carbohydrate intake by lowering your *refined* carbohydrate intake (foods that are highly processed and pre-packaged like chips, cookies, cakes, breads, rice, and pasta), you'll lose weight, have more energy, improve your mental outlook, and gain better health. If you stay with it long enough, you'll lose weight until your body achieves a weight that is best for you. Chapter 6 provides information on controlling your intake of refined carbs.

Understanding genetics and their effect on your body shape

Choose your parents well, because the link between genetics and health is a powerful one. However, you don't have that choice, so the next best thing is being armed with the right type of information. Chapter 4 talks about the importance of knowing your family medical history. Not only are some medical problems passed down through the family, but physical characteristics are passed on as well. You don't even have to know the details to gather some important information. Look around your family and see what body shape is most common; chances are, you look like your family looks. That doesn't mean you can't counteract the genetic hand you're dealt. All body types can become overweight and all body types can become fit.

Some people are genetically predestined to be tall and lanky, round and soft, muscular and strong — and most people are a lot of variations in between. Muscular and strong is the politically correct body type that many people want to be, but that's not the real world. No matter how hard they try, round and soft will never make tall and lanky and neither type will be muscular and strong. Even though you can and should strengthen the muscle mass that you do have, there will be a genetic limit to what you can achieve. A person with a tendency to be round and soft can be extremely fit and healthy even though they don't have the ideal body type they want. Develop an understanding of your own body and then devise a fitness plan that suits it.

Setting Benchmarks beyond the Scale

The scale is a mechanical device, but most people let it determine their health and their self-worth. Don't fall in that trap. Take ownership of your own personal body and discover what makes it feel good and what makes it feel bad. Use your waistline to judge if you're gaining or losing weight. If your clothes are tight and uncomfortable, lose weight until they fit.

You won't be able to get completely away from the scale, but don't let it be the only measure of your progress. The scale is useful to assess your weight and to measure your progress. It's normal for weight to fluctuate 3 or 4 pounds during the course of the day. Fluid retention can greatly affect your weight on the scale.

TIP

Use the scale as one source of assessment, but not the total assessment. Here are some tips:

>> **Don't weigh every day or even once a week if you can avoid it.** If you do weigh daily, accept small fluctuations in weight.

>> **Weigh first thing in the morning, after you go to the bathroom, and before you dress and eat.** Try not to weigh again for a couple of weeks unless you find it useful.

>> **Don't compare weights on different scales.** You're dooming yourself to disappointment. The scale in your bathroom, the doctor's office, and the gym won't synchronize.

>> **Don't compare weights from different times of day.** You naturally weigh less in the morning and steadily gain through the day as you drink and eat. You don't instantly get fatter, but you ingest several pounds of liquid and food each day.

>> **Don't expect your weight to maintain an exact number all the time.** It's normal for your weight to fluctuate a few pounds. Having a salty meal like pizza one night can contribute to water retention and cause you to gain a pound or two, even if you've followed the plan. You'll notice the water weight disappear in a day or two if you follow the plan.

>> **Forget the actual number on the scale.** The main purpose of the scale is to tell you if you're gaining weight, staying the same, or losing weight. Use other measures besides the scale to evaluate your progress. Look for improvements in blood pressure, blood sugar, cholesterol levels, less hip and knee pain, or easier breathing.

Appreciate the benefits of a low-carb eating plan other than just the number on the scale. You'll start reaping these benefits as soon as you start improving your diet. The following sections identify some of those benefits.

More energy

If you want more energy:

>> Lower the total amount of refined carbohydrate in your diet.

>> Eat less food but more often; avoid skipping meals and heavy dinners.

>> Enjoy a variety of exercise, including strength training.

>> Adopt a healthy, self-promoting attitude.

Better sleep

Diet factors can interfere with sleep. A big meal at night causes your body to stay up digesting it just when you want your body to calm down. Blood gets directed away from the brain and into the digestive tract, which can interfere with sleep. Diets low in iron, calcium, and magnesium can cause poor sleep. Avoid caffeine at least four to six hours before bedtime if it's a problem for you. Caffeine is a stimulant and is found in coffee, soda, tea, chocolate, and some over-the-counter medicines. Yes, carbohydrates can increase serotonin levels, which can contribute to sleep, but it doesn't have to be crackers — a piece of fruit or a glass of skim milk will do the same thing. The milk also contains an amino acid that some studies show helps people go to sleep.

WARNING

Even though 20 percent of American adults depend on alcohol to help fall asleep, nothing can be further from the truth. Drinking alcohol regularly — even moderate drinking — is much more likely to interfere with sleep than to assist it. Alcohol disrupts circadian rhythms interfering with liver function and suppressing the sleep aid facilitator melatonin. Develop a smart, sleep-friendly lifestyle by avoiding excessive or regular alcohol consumption. Refer to Chapter 4 for more information on moderate drinking.

TIP

If frequent trips to the bathroom are disturbing your sleep, drink less water two to four hours before bedtime. Although drinking lots of fluids is healthy, it shouldn't disturb your sleep. You need 6 to 8 glasses per day and that includes the water in fruit, soups, and other foods.

Improved mood

Eating a well-balanced diet and exercise makes your body feel good. Your body is able to thrive on the good nutrients you're feeding it because the good nutrients aren't being diverted into handling excessive processed foods and unhealthy fats. When your body feels good, you feel good all over, and it translates into a better mood. You're sleeping well, and you feel rested when you awaken in the morning. You have more energy, which automatically gives you a more positive mental outlook.

More self-confidence

As you gain control of your eating and start exercising you'll be able to gain control of other aspects of your life, which can result in more confidence. Praise yourself for the healthy choices you make throughout the day. Don't focus on an occasional slip-up.

Getting Up and Moving

Less than 30 percent of American adults are sufficiently active in their leisure time to achieve health benefits. Lifestyles today aren't conducive to a lot of physical activity. People are active, but not *physically* active. Today you can take the kids to school, drop off the dry cleaning, grab a coffee, pick up your medicine, and never get out of the car until you're back home.

TIP

Here are some ideas for making those errands add up to true physical activity:

>> **Park farther from the school and walk the kids to the door.** If the kids are too big to be seen with Mom or Dad, you can still park farther away and let them walk. (Activity: 10 minutes)

>> **At the cleaners, park farther away and carry the clothes inside.** (Activity: 3 minutes)

>> **At the coffeeshop, park outside and walk inside to grab your drink.** (Activity: 3 minutes)

>> **At the pharmacy, park outside and walk in to pick up the prescriptions.** Those prescriptions are all probably for something that walking will help. Get the best remedy around: exercise! (Activity: 3 minutes.)

If you follow these tips, you gain a total of 19 minutes of physical activity, just by making a few small changes in running your daily errands.

If you're thinking, "This will take so much time!" Well, what are you going to do with that extra time? If you'd instead use the time to go to the gym or take a walk, by all means do it. But if you're going to watch TV, upload photos to social media, or do other activities that aren't so active, at least work these ideas into your lifestyle part of the time.

TIP

If you really do have a time crunch, divide up the errands. Who says they have to be done at the same time? Do part of them when you take the kids to school and the other part before you pick them up in the afternoon.

Everyone is different and each person has different demands on their time. So, what works for one person may not work for another. The point is to take a look at your lifestyle and find ways to be more active. That's often a lot more practical than finding the time to go to the gym for an hour. Don't dismiss the importance of these small changes. Before you know it, you'll always take the long way around and be thankful for the opportunity to do it.

Knowing how much exercise is enough

In 2018, the U.S. Department of Health and Human Services (DHHS) published its second edition of *Physical Activity for Guidelines for Americans,* which provides science-based guidance to help Americans improve their health through participation in regular physical activities. Scientific evidence continues to build that physical activity is linked with even more positive health outcomes than researchers previously thought. New evidence links benefits of physical activity to brain health including possible improved cognitive function, reduced anxiety and depression risk, improved sleep and quality of life, reduced risk of cancer at a greater number of sites, and improved management of chronic medical conditions.

Adults should move more and sit less throughout the day. Even if you have some mobility concerns, some physical activity is better than none. Adults who sit less and do any amount of moderate-to-vigorous physical activity gain some health benefits. In fact, adults need a mix of moderate-intensity aerobic activity at least 150 minutes up to 300 minutes a week and muscle-strengthening activity at least two days a week. Moderate-intensity aerobic activity is any activity that gets your heart beating faster counts, such as biking, swimming, gardening, or even walking the dog. Muscle-strengthening activity is activity that makes your muscles work harder than usual such as lifting weights, wearing ankle weights, or working with resistance bands. If those activities are more than you can do right now, then do what you can. Even five minutes of physical activity has real health benefits.

These guidelines are for an average-weight person. If you're overweight, first decide how active you currently are and then increase from there. Always check with your healthcare provider before starting any exercise program.

TIP

The most practical way to achieve 150 minutes of exercise per week is to incorporate them into your daily activities and let them add up. Many consumer groups have promoted 10,000 steps as the gold standard for daily walking. However, recent research doesn't support that recommendation. Actually, many health benefits result from 4,500 to 5,000 steps per day. If you can achieve that amount on a regular basis, you'll be on your way to being fit. Also, prior guidelines stated that bouts of exercise needed to be at least 10 minutes long to be beneficial. Researchers now recognize that any bout of exercise is beneficial.

REMEMBER

Getting sufficient exercise helps with the control of your appetite. People who exercise regularly report fewer cravings for fat and fewer cravings for sugar than inactive people. Getting enough exercise also gives you more energy. If you're tired all the time, try a ten-minute walk. A ten-minute walk can refresh and energize you better than a ten-minute nap. Taking walks regularly will give you more energy overall. Exercise begets energy and energy begets exercise.

Using fitness trackers

If you're into gadgets, a proliferation of tools is available to help you measure your fitness. Here are a couple that you can use in tracking your fitness:

» **Pedometer:** This simple tool records the number of steps you take based on your body's movement.

» **Smartwatches:** They not only tell the time, but they also track all sorts of information in addition to connecting to your cellphone, allowing you to text, send emails, and make/answer phone calls.

» **Smartphones:** Most smartphones come with a built-in fitness tracker or at least a step counter. These built-in apps are on par with most other digital fitness tools.

The device you choose to use depends on how much technology you can handle. The accuracy of these devices is highly variable, and the consistency of the results between devices is practically nonexistent. Depending on what you choose, using a fitness tracker can help you measure your current physical activity and also motivate you to walk more and be more active.

Checking your steps throughout the day can be motivating. If you're behind the day before, you can plan a short walk to make up the difference. If you're at the same or greater than the day before, be proud of yourself. Just use the trackers to evaluate yourself and not compare yourself to someone else.

Accumulating exercise and letting it add up

Research shows that your exercise activity can be cumulative. In other words, two 15-minute walks can equal one 30-minute walk. With the current guidelines recommending 150 minutes of exercise per week, you need to develop a more active lifestyle overall and find ways to build exercise into your daily activities. Start maximizing opportunities in your life to move more. Small changes can add up to large increases in your daily activity level.

TIP

Here are just a few ideas to get you started:

>> **Walk, run, and play actively with your children or grandchildren.** A good tickle session can get your heart rate up.

>> **Mow your yard using a push mower.** If you have a self-propelled mower, alternate between using this feature and just pushing it with good old-fashioned elbow grease. If you don't have the option to turn it off, add ankle weights for an extra strength-training push.

>> **Take the stairs instead of the elevator.** Even just a few flights a day can make a huge difference. Spend five minutes of your lunch hour going up and down some stairs to increase your heart rate in a hurry.

>> **Clean your house.** You'd be surprised how many calories you can burn this way. Depending on your weight and age, you can burn 200 to 350 calories per hour with this activity.

>> **Wash your car.** Do some extra detailing and maybe waxing to get some extra activities in.

>> **Take up dance — ballroom, square-dancing, line dancing, clogging, you name it.** Most people love music, and dancing is fun!

TIP

Whether you're watching television or streaming movies, shut it down! A recent study found that for each two hours per day increase in time spent watching television, there was a 23 percent increase in obesity risk. You won't be bombarded with food commercials and you may be surprised at how much more time you have. Use that time to be more active.

Walking your way to fitness

Walking is one of the easiest ways to add physical activity to your day. It's simple, convenient, and almost everyone can do it. It requires comfortable, but not special, clothes and a sturdy pair of walking shoes. Keep the following tips in mind:

>> **Dress for the weather.** Wear layers that allow you to cool off or warm up as needed. Take sunscreen, a hat, a water bottle, keys to your house, your ID, and your cell phone.

>> **Choose walking shoes with a low, rounded heel, a flexible sole, and plenty of toe room.** They should support your arches and cushion your feet.

Look for shoes that are lightweight and ventilated. Walking shoes don't have to be expensive. Shop at a discount shoe store or look for markdowns at department stores. Last season's shoes walk just as well as the latest model. Wear your shoes only for walks to help them last longer.

>> **Keep safety in mind.** Choose streets with level sidewalks, a park with a well-worn path, or even an outdoor track at a local school or college. If you walk at night, walk with a companion. Make sure the area is well lit. Wear light-colored, reflective clothing or shoes to make you more visible to drivers. If you're in an area with traffic, skip the headphones or earbuds and turn off the cell phone so you can hear traffic. Stay aware of your surroundings.

>> **For indoor walking, look for malls, museums, or convention centers.** Look at the place where you work. Walk to your coworkers' desks instead of using email or the phone. Take the stairs at work and in public buildings.

Fitness for Life: It's Never Too Late

Do you know the saying, "Today is the first day of the rest of your life"? Don't bemoan the fact that you haven't had the healthiest lifestyle. Start today and begin reaping benefits. You may be suffering consequences from poor habits in the past, but why add to that load?

Studies show that elderly people confined to wheelchairs or walkers can improve their strength, stamina, and endurance with regular exercises. Some in wheelchairs can move up to walkers and some using walkers can switch to canes.

Step up the workload as you get older. The 30-minute mall walk you've faithfully trekked three times a week may not cut it any more. Because your metabolic rate is slowing down, you may need 45 to 60 minutes of aerobic activity four or five times a week to reduce your body fat. Or better yet, if you're younger, get rid of the fat now, so you'll just need to maintain (rather than reduce) as you get older.

Middle-aged and older people of today grew up in a very youth-oriented society. Accepting the fact that they're aging is often difficult. But why hold on to the past? Today, aging is the new "prime of life." The over-50 crowd is breaking all the rules (just like they did in the '60s) for growing older but not old. They're the role models for the future generation and are making aging an enviable state to be in.

To join this hip crowd, change the way you think about food, fitness, and your own body image, which the following sections discuss.

Changing your attitude

Start by adjusting your attitude:

>> **Act your age.** That's to say, accept yourself and your age and move forward, not backward. One day you'll see the age you are today as being very young. Don't waste it by thinking of yourself as old.

>> **Remember that fitness is the goal — forget about looking like a runway model or ballerina.** In fact, the more meat on your bones in the form of lean, toned muscle, the higher your metabolism, which means the faster you'll burn calories. And no matter what you weigh, the more muscle mass you have, the better off you are.

>> **Forget the scale as your primary assessment tool.** Concentrate on how you feel in your clothes.

>> **Focus on progress not perfection.** Celebrate minor victories, like every improvement on your BMI rating. Or start smaller: Celebrate the first week you stay within your five carb choices every day. Find something to celebrate every week. Don't dwell on setbacks. Learn from them and move on.

>> **Empower yourself.** Remind yourself that you have the power to improve your health — whatever your age.

Altering what you eat

Then begin adjusting your plate:

>> **Eat smaller meals, several times a day.** Afraid of between-meal snacks? Just make smart choices, and you're on your way to healthy eating. Eat smaller portions more frequently to help burn more for energy and store less as fat. Never skip meals; it's energy draining and can lead to bingeing.

>> **Enjoy a power lunch.** Make lunch the main meal by enjoying some of your carb choices for the day, and taper off in the evening. Try to stick to mostly Green Light foods as the day progresses. (Check out Chapter 5.)

>> **Remember that variety is the spice of life.** Choose from the different food groups, fruits, vegetables, lean protein, and low-fat dairy.

>> **Don't give up your favorite foods.** Allow yourself an occasional indulgence.

>> **Drink more water.** Drink at least 6 to 8 glasses a day. Try to carry a water bottle wherever you go (in your car, at your desk, in your diaper bag, and so on) so that you'll always have it with you.

>> **Limit your alcohol intake.** See Chapter 4.

Modifying your workouts

Adjust your workouts by:

>> **Extend your cardio workout.** By spending just five more minutes at your peak exercising rate, you can burn more calories per workout. That's a good investment in your own good health.

>> **Try strength training.** This can be as simple as adding ankle or hand weights to your walk, or as complicated as working with a personal trainer to develop a personalized plan. Wherever you start, strive to work up to at least two sessions each week. Each session should last 30 to 40 minutes. Building muscle mass helps improve your metabolism, helps you lose weight, and slows or prevents bone loss as you age.

>> **Vary your activity.** Try walking, swimming, golfing, whatever activity sounds fun to you. Even if walking is your only cardio activity, you can vary where you walk, and with whom you walk. Walk with your dog. Walk with friends. Walk with ankle or hand weights. You get the picture.

>> **Remember that patience is a virtue.** Don't expect to be able to do 60 minutes each of the first seven days you start the program. Aim for every other day for the first few weeks, and then increase from there. Don't burn out or get so sore that you're unable to maintain the activity. Remember, living a low-carb lifestyle is a marathon, not a sprint, so take it slow, but be consistent.

6

The Part of Tens

IN THIS PART . . .

Discover ten benefits of low-carb dieting and how to maintain them.

Answer frequently asked questions about low-carb dieting to better understand the plan.

Recognize sources of dietary antioxidants and appreciate their importance to your health.

Chapter **23**

Ten Benefits of Low-Carb Dieting

Eating a healthy diet and exercising have many benefits. In fact, these two activities alone are the most important things you can do to improve your health. But don't shortchange yourself when you evaluate your progress. Don't put the whole focus on the number of pounds you've lost or what you weigh. If you do, you'll be missing some of your greatest rewards. And if you give up the plan because you didn't reach the magic number on the scale, you're throwing out your greatest benefits. In this chapter, I list ten very gratifying ways to discover that you're on the right track.

Improved Glucose Control

One of the first benefits of reducing the total amount of carbohydrate (especially the refined carbohydrate foods) in your diet is usually an improvement in your *blood glucose* (blood sugar) level. Let the carbohydrate foods that you do choose to eat be fruits, vegetables, and whole-grain or unrefined grain foods. You'll notice fewer sugar highs and sugar lows, which create hunger.

Quality whole foods sustain you, are easier for your body to process, and are chock-full of vitamins and minerals you can't get in a pill.

REMEMBER

Better Appetite Control

Another benefit of low-carb dieting is an improvement in your appetite. You'll have a normal hunger at mealtimes, but it will be easily satisfied by the foods on the Whole Foods Weight Loss Eating Plan. You'll no longer have periods of ravenous hunger. On those days when you *are* hungrier, you have a variety of Green Light foods to satisfy that hunger and still maintain your healthy eating plan. Check out Chapter 10 for planning tips and Chapter 5 for the full list of Green Light foods.

Improved Concentration

As your blood sugar becomes more stable, you'll notice that you can concentrate better. You'll no longer feel lethargic and barely able to hold your eyes open after lunch. Your focus will improve. (If you've ever found yourself reading and re-reading the same section of the newspaper, an email, or a book, you know what I'm talking about.) You'll be better able to start and complete tasks quickly, with fewer interruptions.

Weight Maintenance

On the Whole Foods Weight Loss Eating Plan, you'll notice that you feel more comfortable in your clothes and your body feels lighter. Your weight won't increase; in fact, you'll probably lose a few pounds. Your weight loss will be slow and healthy and will continue, but remember that no weight gain is always progress. If you're on a cycle of weight gain, stopping it is extremely important to your future health.

Improved Blood Pressure

The Whole Foods Weight Loss Eating Plan provides low-fat dairy products, protein, calcium, potassium, magnesium, and fiber — all nutrients proven to lower your blood pressure. The Whole Foods Weight Loss Eating Plan allows you to rid yourself of extra water you may be retaining. This loss of excess water not only makes you feel better, it also helps to lower your blood pressure. You'll notice your blood pressure is improving if you check it regularly. If you require medication to control your blood pressure, your family doctor may eventually be able to decrease the amount, or eliminate it completely.

TIP

Blood-pressure monitors in pharmacies are good places for periodic checks between doctor visits.

Improved Cholesterol

The Whole Foods Weight Loss Eating Plan significantly lowers your intake of saturated fat and trans fatty acids as well as lowers your overall carbohydrate intake. You're encouraged to choose monounsaturated fats and to increase your intake of fish supplying omega-3 fatty acids. These dietary changes are important in lowering your total cholesterol, LDL cholesterol, and triglyceride levels in your blood. When your physician repeats your cholesterol blood tests, you should notice an improvement in your cholesterol and triglyceride levels. Discuss this with your healthcare provider.

Improved Sleep

Lowering the amount of carbohydrate and the amount of food that you eat in the evening will allow you to sleep better. Your body is able to fully relax because it isn't up digesting a heavy meal. Stabilizing your blood sugar and getting rid of excess water cuts down on your number of trips to the bathroom. You'll be able to sleep longer without being disturbed. You'll feel rested when you awaken in the morning because you had a good night's sleep.

And with increased physical activity, your body will become more physically tired and relaxed. You're likely to be able to more quickly settle in at night and fall asleep faster.

More Energy

You'll definitely notice that you have a lot more energy. That's partly because you'll be getting good sleep. The Whole Foods Weight Loss Eating Plan provides nourishment to the cells of your body. You'll get rid of surplus water that was weighing you down. If you add exercise to the program, it will energize you. If you add strength training, you'll be burning more fuel all the time and reduce lethargic episodes.

Better Mood

When you just feel better all over, your mood improves. You'll be happier and you'll respond to people with a more positive attitude. You'll feel stronger, better, rested, and healthy. You'll be amazed at how quickly this happens, when you simply remove the stress of trying to decide how to get fit and healthy.

More Self-Confidence

It all comes together with a more confident you. Your health will improve, your appetite will be controlled, your concentration will be better, you'll be controlling your weight, you'll be sleeping better, you'll be getting more done because you have more energy, and you'll be happier and more confident. And all you'll have done was change your diet and started getting a little more exercise.

Chapter **24**

Ten Questions about Low-Carb Dieting

When you start a low-carb eating plan, you're bound to have some questions. In this chapter, I specifically answer ten questions that I hear frequently from people who are following the Whole Foods Weight Loss Eating Plan.

Do I Count the Carbohydrate in Fruits and Vegetables?

Fruits and vegetables contain carbohydrate, but this is good carbohydrate that your body thrives on. Don't count the carbohydrate in fruits (except bananas). And don't count the carbohydrate in vegetables if they're nonstarchy. Starchy fruits and vegetables — such as bananas, potatoes, corn, dried beans (pinto, garbanzo, navy, limas, butterbeans), English peas, and black-eyed peas — all count in your carbohydrate allowance.

Can I Use Dried Beans and Peas as Meat Substitutes?

Dried beans and peas are a good source of protein and are often referred to as a substitute for meat, which they can be. However, they also contain carbohydrate — but this carb is good carb. If your meal includes meat, count the dried beans and peas as a carbohydrate. If your meal doesn't include meat, count about 1 to 1½ cups of the beans as a portion of meat and not as a carb — this serving of beans would be free as a lean protein. Count any additional beans or peas beyond this amount as a carb. Check out Chapter 14 for other vegetarian protein sources. If the meal doesn't have any meat, count your vegetable protein as meat and not as a carb.

How Do I Follow a Lower-Carbohydrate Diet If I'm a Vegetarian?

If you're a vegetarian, lower your intake of processed carbs and reduce your portion sizes of the other carbohydrates. The important thing to remember is that you want the carbohydrates you eat to be good ones.

Chapter 14 discusses the different vegetarian options in greater detail.

What If I Just Eat Green Light Foods?

If you eat just the Green Light foods, you won't get enough carbohydrate, plus you'll be omitting milk, monounsaturated fats, and whole grains and starchy vegetables. If you eat only the Green Light foods, you're following a very-low-carbohydrate diet and you can end up in *ketosis* (the process of burning fat for fuel). Ketosis for extended periods of time can lead to problems in some people. That's one of the significant drawbacks to the Keto Diet.

Do I Need to Take a Supplement?

If you follow the Whole Foods Weight Loss Eating Plan exactly as recommended, you may not need a vitamin/mineral supplement. You should be able to get all your nutrients from the food in your diet. However, if you have a chronic illness like diabetes or high blood pressure or heart disease, you may want to add some supplements to your diet to prevent worsening of the disease. Also, if you're at risk for osteoporosis, you may want to start taking a calcium supplement to lessen the disease's impact. Certain age groups need more of some vitamins or minerals. See Chapter 21 for more information.

How Much Weight Can I Expect to Lose?

Weight loss varies among individuals. The more overweight or obese you are, the greater your initial weight loss will be. The initial weight loss is usually the greatest weight loss because you're losing water. You won't continue to lose at this same rate for the duration of the diet. After a few weeks on the diet, your weight loss will level off to 1 to 2 pounds per week. The closer you get to your desirable weight, the slower the weight loss.

TIP

Don't focus on a number on a scale to evaluate your progress. Concentrate on eating a healthy, satisfying diet and let the weight loss just be a side effect.

Is a Low-Carb Diet Safe for Kids?

The Whole Foods Weight Loss Eating Plan wasn't designed for kids, and a very-low-carb diet is totally inappropriate for children. Children and teenagers need the nutrients provided by milk and starchy foods. At a minimum, children older than the age of 2 years need four 8-ounce servings of low-fat or skim milk per day. Carbohydrate foods are necessary for growth and energy. Five servings a day is too few for active children. Six to eleven servings of breads, cereals, and starchy vegetables are more appropriate. The concept of free lean protein, fruits, and vegetables still applies. If your child's diet consists of a lot of soft drinks, cookies, candy, or other refined carbohydrate or fast food, reducing the intake of those foods is a good idea.

What Can I Keep in the House for When I'm in a Hurry?

A quick change in plans can easily cause you to grab fast food. Plan for these events because they'll happen — it's part of life. If you think a situation through and plan what you will do before it happens, you've won the battle. Plan to have quick meals in the freezer or a meal you can whip up from canned goods in the pantry. Many good-quality frozen dinners or entree items are suitable for a lower-carb eating plan. Keep a few of those in the freezer. You can zap one in the microwave and prepare a side salad, have a piece of fruit, and add a glass of skim milk faster than you can go pick something up. You'll feel better physically and mentally by doing this. And you'll be better prepared to deal with the crisis.

How Do I Control Cravings?

In the early stages of a low-carb diet, you may crave carbs. That's why planning some between-meal snacks is smart. Try a protein food combined with a fruit or vegetable (for example, mozzarella string cheese and grapes or cottage cheese and tomatoes). Chapter 13 gives you plenty of ideas for healthy snacks. If you notice the craving occurs about the same time every day, intervene with a snack 30 minutes earlier. Cravings can occur from erratic eating patterns, skipped meals, and diets high in refined carbohydrate. Overall, when you adapt to a lower-carbohydrate eating plan, you'll have better appetite control and fewer cravings.

If you just can't resist an urge for something sweet, then don't bake a cake or bring home a gallon of ice cream. Purchase a single portion of the food. Eat it slowly. Savor the taste. And then get back on your plan. You may save two or three of your carbohydrate choices to spend that way on occasion. Just compensate for the splurge by eating wisely at your other meals. If you just have a sweet tooth, satisfy it with the natural sweetness of fruit.

What Do I Do When I Just Can't Keep to the Five Carbohydrate Choices per Day?

When you're in a situation that prevents following the five carb choices, always practice portion control. Try as much as possible to concentrate on foods that meet your eating plan, but if you're in a situation that just won't work, eat smaller portions. Doing so will get you through the meal or situation. You can always balance the extra carbohydrate intake by just choosing lean protein, fruits, and vegetables at the next meal. Don't skip the meal just because the food choices aren't right. Meal skipping can do more harm in the long run.

Chapter **25**

Ten (Plus Two) Best Sources of Dietary Antioxidants

Dietary antioxidants are part of a larger class of nutrients known as *phyto-chemicals. Phyto* means plant; therefore, phytochemical refers to any of the various biologically active compounds found only in plants. Check out Chapters 3 and 5 for more information on phytochemicals.

Listing only ten sources of dietary antioxidants isn't easy because they're so abundant in the plant kingdom, and all are good. The Whole Foods Weight Loss Eating Plan allows generous amounts of vegetables and fruits and regular amounts of cereal grains and starchy vegetables. This chapter identifies ten plus two additional sources (from the organization Heath Research Funding (www.healthresearchfunding.org), but don't let that diminish the antioxidants not mentioned. Include these food sources frequently in your daily food intake.

Berries

Berries like strawberries, blueberries, blackberries, cranberries, and raspberries are overflowing with antioxidants called *anthocyanins.* Anthocyanins, which are in the flavonoid category of phytochemicals, can protect against cardiovascular and heart disease, improve immune function, protect against cancer, improve cognitive function, enhance exercise performance and recovery, and enhance vision and eye health. Berries are also a good source of vitamin C (ascorbic acid), which is also an antioxidant.

Broccoli

Broccoli contains more vitamin C than an orange and has more calcium than a glass of milk. Broccoli, which is collectively referred to as *cruciferous,* is closely related to cabbage, Brussels sprouts, kale, and cauliflower. This family of vegetables takes its name from the Crucifix meaning fixed to a cross as is the image of Jesus himself on the cross. The flowers of these plants have four petals resembling a cross.

REMEMBER

Cruciferous vegetables are rich in nutrients, including several carotenoids (beta-carotene, lutein, and zeaxanthin), vitamins C, E, and K; folate; and minerals. They're also a good fiber source. Researchers have investigated possible associations between intake of cruciferous vegetables and the risk of prostate cancer, colorectal cancer, lung cancer, and breast cancer.

Garlic

Garlic contains antioxidants in the allium compounds category of antioxidants, whereas aged garlic extracts contain a high amount of an antioxidant called *kyolic acid.* This powerful antioxidant may help protect the brain from damage due to aging and disease.

Garlic is also useful for decreasing blood pressure and cholesterol and removing heavy metals from the body. Garlic contains a lot of antioxidants that have an anti-inflammatory function. Plus, garlic also has antibacterial properties, which means it has a disinfectant and healing function. Garlic promotes heart health, contains cancer-fighting characteristics, potentially combats the common cold, acts as a natural antibiotic, and clears your skin.

Green Tea

Green tea contains high concentrations of catechin polyphenols, which seem to be responsible for many of green tea's health benefits, and also has been shown to be preventive against cancer, heart disease, and high cholesterol. *Catechins* are antioxidants in the flavonoids category that fight and may even prevent cell damage. Green tea isn't processed much before it's poured in your cup, so it's rich in catechins. Green tea has been shown to improve blood flow and lower cholesterol. Green tea contains 2 to 4 percent caffeine, which affects thinking and alertness and increases the release of certain chemicals in the brain called *neurotransmitters.*

Tomatoes

Tomatoes are brimming with the antioxidant *lycopene,* which is more potent in cooked tomatoes. Lycopene gives tomatoes their bright red color and helps protect them from the sun's ultraviolet rays. In much the same way, it can help protect your cells from damage. Tomatoes also have potassium, vitamins B, C, and E, and other nutrients such as alpha-lipoic acid, choline, beta-carotene, and lutein.

REMEMBER

Lycopene fights free radicals that can damage your cells and affect your immune system. Because of that, foods high in lycopene, like tomatoes, may make you less likely to have lung, stomach, or prostate cancer. Some research shows tomatoes may help prevent cancer in the pancreas, colon, throat, breast, and cervix as well.

Corn

Corn has a handful of antioxidants including *zeaxanthin,* which helps protect your eyes. Corn is also a good source of the phenolic flavonoid antioxidant, ferulic acid. Corn has higher amounts of ferulic acid than other cereal grains like wheat, oats, and rice.

Several research studies suggest that ferulic acid plays a vital role in preventing cancer, aging, and inflammation in humans. Furthermore, studies show corn may prevent chronic heart conditions, lower blood pressure, and reduce neural-tube birth defects.

Bell Peppers

A bell pepper has more vitamin C than an orange. Red bell peppers have even more vitamin C than the green ones. Other vitamins and minerals in bell peppers include vitamin K_1, vitamin E, vitamin A, folate, and potassium. Bell peppers contain many healthy antioxidants, including capsanthin, violaxanthin, lutein, quercetin, and luteolin. The plant compounds are associated with many health benefits, such as improved eye health and reduced risk of several chronic diseases.

Spinach

This green leafy bunch of goodness is one of the top sources of the antioxidant *lutein,* which helps protect your eyes from macular degeneration. Raw spinach is a source of potassium, magnesium, B vitamins, and low in sodium.

In addition to its many vitamins and minerals, spinach provides antioxidants tied to anti-inflammation and disease protection. These include *kaempferol,* a flavonoid shown to reduce the risk of cancer, as well as slow its growth and spread. Another antioxidant called *quercetin* has been linked to possible protective effect on memory as well as heart disease and type 2 diabetes.

Cherries

Cherries are high in two inflammation-fighting phytochemicals, *anthocyanin* and *quercetin.* The anti-inflammatory effect of cherries not only keeps your body healthy, but cherries also rank lower than many fruits on the glycemic index. That means they don't trigger spikes and crashes in your blood sugar and insulin.

REMEMBER

Cherries are a well-known brain food and can help to strengthen cognitive function by helping improve memory, focus, and concentration and by helping reduce brain fog. They're also a fantastic food for cardiovascular health and can help reduce the risk of heart disease, stroke, and heart attack. Cherries may help keep your heart healthy by protecting against cellular damage and reducing inflammation.

Peaches

Peaches are high in the antioxidant lutein, which gives this fruit its gorgeous hue. Lutein helps keep your heart, skin, and eyes healthy. In addition to lutein, peaches contain health promoting flavonoid polyphenolic antioxidants such as *zeaxanthin*, and *beta-cryptoxanthin*. These compounds help act as protective scavengers against oxygen-derived free radicals and reactive oxygen species (ROS) that play a role in aging and various disease processes. Even though you can find all the antioxidants, anti-inflammatory nutrients, and other vitamins and minerals in peaches in other foods, researchers believe the fusion of the specific levels of these nutrients is what makes peaches so special.

Dark Chocolate

Dark chocolate contains 50 to 90 percent cocoa solids. Cocoa is rich in flavanols that may help to protect the heart. According to the Harvard Nutrition Source, dark chocolate contains up to two to three times more flavanol-rich cocoa solids than milk chocolate.

Flavanols have been shown to support the production of nitric oxide (NO) in the *endolethium* (the inner cell lining of blood vessels) that helps to relax the blood vessels and improve blood flow, thereby lowering blood pressure. Flavanols in dark chocolate can increase insulin sensitivity in short-term studies; in the long run this increase can reduce the risk of diabetes.

Red Grapes

Grapes contain powerful antioxidants known as polyphenols, which are thought to have anti-inflammatory and antioxidant properties. One of these polyphenols is *resveratrol* found in the skins of red grapes, red wine, grape juice, peanuts, and mulberries. Resveratrol is the key nutrient in grapes that may offer health benefits. It has been promoted to have many health benefits such as protecting the heart and circulatory system, lowering cholesterol, and protecting against clots that can cause heart attacks and stroke.

7

Appendixes

Understand what the glycemic index and glycemic load of carbohydrate foods are and how to use them to evaluate carbohydrate quality.

Use a grocery list to target whole foods so you're prepared the next time you go to the supermarket.

Review the Dietary Reference Intakes (DRI) to evaluate your dietary and supplement intake.

Convert recipe measurements from English to metric.

Appendix A

The Glycemic Index and Glycemic Load of Foods

C arbohydrate provides energy in the form of glucose to the body. Carbohydrate foods are foods rich in carbohydrate usually in the form of sugar or starch. These foods can be digested or converted into glucose for the body. Fruits, vegetables, beans, corn, potatoes, bread, cake, cookies, sugar, and rice are easily recognized as carbohydrate foods.

Traditionally, carbohydrate foods have been divided into two categories based on their chemical structure — simple and complex. It was generally accepted that the effect on blood sugar levels was tied to a carbohydrate's chemical structure. Simple carbohydrate foods such as orange juice and apple juice were thought to raise blood sugar levels quickly, whereas complex carbohydrate foods such as bread and potatoes were thought to raise blood sugar levels more slowly.

This thinking was fully accepted and unchallenged until 1981 when researchers David Jenkins and Thomas Wolever of the University of Toronto published a study suggesting glycemic index be used to classify carbohydrate foods rather than the two-category system of simple and complex. This revolutionized current thinking because complex carbohydrates such as bread and potatoes were found to be digested quickly with a quick rise in blood sugar, whereas simple carbohydrate foods like orange juice and apple juice were digested more slowly with a moderate rise in blood sugar levels. As enlightening as this research was, the issue continued to be controversial in the United States. However, since then hundreds of research studies and investigations have established a solid foundation for understanding why a high glycemic index diet can be harmful to your health. The glycemic index is very useful in determining the *quality* of carbohydrate foods.

In this appendix, I tell you what you need to know about the glycemic index and glycemic load, clearing up some of the confusion.

What Is the Glycemic Index?

The *glycemic index (GI)* describes the type of carbohydrate in a food and its ability to raise your blood sugar. The glycemic index is a value that tells how fast a particular food will raise your blood sugar. A high glycemic index value is 70 or more; moderate is in the 40 to 69 range; and low is 39 or less.

The *glycemic index value* is based on 50 grams of carbohydrate in the food without consideration for how much of the food it takes to supply 50 grams of carbohydrate. For example, a slice of bread has a high glycemic index value of 73. It takes slightly more than three slices of bread to supply 50 grams of carbohydrate. On the other hand, a carrot has a high glycemic index value of 92, but it takes about a dozen raw carrots to give you 50 grams of carbohydrate.

What Is the Glycemic Load?

The *glycemic load (GL)* is a value of how much a standard *serving* of a food will raise your blood sugar. The lower the glycemic load value, the less a *serving* will spike your blood sugar. A high glycemic load value is 20 or more; moderate is in the 11 to 19 range; and low is 10 or less. When you're choosing which foods to eat, you want to shoot for foods with a lower glycemic load.

The glycemic load value is calculated by multiplying the amount of carbohydrate in a serving by the glycemic index of the food divided by 100. For example, an apple has a GI of 38, which puts it in the low category for GI. A serving of an apple (1 medium apple) contains 15 grams of carbohydrate. So $38 \times 15 = 570$, and $570 \div 100 = 5.7$ (rounded to 6). So, the apple has a low glycemic index and a low glycemic load.

On the other hand, a piece of chocolate cake with chocolate frosting also has a GI of 38, which puts it in the low category for GI. So, you may think, "Hey, chocolate cake is low glycemic, and I can eat a lot of it." But an average 4-ounce serving of chocolate cake with frosting contains 52 grams of carbohydrate. So, 38 × 52 = 1,976, and 1,976 ÷ by 100 = 19.76 (rounded to 20). This puts chocolate cake in the high glycemic load category. This should tell you to be careful about your portion size of chocolate cake and not to eat it too frequently. (Eat the apple instead.)

Remember those carrots with a GI of 92 (really high). Well, there are only 5 grams of carbohydrate in a 4-ounce serving, making the glycemic load 4.6 (rounded to 5, which is really low).

This helps explain why the glycemic load value is better than the glycemic index value in evaluating the foods you eat.

What Alters the Glycemic Value of a Food?

The glycemic value of a food is affected by how the carbohydrate in the food is changed during cooking, how much processing the carbohydrate in the food has undergone, and the amount of fiber in the food. Adding a small amount of fat or oil to a food (such as soft margarine or olive oil) or a little acid (such as lemon juice or vinegar) will lower the glycemic effect of the food.

Why Are Glycemic Values Important?

Food plans that incorporate low-glycemic foods over high-glycemic foods aren't based on starvation and deprivation. These plans consider the *kind* of carbohydrate you eat, not the amount. Low-glycemic foods don't stimulate food cravings, don't elevate blood sugar or insulin, and don't promote fat storage.

Eating *only* low-glycemic foods isn't necessary. You can eat high-glycemic foods occasionally, as long as you keep your intake of low-glycemic foods greater than your intake of high-glycemic foods. Also watch your portion sizes of higher glycemic foods. Coca-Cola has a GI of 63 and a GL of 16. This may make you think that Coke has a moderate GI and a moderate GL. But the GL is calculated on an 8-ounce serving. That 12-ounce can of Coke has a GL of 25 and a 20-ounce bottle has a GL of 38! (Don't even ask what the GL of a 32-ounce Coke at your favorite fast-food restaurant is.)

Where Can I Get More Information?

You can find more information on glycemic index and glycemic load as well as an online database of the GI and GL of foods at www.glycemicindex.com. This website from the University of Sydney, Australia, is where considerable research is being conducted on the glycemic value of foods. In addition to the database, the site provides the latest information on new GI data and research. You can also sign up for their newsletter on the website.

Appendix **B**

Sample Grocery List

n this appendix, I provide you with a sample grocery list, which you can photocopy and use again and again as you go to the store. Check out Part 2 for the full details and definitions of Green Light and Yellow Light foods.

Green Light Fruits

Fresh fruits

____ Apples

____ Apricots

____ Blackberries

____ Blueberries

____ Cantaloupe

____ Cherries, sweet

____ Figs

____ Grapefruit

____ Grapes

____ Honeydew melon

____ Kiwi

____ Lemon

____ Lime

____ Mango

____ Nectarine

____ Orange

____ Papaya

____ Peach

____ Pear

____ Pineapple

____ Plums

____ Raspberries

____ Strawberries

____ Tangerines

____ Watermelon

Dried/canned fruits

____ Apples, dried

____ Applesauce, unsweetened

____ Apricots, dried

____ Cherries, sweet, canned, light

____ Dates

____ Figs, dried

____ Fruit cocktail, light

____ Grapefruit sections, canned, light

____ Mandarin oranges, canned, light

____ Peaches, canned, light

____ Pears, canned, light

____ Pineapple, canned, chunks, in own juice

____ Pineapple, canned, crushed, in own juice

____ Plums, canned, light

____ Prunes, dried

____ Raisins

Fruit juices

____ Apple juice/cider

____ Cranberry juice cocktail, reduced-calorie

____ Fruit juice blends, 100-percent juice

____ Grape juice

Other fruits

_____

_____

Green Light Vegetables

Fresh veggies

____ Artichoke

____ Asparagus

____ Bean sprouts

____ Beans (green, wax, Italian)

____ Beets

____ Broccoli

____ Brussels sprouts

____ Cabbage

____ Carrots, mini bags of baby carrots

____ Cauliflower

____ Celery

____ Cucumber

____ Eggplant

____ Green onions or scallions

____ Greens (collard, kale, mustard, turnip)

____ Kohlrabi

____ Leeks

____ Mushrooms

____ Okra

_____ Onions

_____ Peppers, bell, any color, mini snacking peppers

_____ Peppers, hot, any variety

_____ Radishes

_____ Salad greens (endive, escarole, lettuce, romaine, spinach)

_____ Snow peas

_____ Spinach

_____ Squash, summer

_____ Tomatoes

_____ Turnips

_____ Watercress

_____ Zucchini

Canned veggies

_____ Artichoke hearts

_____ Asparagus

_____ Beans (green, wax, Italian)

_____ Beets

_____ Carrots

_____ Mushrooms

_____ Salsa or picante sauce

_____ Sauerkraut

_____ Spinach

_____ Tomato sauce

_____ Tomato/vegetable juice

_____ Tomatoes

_____ Water chestnuts

Other vegetables

_____

_____

_____

Green Light Proteins

Beef

____ Corned beef

____ Flank steak

____ Ground beef, lean

____ Ground beef, regular

____ Prime rib

____ Roast (rib, chuck, rump)

____ Round

____ Short ribs

____ Sirloin

____ Steak (T-bone, porterhouse)

____ Tenderloin

Pork

____ Boston butt

____ Canadian bacon

____ Center loin chop

____ Cutlet, unbreaded

____ Ham, canned

____ Ham, cured

____ Ham, deli-style

____ Ham, fresh

____ Tenderloin

Lamb

____ Chop

____ Leg

____ Roast

Eggs

_____ Eggs, white

_____ Eggs, brown

Cheese

_____ Cheddar, reduced-fat

_____ Colby, reduced-fat

_____ Cottage cheese

_____ Feta

_____ Mozzarella, string cheese

_____ Parmesan

_____ Ricotta

Fish

_____ Catfish

_____ Cod

_____ Flounder

_____ Grouper

_____ Haddock

_____ Halibut

_____ Herring

_____ Mahimahi

_____ Mackerel

_____ Pompano

_____ Orange roughy

_____ Salmon

_____ Scrod

_____ Snapper

_____ Sole

_____ Swordfish

____ Trout

____ Tuna, ahi

____ Tuna, albacore

____ Tuna, yellowfin

Poultry

____ Chicken, breast, bone-in

____ Chicken, breast, boneless,

____ Chicken, fryer, whole

____ Chicken, ground

____ Chicken, legs

____ Chicken, pieces, pick of chick

____ Chicken, stuffer, whole

____ Chicken, tenders

____ Chicken, thighs, boneless

____ Chicken, wings

____ Cornish hen

____ Duck

____ Goose

____ Turkey, breast

____ Turkey, legs

____ Turkey, ground

____ Turkey, whole

Veal

____ Chop

____ Cutlet, unbreaded

____ Roast

Game

____ Alligator

____ Buffalo

____ Emu

____ Ostrich

____ Rabbit

____ Venison

Canned proteins

____ Anchovies

____ Chicken, canned

____ Crab meat

____ Ham, canned

____ Salmon

____ Sardines

____ Shrimp

____ Tuna, canned or dried

Shellfish and mollusks

____ Clams

____ Crab

____ Crawfish

____ Lobster

____ Mussels

____ Oysters

____ Scallops

____ Shrimp

Other proteins

_____

_____

Dairy Foods

REMEMBER

Choose 2 to 3 servings from this list and don't forget to look at the cheese part of the Green Light protein list for extra calcium.

_____ Buttermilk

_____ Milk, lactose-free, low-fat

_____ Milk, 1%

_____ Milk, skim

_____ Yogurt, fruited, fat-free

_____ Yogurt, fruited, low-fat

_____ Greek yogurt

_____ Yogurt, plain, fat-free

_____ Yogurt, plain, low-fat

Dairy alternatives

_____ Almond milk

_____ Cashew milk

_____ Coconut milk

_____ Hemp milk

_____ Macadamia milk

_____ Oat milk

_____ Quinoa milk

_____ Rice milk

_____ Soy milk

Yellow Light Carbs

You get five carbohydrate choices each day from this list. Look for total carbohydrate on the food label to be about 15 grams per serving for one carbohydrate choice. You can subtract the fiber from the total carbohydrate value.

Breads

_____ Bagel

_____ Bread, reduced-calorie

_____ Bread, white

_____ Bread, whole-wheat

_____ Bread, pumpernickel

_____ Bread, rye

_____ Breadsticks, crisp

_____ English muffin

_____ Hamburger buns

_____ Hot dog buns

_____ Pita

_____ Raisin bread, unfrosted

_____ Roll, plain

_____ Tortilla, corn

_____ Tortilla, flour

_____ Waffle, reduced-fat

Vegetables and fruits

_____ Avocado, guacamole

_____ Banana

_____ Corn

_____ Mixed vegetables

_____ Peas

_____ Plantain

_____ Popcorn

_____ Potato

_____ Squash, acorn or butternut

_____ Sweet potato

Legumes

____ Black beans

____ Black-eyed peas

____ Garbanzo beans

____ Hummus packets

____ Kidney beans

____ Lentils

____ Lima beans

____ Peanuts

____ Pinto beans

____ White beans

Grains and cereals

____ Bran cereals

____ Bulgur

____ Cereal, cooked

____ Cereal, sugar-frosted

____ Cereal, unsweetened

____ Cornmeal, dry

____ Couscous

____ Flour, dry

____ Granola, low-fat

____ Grape-Nuts

____ Grits

____ Kasha

____ Millet

____ Muesli

____ Oats

____ Pasta

____ Puffed cereal

____ Quinoa

_____ Rice, brown

_____ Rice, white

_____ Shredded Wheat

_____ Wheat germ

Soy products

_____ Edamame (green soybeans)

_____ Miso

_____ Soy milk

_____ Soy nuts

_____ Tempeh

_____ Tofu, extra firm

_____ Tofu, silken

Other Elements of a Low-Carb Lifestyle

_____ Broth, beef

_____ Broth, chicken

_____ Broth, vegetable

_____ Brown Sugar sweetener

_____ Cake mix, sugar-free

_____ Colas sweetened with natural sweeteners

_____ Cooking spray, nonfat

_____ Crystal Light

_____ Flavored waters (non-calorie, non-carbonated)

_____ Gelatin, sugar-free

_____ Jerky, no sugar added

_____ Mayonnaise, reduced-fat

_____ Natural sweeteners, such as allulose, erythritol, monk fruit, stevia leaf extract, xylitol

_____ Pudding, sugar-free, fat-free

_____ Salad dressing, reduced-fat

_____ Sour cream, reduced-fat

Appendix C
Dietary Reference Intakes

Y ou may be familiar with Recommended Dietary Allowances (RDAs), but you may not have heard of Dietary Reference Intakes (DRIs). DRIs were established in 1997 by the Food and Nutrition Board, and they're based on several factors, including the RDAs. Put simply, the RDAs are a part of the DRIs, but they aren't the whole story.

The DRIs don't just talk about how much of the various vitamins and minerals you should have. They also address issues such as exercise and sugar consumption, and how many of your calories should come from protein versus carbohydrates. In this appendix, I sort through the report and give you only the information you need.

Vitamins and Minerals

The DRIs represent a shift in focus from preventing vitamin and mineral deficiency to decreasing the risk of chronic disease. The levels recommended in the DRIs may reduce your risk of cardiovascular disease, osteoporosis, certain cancers, and other diet-related diseases.

If you take vitamin and mineral supplements, pay particular attention to the RDAs as a goal for your average daily intake from food and supplements and the ULs (Tolerable Upper Intake Level) as an indicator of the highest amount you can take safely.

Table C-1 lists the 2011 RDAs that are part of the current DRIs. (Yes, 2011 is right. The RDAs haven't been updated since then.) Table C-2 lists the ULs (the maximum you can take safely).

TABLE C-1

RDAs for Men and Women Ages 19 to 50

Vitamin or Mineral	Men	Women
Vitamin A µg/d	900	700
Vitamin C (mg/d)	90	75
Vitamin D (µg/d)	15	15
Vitamin E (mg/d)	15	15
Vitamin K (µg/d)	120	90
Thiamin (mg/d)	1.2	1.1
Riboflavin (mg/d)	1.3	1.1
Niacin (mg/d)	16	14
B6 (mg/d)	1.3	1.3
Folate (µg/d)	400	400
B12 (µg/d)	2.4	2.4
Calcium (mg/d)	1,000	1,000
Phosphorus (mg/d)	700	700
Magnesium (mg/d)	420	320
Iron (mg/d)	8	18
Zinc (mg/d)	11	8
Selenium (µg/d)	55	55

TABLE C-2   ## ULs for Men and Women Ages 19 to 70

Vitamin or Mineral	Upper Limit
Vitamin A (μg/d)	3,000
Vitamin C (mg/d)	2,000
Vitamin D (μg/d)	100
Vitamin E (mg/d)	1,000
Niacin (mg/d)	35
B6 (mg/d)	100
Folate (μg/d)	1,000
Calcium (mg/d)	2,500 for ages 19–50; 2,000 for ages >51
Phosphorus (g /d)	4
Magnesium (mg/d)	350 (non-food)
Iron (mg/d)	45
Zinc (mg/d)	40
Selenium (μg/d)	400

Carbohydrate, Protein, and Fat

In 2019, a DRI report addressed the question of how much carbohydrate, fat, and protein you need to consume on a daily basis to ensure good health. The ranges are geared toward achieving a nutritionally adequate diet while minimizing your risk of developing chronic disease.

Here are the recommended percentages for adults:

» **Carbohydrate:** 45 to 65 percent of calories

» **Fat:** 20 to 35 percent of calories

» **Protein:** 10 to 35 percent of calories

An amount of 130 grams of total carbohydrate was set as a minimum amount for both children and adults. This DRI is based on the amount of carbs your body needs in order to provide enough glucose for the brain to function, enough glucose to fuel red blood cells and the central nervous system, and enough glucose to prevent loss of lean body mass. Very-low-carbohydrate diets of 20 to 30 grams of total carbohydrate fall far short of this goal. (The Whole Foods Weight Loss Eating Plan outlined in this book falls well within the current DRI.)

Sugar

According to the 2020–2025 Dietary Guidelines for Americans report, no more than 10 percent of your total calories should come from foods with added sugars (soft drinks, pastries, cookies, candies, and other foods and beverages to which sugar is added during production). This maximum amount of sugars was based on evidence that people whose diets are high in added sugars have lower intakes of essential nutrients. In general, the 10 percent of total calories is usually based on a 2,000 calorie diet. That would be 200 calories of added sugars or no more than 50 grams of sugar per day. (Remember: Carbs have 4 calories per gram – 200 ÷ 4 = 50 grams).

Dietary Fiber

Studies show that people with low-fiber diets have an increased risk of developing heart disease. There is additional evidence to suggest that more fiber in the diet helps prevent colon cancer and promotes weight control, but the findings are unconfirmed at this point.

The dietary fiber recommendations are as follows:

>> **Men:** 38 grams up to age 50, and 30 grams older than 50

>> **Women:** 25 grams up to age 50, and 21 grams older than 50

>> **Children 1 to 3 years:** 19 grams per day

>> **Children 4 to 8 years:** 25 grams per day

>> **Boys 9 to 13 years:** 31 grams per day

>> **Boys 14 to 18 years:** 38 grams per day

>> **Girls 9 to 18 years:** 26 grams per day

Appendix D

Metric Conversion Guide

The recipes in this book weren't developed or tested using metric measurements. There may be some variation in quality when converting to metric units.

Common Abbreviations

Abbreviation(s)	What It Stands For
cm	Centimeter
C., c.	Cup
G, g	Gram
kg	Kilogram
L, l	Liter
lb.	Pound
mL, ml	Milliliter
oz.	Ounce
pt.	Pint
t., tsp.	Teaspoon
T., Tb., Tbsp.	Tablespoon

Volume

U.S. Units	Canadian Metric	Australian Metric
¼ teaspoon	1 milliliter	1 milliliter
½ teaspoon	2 milliliters	2 milliliters
1 teaspoon	5 milliliters	5 milliliters
1 tablespoon	15 milliliters	20 milliliters
¼ cup	50 milliliters	60 milliliters
⅓ cup	75 milliliters	80 milliliters
½ cup	125 milliliters	125 milliliters
⅔ cup	150 milliliters	170 milliliters
¾ cup	175 milliliters	190 milliliters
1 cup	250 milliliters	250 milliliters
1 quart	1 liter	1 liter
1½ quarts	1.5 liters	1.5 liters
2 quarts	2 liters	2 liters
2½ quarts	2.5 liters	2.5 liters
3 quarts	3 liters	3 liters
4 quarts (1 gallon)	4 liters	4 liters

Weight

U.S. Units	Canadian Metric	Australian Metric
1 ounce	30 grams	30 grams
2 ounces	55 grams	60 grams
3 ounces	85 grams	90 grams
4 ounces (¼ pound)	115 grams	125 grams
8 ounces (½ pound)	225 grams	225 grams
16 ounces (1 pound)	455 grams	500 grams (½ kilogram)

TABLE D-4

Length

Inches	Centimeters
0.5	1.5
1	2.5
2	5.0
3	7.5
4	10.0
5	12.5
6	15.0
7	17.5
8	20.5
9	23.0
10	25.5
11	28.0
12	30.5

TABLE D-5

Temperature (Degrees)

Fahrenheit	Celsius
32	0
212	100
250	120
275	140
300	150
325	160
350	180
375	190
400	200
425	220
450	230
475	240
500	260

Index

Numbers

2-40-140 rule, 330

A

acesulfame-potassium (Ace-K), 106
action stage (Stages of Change model), 318
Adult Family History Form, 47
adult-onset diabetes, 51
age, 47–49
alcohol, 62, 359
almonds
  Chocolate-Almond Crisps, 289
  as dairy alternative, 122–123
  Poached Pears with Raspberry Almond Purée, 281
American College of Cardiology, 55
American Heart Association (AHA), 25, 55, 131
American Medical Association (AMA), 47
amino acids, 80
antioxidants. *See also* nutrients and nutrition
  benefits of, 88
  dietary sources of, 377–381
  in monk fruit, 105
  supplements, 345–346
appetizers
  Artichoke-Ham Bites, 211
  Bell-Pepper Nachos, 209
  Crunchy Stuffed Mushrooms, 206
  Deviled Eggs, 214
  Fruit and Brie Kabobs, 207
  Marinated Mushrooms, 205
  Mushroom Cocktail, 212
  Spicy Meatballs, 210
  studying menus in advance, 305
  Tasty Chicken Roll-Ups, 213
  Zucchini-Shrimp Canapés, 208
apples
  Apple Treats, 219
  Apple-Cheese Spread, 227
  as Green Light foods, 70, 73
  Maple Apple Rings, 283
  Pimiento Cheese–Apple Wedges, 220
  Pork Chops with Apples, 250
apricots, 71
arthritis, 29
artichokes
  Artichoke-Ham Bites, 211
  as Green Light food, 74
arugula, 78
asparagus
  Asparagus with Lemon Sauce, 267
  as Green Light foods, 74
  Stir-Fried Asparagus, 268
aspartame, 108
atherosclerosis, 27, 48
Atkins Diet, 12
avocados
  Avocado Salsa, 229
  Avocado-Orange Salad, 197

B

Baked Catfish Delight, 233
Baked Chicken with Winter Vegetables240
Baked Crimson Pears, 288
Baked Stuffed Potatoes, 271
Banting, William, 20
beans
  bean sprouts, 74
  buying, 148
  Navy Bean Soup, 191
  as source of protein, 251
beef
  alternatives, 278
  Beefy Chili, 192
  Bertie Jo's Company Chicken, 241
  Betty's Busy-Day Roast, 244
  Bun-Less Bacon Cheeseburgers, 249
  as Green Light foods, 81
  No-Fail Meatloaf, 246
  purchasing, 146

lentils, 96–97, 277

lettuce

  as Green Light foods, 78

  Low-Carb Crunchy Coleslaw, 272

  Pinto Bean Salad, 259

  South-of-the-Border Salad, 195

  Sweet Potato Salad, 200

  Vegetable Salad, 198

limes

  as Green Light foods, 74

  Key Lime Pudding Cakes, 291

Link, Rachel, 88

linoleic acid, 156

lipids, 53–54

Lo-Cal Salad Dressing, 201

Low-Carb Crunchy Coleslaw, 272

low-carb diet. *See also* carbohydrates; diets; Green Light foods; health

  analyzing eating habits, 314

  benefits of, 34, 369–372

  children and, 375

  cholesterol and, 371

  committing to, 16, 313–321, 339

  concentration and, 370

  controlling hunger with, 370

  energy and, 371

  evaluating, 29–31, 63

  factors for overall health

    exercise and, 15

    vitamins and, 15, 374

  frozen desserts and, 282

  health and, 14–15

  high-protein diet with, 20–21

  history of, 20

  as lifestyle, 13

  mood and, 372

  overview, 8–13

  planning, 16

  pork and, 250

  questions about, 373–376

  self-confidence and, 372

  side-effects, 43–44

  sleep and, 371

  special occasions and, 156–157

  supplements and, 15

  trade-offs and, 102–103

  vegetarians and, 374

  visualizing success, 315

  weight, 370, 374

  Yellow Light foods, 32–33

low-density lipoprotein (LDL) cholesterol, 54, 129–130, 132, 137

low-fat, high-carb diet, 19–20

low-glycemic-load of carbohydrates, 100

lunch

  Avocado-Orange Salad, 197

  Beefy Chili, 192

  Chicken-Vegetable Salad, 199

  Gazpacho, 193

  Green Wonder Salad, 196

  Hearty Vegetable Soup, 189

  Honey-Lime Dressing, 202

  Jim's Sausage Soup, 190

  Lo-Cal Salad Dressing, 201

  Navy Bean Soup, 191

  overview, 164–168

  South-of-the-Border Salad, 195

  Sweet Potato Salad, 200

  Vegetable Salad, 198

M

macadamia milk, 124

macular degeneration, 351

magnesium, 112

maintenance stage (Stages of Change model), 318–319

mangoes

  as Green Light foods, 72

  Mango Salsa, 228

mannitol, 105

Maple Apple Rings, 283

Marilyn's Orange-Pineapple Delight, 221

Marinated Mushrooms, 205

MCTs (medium-chain triglycerides), 123, 134

meals

  breakfasts, 160–164

  dinner, 168–171

  lunch, 164–168

  planning

    busy lifestyle and, 376

    developing strategies, 154–156

    grocery lists, 158–159

About the Author

Katherine Chauncey, PhD, RDN, is an Emeritus Professor in the Department of Family Medicine at Texas Tech University School of Medicine and is a Fellow of the Academy of Nutrition and Dietetics. She received her BS degree from the University of Arkansas and her MS and PhD degrees from Texas Tech University. Dr. Chauncey is a licensed registered dietitian nutritionist (RDN). She has more than 35 years of experience in medical and resident nutrition education and in providing medical nutrition therapy to patients with chronic illnesses. Her research focused on medical student and resident education and clinical nutrition interventions for diabetes, metabolic syndrome, and obesity. She has a long-time interest in low-carb diets and developed the Whole Foods Weight Loss Eating Plan for use with patients in family medicine clinics. Dr. Chauncey enjoys time with family and friends and loves to travel.

Dedication

To all of those who are frustrated and confused with all the media hype about the latest dieting fads and are looking for a healthier and permanent way to do low-carb.

Author's Acknowledgments

I want to extend a sincere thanks to the hard-working team at John Wiley and Sons. A special thanks to Kelsey Baird, Acquisitions Editor, for giving me the opportunity to write this second edition and for starting me in the right direction. I greatly appreciate Project Manager and Development Editor, Chad Sievers, for his attention to detail, for his sense of organization, and for keeping the project on track. I wish to thank Emily Nolan for her careful testing of the recipes and for her nutritional analysis.

A special thank you goes to Kristina LaRue, RDN for her technical review of the book. Thanks to my agent, Grace Freedson, for her warm support and guidance. A big thank-you goes to Marilyn Beavers, Carol Chauncey, Jim Chauncey, Mildred Chauncey, Betty Kendrick, Sharon Mandrell, and Harold and Bertie Jo Priddy for allowing their great recipes to be included in this book.

And, of course, last but definitely not least, I'm grateful to my family and friends for their patience and encouragement during the writing of this book.

Publisher's Acknowledgments

Acquisitions Editor: Kelsey Baird

Project Manager and Development Editor:
Chad R. Sievers

Technical Editor: Kristina M. LaRue, RDN

Production Editor: Tamilmani Varadharaj

Cover Photo: © Wendy Jo Peterson

Color Insert Photos: Wendy Jo Peterson